Sibling Relations and the Horizontal Axis in Theory and Practice

This book explores the interpersonal world of sibling relationships, explaining how these relationships are central to the development of the psyche of the individual, of the group, of society and of the organisation.

Sibling Relations and the Horizontal Axis in Theory and Practice considers four key areas: sibling relations, sibling trauma, the law of the mother and the horizontal axis. The contributors journey through examples from the psychological, philosophical, organisational, social and cultural realms, giving a new perspective on the psychic world and the importance of sibling relationships as an empowering and therapeutic component for building relationships. While we are used to looking at the individual, the group and at society through the vertical, hierarchical relationship that results from parent–child relationships, this book discusses and reveals the impact of the horizontal axis.

Sibling Relations and the Horizontal Axis in Theory and Practice will be important reading for psychoanalysts, group analysts and psychoanalytic psychotherapists in practice and in training.

Smadar Ashuach is a clinical psychologist, supervisor, training psychoanalyst and group analyst based in Israel.

Avi Berman is a clinical psychologist, psychoanalyst, training psychoanalyst and group analyst. He is the founder of the Israeli Institute of Group Analysis.

The New International Library of Group Analysis (NILGA)
Series Editor: Earl Hopper

Drawing on the seminal ideas of British, European and American group analysts, psychoanalysts, social psychologists and social scientists, the books in this series focus on the study of small and large groups, organisations and other social systems, and on the study of the transpersonal and transgenerational sociality of human nature. NILGA books will be required reading for the members of professional organisations in the field of group analysis, psychoanalysis, and related social sciences. They will be indispensable for the "formation" of students of psychotherapy, whether they are mainly interested in clinical work with patients or in consultancy to teams and organisational clients within the private and public sectors.

Recent titles in the series include:

Addressing Challenging Moments in Psychotherapy
Clinical Wisdom for Working with Individuals, Groups and Couples
Edited by Jerome S. Gans

Psychoanalysis, Group Analysis, and Beyond
Towards a New Paradigm of the Human Being
Juan Tubert-Oklander and Reyna Hernández-Tubert

An Introduction to Psychotherapeutic Playback Theater
Hall of Mirrors on Stage
Ronen Kowalsky, Nir Raz and Shoshi Keisari with Susana Pendzik

Psycho-social Explorations of Trauma, Exclusion and Violence
Un-housed Minds and Inhospitable Environments
Christopher Scanlon and John Adlam

Sibling Relations and the Horizontal Axis in Theory and Practice
Contemporary Group Analysis, Psychoanalysis and Organization Consultancy
Edited by Smadar Ashuach and Avi Berman

Sibling Relations and the Horizontal Axis in Theory and Practice

Contemporary Group Analysis, Psychoanalysis and Organization Consultancy

Edited by Smadar Ashuach and Avi Berman

Routledge
Taylor & Francis Group
LONDON AND NEW YORK

Cover image: beastfromeast / Getty Images

First published 2022
by Routledge
4 Park Square, Milton Park, Abingdon, Oxon OX14 4RN

and by Routledge
605 Third Avenue, New York, NY 10158

Routledge is an imprint of the Taylor & Francis Group, an informa business

British Library Cataloguing-in-Publication Data
A catalogue record for this book is available from the British Library

Library of Congress Cataloging-in-Publication Data
A catalog record for this book has been requested

ISBN: 978-1-032-11476-7 (hbk)
ISBN: 978-1-032-11478-1 (pbk)
ISBN: 978-1-003-22006-0 (ebk)

DOI: 10.4324/9781003220060

Contents

Contributors

Smadar Ashuach is a clinical psychologist, supervisor, training psychoanalyst and group analyst. She is a member teacher and supervisor at the Israeli Institute of Group Analysis and at Tel-Aviv Institute for Contemporary Psychoanalysis. She is a member of the OFEK-group relations organisation, and lives and practices in Israel. smadar.ashuach@gmail.com

Limor Avrahami-Reshef, MsC, is an occupational therapist and mental health, group analyst and psychotherapist. She is a student of philosophy at Tel Aviv University, and a lecturer in group therapy in Haifa University.

Avi Berman, PhD, is a clinical psychologist, psychoanalyst, training analyst and a group analyst. He is a member of the Tel-Aviv Institute of Contemporary Psychoanalysis, and the initiator and co-founder of the Israeli Institute of Group Analysis as well as its first chairperson. He is a co-founder of the Be'Sod Siach organisation for conflict resolution in Israel. He is the head of the group psychotherapy track at Tel-Aviv University (within the psychotherapy program of Sackler School of Medicine). He is an active teacher and a supervisor in these institutes. His professional experience includes post-traumatic therapy and supervision in Amcha (an association for treating holocaust survivors and their second generation's siblings. He is a co-author (with Ivan Urlić and Miriam Berger) of *Victimhood, Vengefulness, and the Culture of Forgiveness*, recently published. avi@berman-psychology.com

Richard M. Billow, PhD, is a clinical psychologist certified in psychoanalysis and group psychotherapy. He has been affiliated with the Derner Institute of Adelphi University for more than 40 years, and has served as associate professor in the doctoral program and as faculty in the postgraduate programs in psychoanalysis and child psychotherapy. Until recently, he directed the Adelphi Postgraduate Program in Group Psychotherapy. Billow has published more 50 peer-reviewed journal articles and four books: *Relational Group Psychotherapy: From Basic Assumptions to Passion* (2003); Resistance, *Rebellion, and Refusal in Groups*: *The 3 R's* (2010); *Developing Nuclear Ideas: Relational Group Psychotherapy* (2015); and *Richard M. Billow's Selected Papers on Psychoanalysis and Group Process: Changing Our Minds* (T. Slonim, Ed.) (2021). He lives and practices in Great Neck, New York.

Maria-José Blanco, PhD, is a psychodynamic psychotherapist, group analyst (IGA, London) and academic. Her academic interests lie in therapeutic writing, life-writing and autobiography. She has co-edited (with Ricarda Vidal) *The Power of Death: Reflections on Death in Western Society* (Berghahn, 2014 and 2017), and written *Feminine Singular: Women Growing Up Through Life-Writing in the Luso-Hispanic World* (Peter Lang, 2017) and *Women in Transition: Crossing Boundaries, Crossing Borders* (with Claire Williams; Routledge, 2021). She guest co-edited two special issues of the *Journal of Romance Studies* on autobiographical writing and women's aging and a special issue of *Contexts* (GASi) on "group analysis in Spanish" (Summer 2021).

Shoshi Breiner, MA in creative writing, is an author and literary editor. She leads book clubs and teaches creative writing and has published the following novels: *Ariadna* (Hakibutz Hameuhad Publishers, 1990), *Hebrew Love* (Am Oved Publishers, 2006; one of five finalists for the Sapir prize), *The Book of Farewell* (Am Oved Publishers, 2009; translated into Dutch and German), and *Secret Scrip* (Am Oved Publishers, 2016). She currently resides in Herzliya, Israel.

Prophecy Coles is a retired psychotherapist. In all she has written she has been pursuing the idea that the relationships we have with those other than our parents can leave a lasting impression on the patterns of our relationships in later life. Her publications include *The Importance of Sibling Relationships in Psychoanalysis*; *Sibling Relationships, the Uninvited Guest from the Unremembered Past*; *The Shadow of the Second Mother, Psychoanalytic and Psychotherapeutic Perspectives on Stepfamilies and Stepparents*; and *Psychoanalytic Perspectives on Illegitimacy, Adoption and Reproductive Technology*.

Rina Dudai, PhD, is a researcher of literature and a member of the Interdisciplinary Group at the Tel Aviv Institute for Contemporary Psychoanalysis. Her work focuses on patterns in poetic processing of extreme experiences in the space between literature, film and psychoanalysis. Her forthcoming book is *Tongue of Fire: Poetic Testimony to the Holocaust*.

Robi Friedman, PhD, is a clinical psychologist, group analyst in private practice in Haifa, Israel. He is former president of the International Group Analytic Society (GASi), was the Foulkes Lecturer (2018), and is a co-founder and former chair of the Israel Institute for Group Analysis. He is also former chair of the Israel Association for Group Psychotherapy, and co-founder of the International Dialogue Initiative. His published books include *Dreamtelling, Relations Disorders and Large Groups* (2019); *Dreams in Group Psychotherapy* (with Neri and Pines; 2002); *Desire, Passion and Gender, Clinical Implications* (with Navarro and Schwartzberg; New York, Nova, 2011); and *Group Analysis in the Land of Milk and Honey* (with Yael Doron; Karnac, London, 2017).

Einar Gudmundsson, MD, group analyst, worked as a psychiatrist at different hospitals and outpatient clinics in Iceland, Norway and Sweden for more than 30 years. He was in private practice in Oslo, Norway, from 1989 to –1995 and in Reykjavik, Iceland, from 1995 to 2021. Since April 2021, he has been part-time senior consultant psychiatrist at Landspitalinn National University Hospital, in Reykjavik, Iceland. He is a member of the board of directors at IAGP (International Association of Group Psychotherapy; 2003–2009), and president of IGTA (Icelandic Group Therapy Association; 2005–2010) and a member of the executive committee since 2014.

R.D. Hinshelwood is a Fellow of the British Psychoanalytical Society and a Fellow of the Royal College of Psychiatrists. He has a number of publications on Kleinian psychoanalysis, on the dynamics of organisations and groups, and on the organisational dynamics of psychiatry in the NHS. He was a consultant psychotherapist in the psychiatry service for many years and clinical director of the Cassel Hospital in the 1990s. Subsequently, he was professor in the Centre for Psychoanalytic Studies at the University of Essex, UK, and is now Professor Emeritus.

Earl Hopper, PhD, is a psychoanalyst, group analyst and organisational consultant in private practice in London. He is a Fellow of the British Psychoanalytical Society, an honorary member of the Institute of Group Analysis, an honorary member of the Group Analytic Society International and a Distinguished Fellow of the American Group Psychotherapy Association. He is the editor of *The New International Library of Group Analysis* for Routledge.

Gita Kiper, MA, is a psychologist and a PhD candidate in the Department of Politics and Government at Ben-Gurion University of the Negev, Israel. Her academic career focuses on the social and political aspects of psychotherapy. Kiper has co-authored the paper "'Good residents' for Themselves: Psychological Screening and Cultural Imagination of Future Citizenship in Contemporary Israel", and has presented her research at international conferences.

Martin Mahler is a training and supervising analyst of the IPA, a past president of the Czech Psychoanalytic Society and Director of the Czech Psychoanalytic Institute. He is also a co-founder and past president of Rafael Institute in Prague. He works as an individual and a group therapist in private practice in Prague.

Gila Ofer, PhD, is a clinical psychologist, training psychoanalyst and group analyst. Dr Ofer is a founding member and past president of the Tel-Aviv Institute of Contemporary Psychoanalysis (TAICP) and a founding member of the Israeli Institute of Group Analysis (IIGA), and she serves on the faculty of both institutes and at the Post-Graduate School for Psychoanalytic Psychotherapy, Tel-Aviv University. Dr Ofer has been the chair of the group analytic section and board member of the EFPP, and later a conjoint member of the board as the coordinator of Eastern European countries of the EFPP. Currently, she is the editor of the EFPP *Psychoanalytic Psychotherapy Review*. She has published her work in leading journals and presented her work and taught in Israel, Europe and the United States. Her edited book *A Bridge over Troubled Water: Conflicts and Reconciliation in Group and Society* was published in 2017.

Esther Rapoport, PsyD, is a clinical psychologist and a psychoanalytic candidate (Academy of Clinical and Applied Psychoanalysis, Livingstone, New Jersey). She writes and teaches on topics related to gender, sexuality, race, clinical work with LGBT populations, history of psychoanalysis and critical psychology. Her book *From Psychoanalytic Bisexuality to Bisexual Psychoanalysis: Desiring in the Real* (Routledge, 2019) won the Bisexual Book Award. Until recently, she served as a board member of the Israeli Forum of Relational Psychoanalysis and Psychotherapy.

Pnina Rappoport, PhD Psychologist and Group Analyst, is an individual and couples therapist. She was a member of the board of the Israeli Institute of Group Analysis. She has specialised in the treatment of "stage fright" and organisation development, and has taught and lectured in many universities in Israel and the United States.

Suzi Shoshani, PhD, is a clinical psychologist and supervisor of individual, couple and group therapists. She is a former co-chair of the Israeli Institute of Group Analysis (IIGA) (2005–2010) and was the convener of the Training Program for Group Analysts at the Israel Institute (2010–2016).

Joanna Skowronska is a training group analyst, supervisor and teacher at the Institute of Group Analysis, Rasztów, Warsaw. She runs small analityk groups in private practice and staff support groups for health institutions as well as individual and family psychotherapy. She is interested in factors shaping relationships in group analytic psychotherapy and the applicability of groups in different contexts and has published on these subjects in both Polish and English. Address: Joannagrazynaskowronska@gmail.com; Poland; 04–859 Warsaw, 20c Ulanowska st.

Ella Stolper, MA, is a psychoanalytic psychotherapist and group analyst, and is a member of the Israel Institute for Group Analysis (IIGA). She is a faculty member at the Group Facilitation Programs at Tel Aviv University (TAU), at the Moscow Institute for Group Analysis (MIGA) and at the Kiev International School of Relational Psychoanalysis and Psychotherapy (KISRPP). She is chair and lecturer at the central School of Social Work of the Ministry of Labor and Social Affairs, and she conducts private practice (individual, group and pair) and supervises organisations. ellastolper@gmail.com

Simi Talmi, MSW, is a training psychoanalyst and organisational consultant. She is a former co-director of the program in Organization Consultation & Development: A Psychoanalytic-Systemic Approach, and she teaches in the program of psychotherapy at Haifa University. She is currently the president of Tel Aviv Institute for Contemporary Psychoanalysis, OFEK member.

Ivan Urlić, MD, PhD, is neuropsychiatrist, psychoanalytical psychotherapist and group analyst. He teaches at the medical school and the Academy of Arts of the University of Split, Croatia, as well as internationally. He is a founding member of IGA Zagreb and IGA Bologna (Italy), where he is a training group analyst and supervisor.

Liat Warhaftig-Aran is a clinical psychologist, group analyst and a candidate at Tel Aviv Institute for Contemporary Psychoanalysis. She works in individual, couple, and group therapy in a private practice. She is a staff member in the Israeli Institute of Group Analysis and in the Ministry of Welfare School of Social Work. Liat is the co-founder and the academic director of Kiev International School of Relational Psychoanalysis and Psychotherapy.

Gerhard Wilke studied anthropology at King's College, Cambridge, and trained as a group analyst at the Institute of Group Analysis in London. He was for many years an associate of Ashridge Business School and taught at the Institute of Group Analysis and Birkbeck College, London. He is a training analyst on the German postgraduate training GRAS and supervises the work of clinicians and coaches. Over the last 25 years, he has worked across Europe as a consultant in a range of industries and public sector organisations. He also has built up an international reputation as a large group conductor. Gerhard wrote *How to Be a Good Enough GP* (Radcliffe Medical Press, Oxford, 2001) and is the co-author of *Living Leadership – A Practical Guide for Ordinary Heroes* (published by the *Financial Times*, Harlow, 2009). He also published *The Art of Group Analysis in Organisations* (Karnac, London, 2014) and three books in German: *Chaos and Order in Groups*, *The Power of Generations* and *The power of Repetition Compulsion and Rituals*. Most recently, he co-authored *Breaking Free of Bonkers, How to Lead in Today's Crazy World of Organisations* (Brearley, London, 2018).

Foreword

I am pleased to have been asked to write an extended Foreword to this collection of chapters on sibling relations in various settings and related disciplines. The topic continues to be neglected in theory and research, and, I suspect, in clinical work and organisational consultancy. This scotoma may even be an enactment of sibling relations within the peer relations of our professional work. In any case, I welcome the opportunity to try briefly and personally to contextualise the study of sibling relations within contemporary group analysis, psychoanalysis and organisational consultancy.

It is entirely appropriate to acknowledge that Smadar Ashuach and Avi Berman, the co-editors of this volume, are psychoanalysts and group analysts in Israel. They are training analysts, and have a long history of involvement in consulting to organisations and working in them. They also have a long-standing interest in the study of sibling relations, as seen in their respective publications and in their academic and general professional work. Avi is one of the founders of the Israeli Institute of Group Analysis. They have worked with Juliet Mitchell, who has written a Preface for this book. Juliet has made important contributions to the study of sibling relations. As an Independent of the British Psychoanalytical Society, she has drawn on the perspectives of various psychoanalysts, anthropologists and group analysts, and has had training experience in group analysis. Having first met in 1968, we are now siblings in our professional work.

***

Anthropologists have been careful not to call siblings "sibs", and to reserve their use of this term for certain kinds of family groupings, although this caveat is generally ignored. Sibling bonds or relationships have been called "sib-links", which has been taken up in popular culture. Usually, siblings are related to one another through having biological parents in common. However, given the phenomenon of artificial insemination, siblings are not necessarily biologically related to one another. Step-siblings are related to one another through having one parent in common. In some societies, sibling relations are based on patterns of family authority and the ownership of property, which is often based on sex identity and marriage patterns.

A group of siblings differs from a group of peers, that is, a so-called peer group, who differs from a group of colleagues, who may or may not be a group of friends, that is, a so-called friendship group. As is the case for any group, a group of siblings is comprised of at least three of them. Two of them are a pair. The average size of a group of siblings varies among societies, and among classes and ethnic groups within them, although some evidence would suggest that there is a strong correlation between levels of socio-economic development and the average size of sibling groups. A group of siblings becomes a group somewhat slowly, adding a new member from time to time.

Sibling relations are an essential component of the "family complex", a term which (following Freud) Malinowski and Foulkes, among others, have adopted, at least some of the time. Although Freud suggested that after the birth of a sibling the Oedipus complex gives way to the family complex, he was somewhat ambiguous about this, because in his opinion the Oedipus complex is genetically inherited, and the family complex is a matter of the social unconscious. Actually, the family complex is a good example of a set of socio-cultural constraints and restraints of which we are likely to be unconscious (Hopper, 2003).

A person's location in a family must be described in terms of what today we call socio-cultural "intersectionality", with respect at least to sex, ordinal position, and age, in the context of family structures within the foundation matrix of the society. This is likely to be the crucible of our first experience of rivalry with any person other than our fathers, and is likely to be a major determinant of our structures of loving and hating, and of our patterns of cooperation and competition. It is often difficult for a child to distinguish a parent from a sibling, whether younger or older. Of course, older siblings often act like parents. Obviously, these early relations and experiences cast very long shadows, and are templates for later relationships.

★★★

Sibling relations and their vicissitudes are a central theme of creation myths. Many great novels and plays in many languages are concerned with the dynamics of them. My work with trauma, psychic fragmentation and the Incohesion of social systems has been influenced not only by *Julius Caesar* (Shakespeare, 1599), but also by *The Tempest* (Shakespeare, 1611), in which poor Prospero was displaced by his younger brother Alfredo, and the trauma was encapsulated. The group analyst and psychoanalyst Gerald Wooster (2019) was especially interested in *The Winter's Tale* (Shakespeare, 1623). Twins and twining hold a particular fascination, both in folklore and in professional research, especially when they are identical, most probably because they imply questions about nature and nurture. Personal fungibility is a painful insult to our narcissism, which in the context of royalty takes the notion of "an heir and a spare" to a ridiculous extreme. As usual, Shakespeare got there before Freud and many other psychoanalysts and group analysts, as can of course be seen in *Hamlet* (Shakespeare, 1601). On a more positive note, the reference to a "Band of Brothers" occurs in *Henry V* (Shakespeare, 1598). I say "more positive", but this rather depends on the existence of a common enemy.

Although the great parental figures of psychoanalysis, such as Freud, Jung, Abraham, Klein and Winnicott, have all discussed sibling relations, their work on this topic was concerned mainly with trauma, rivalry and even with sadomasochism in perversions. The notable variations on these themes have focused on the fact that sibling relations offer opportunities for the resolution of ambivalent feelings which are not usually available to only children. (This is one reason why dyadic therapies can sometimes overlook important experiences and processes that are located in sibling relations, and why group analysis and other forms of group psychotherapy can sometimes be particularly efficacious.) Of course, sibling relations were of vital importance in the work of Adler, but he soon left the fold.

It is noteworthy that interest in sibling relations seems to have become more marked in the 1990s. There are many reasons for this, including the dictates of fashion and imitation. The success of women in the field of psychoanalysis, often associated with the ascendency of Kleinian thinking, is undoubtedly important. However, this is not unconnected with the fact that many candidates in psychoanalytical training in the post–World War II baby boom generation were non-medical. I wonder if overcoming the Oedipal father of the American medical establishment was associated with the rediscovery of the "family complex". This rebellion – if not revolution – involved both competition and cooperation with a proliferation of new training organisations, and the recognition of sociology, social psychology and literature as the academic qualifications of candidates.

It must be acknowledged that much of the professional literature in the study of sibling relations still begins with statements such as "It is remarkable how little literature exists concerning the topic of sibling relations". It is in this context that I particularly welcome this collection of new and diverse studies of sibling relations within families, groups, organisations and societies. The authors of them include a wide range of references, both in support of their arguments and for further reading and study. The authors are from societies with different linguistic and cultural traditions, which is reflected in their intellectual styles.

The horizontal dimension of sibling relations is more important (or important in particular ways) in a new country than it is in more traditional societies. This was true of the United States during the nineteenth and even twentieth centuries, and it continues to be true of Israel. It is essential to honour the role of parents and grandparents at the same time that major gulfs – if not splits – develop between the generations. This is especially marked when the children speak the language of the new country more proficiently than their parents, and when the children are obliged to help their parents integrate into their new society. This is even more extreme in societies characterised by waves of immigration or by a large number of immigrants in a short period of time.

***

Several topics in which sibling relations are important continue to hold my interest: sibling incest, gender identity, the development of feelings of relative deprivation and drug addiction. I will discuss each of these topics very briefly. In my (Hopper, this volume; 2021, 2022a, 2022b) work on scapegoating, I have learned that although the myths of plagues and the eventual relief from them, often on the basis of sacrifices made by a heroic figure, tend to focus on the punishment of incest with a parent, they have ignored incest with a sibling. Yet, early sexual experience often occurs between siblings. I have had several patients who reported sexual experience with siblings, ranging from sexual exploration to actual sexual intercourse. I have also had students in supervision who neglected this aspect of their patients' experience, largely because they focused on fantasies of incest and on possible incest with parents and step-parents. I have the impression that although incest with step-parents and step-siblings has become more frequent in the context of the contemporary variety of family formations, which go by various names such as "hybrid" and "blended", sibling incest must be one of the best kept open secrets in our private lives. Sibling relations include homosexual experiences, especially in families in which all the siblings are of the same sex. Early sexual exploration and play involve humiliation, subjugation, and denigration. Whether heterosexual or homosexual, sibling incest is often an indication and even an enactment of parental abuse.

Despite ideologies and protestations to the contrary, it must be acknowledged that gender identity is not a matter of sex identity. Gender identity is normative, and these norms vary among societies and among classes, ethnic groups and other groupings within them (Seglow & Hopper, 1973). Whether or not parents value their sons more or less highly than their daughters, they relate to them in different ways and have different expectations of them. This is especially marked among those who have been born first, and those who have been born last. Younger siblings are very often blocked from making the same kind of identifications with their mothers and fathers that were made by their older siblings. Sisters often feel that their brothers as males have special privileges. These resentments and jealousies lead to competitive and rivalrous identifications with their brothers. Among siblings of the same sex, there is often one who provides what he or she perceives that their parents are missing. This can be a source of masculinity or femininity, and some kinds of sexual choices and practices, in fantasy and/or behaviour.

In my (Hopper, 1981) study of feelings of relative deprivation in the context of social stratification and social mobility, I focused on the development of feelings of relative deprivation as a consequence of negative discrepancies between levels of normative expectation and levels of achievement with respect to objects that have been valued as goals. I also considered the power of comparative reference groups and choices of them with respect to the determination of levels of normative expectation. This was of great importance in understanding patterns of entitlement and their vicissitudes, especially as expressed in political action, not to mention mental health and mental illness more generally. In the terminology of the day, "reference groups" were synonymous with "reference groupings", and, therefore, comparative reference groups were not necessarily groups as such. For example, a person might compare himself to members of the same profession, occupation or neighbourhood, and so on, with respect to income or prestige or influence in the community. My data showed that comparisons with these impersonal groupings were a very important source of feelings of relative deprivation and of relative satisfaction. However, even more important was the extent to which a person's income was higher, lower or approximately equal to the average income of his siblings. It also mattered how one's siblings earned their income, for example, through the practice of medicine or the practice of accounting or through trade. Inconsistencies between economic achievements and status achievements were both a manifestation of and a source of tension among siblings and their families. In other words, siblings were a crucial source of a person's comparative reference groups, and this had been entirely neglected in the professional literature.

As I (Hopper, 1991, 1995) noted in my study of drug addiction and encapsulation, sharing needles and taking heroin together in "shooting galleries" with other members of the brotherhood and sisterhood of addicts are hardly rooted only in love. Opposition to a common enemy is also important: a group of generationally specific peers tries to protect themselves from, and ultimately to defeat, what they perceive to be a parental Establishment. By sharing needles, addicts make a kind of suicide pact, ritualising their attack on their internalised parents. Although anti-viral medication may have defeated or at least brought under control HIV and hepatitis viruses, the rebellious refusal of teenagers and young adults to be vaccinated against the new collection of coronaviruses suggests that sibling dynamics continue to be repeated in peer group alliances, perhaps throughout the world.

***

In my experience, not only in England but in other countries as well, organisations in our fields of psychoanalysis and group therapy in general are ridden with the derivatives and residues of sibling rivalry (Hopper, 2012; Limentani, 1989). These organisations and their professional disciplines are marked by the shadows of their own special interests and skills, which become obvious during consultations to these organisations when they are in particular difficulties (Hopper, 2012). This can become associated with the topics of conferences and presentations more generally (Hopper & Garland, 1980/2003; Hopper & Kreeger, 1980/2003), which can also be a way of communicating through enactments their mission statements of the particular events.

It is hardly curious but certainly ironic that the Group Analytic Society International has never been free of patterns of competition, which can really be understood in terms of sibling relations, perhaps magnified and amplified by its large number of immigrants and refugees who were obliged to adopt to the "ways" of meetings of learned societies in England. Having been alerted through the study of this book to the scientific myths of "Totem and Taboo" (Freud, 1913) and to the drama of "Julius Caesar", I am reminded of enactments of sibling relations within the early life of the Group Analytic Society. Dr Walter Schindler, who was one of my first supervisors, developed what he called "group therapy on the family pattern" (1951). He focused mostly on vertical and horizontal transferences. However, he reserved the right to make the ultimate interpretations of them according to a formula in which he was always the father, the group as such was always the mother, and the members of the group were always the children and siblings to one another. During 1974 or 1975, in a Scientific Meeting of the Society, Dr Foulkes said to Schindler that he did not understand that transferences among members of a group were not necessarily about sibling relations, and that males in the group were not always brothers in the transference. Not all peer relations were based on sibling relations, and males in a group could be experienced as sisters. At my next supervision with Walter, he hastened to tell me that in the early days of the Society, perhaps a couple of decades ago, he was in a training group with Foulkes, and he complained that Foulkes was too silent and too passive. This was why Foulkes and his colleagues did not take Walter as seriously as he would have liked, and why he was patronised as a slightly wayward and rebellious sibling. Dr Robin Skynner, who was present at the Meeting of the Society in which Walter felt that he was patronised by Dr Foulkes, was somewhat uncertain about how to participate in the ensuing discussion. On the one hand, Robin was loyal to Foulkes, and was involved in the development of a group analytic style of family therapy; on the other hand, temperamentally, he was not entirely dissimilar to Walter. Men should be men, women should be women and children should be children! This was connected with their ideas concerning the importance of hierarchy and of what they regarded as the healthy differentiation of family roles, which should be derived from sexual identification and classification. This went against the emerging metatheory of socially unconscious processes which were increasingly at the core of Group Analysis. Dr Malcolm Pines, who was also present at the meeting, objected to Robin's habit of raising his index finger in order to make a point, and agreed with Hopper and Seglow, who had recently presented their paper to the Society to the effect that masculinity and femininity were socio-cultural constructions, and that gender was normative, which was consistent with the point of view of Freud himself. Several senior women raised their hands to speak, and in fact began to speak over one another. I had the impression that this was the first and only time that Vivian Cohen, Meg Sharpe and Liesel Hearst formed an intellectual and political alliance. They agreed with Malcolm. Dr Lionel Kreeger continued to sit and to observe in silence. We were lucky to have at least one senior colleague who did not feel the need to speak. Lionel was an only child. I have often wondered about the representation of only children among our colleagues.

This is not the place for a more extended discussion of the enactment of sibling relations among the founders of group analysis in England. However, I will allow myself a couple of further observations. Dr Robin Skynner was a very effective and extremely popular group analyst. Many women seemed to be attracted to him and to his way of thinking and working in groups. At the same time, they complained about his clinical ideology. Perhaps they thought that they could and would change him. In any case, this inconsistency suggested to me that the Oedipus complex tends to linger long after the family complex emerges, and remains at the core of it.

Sibling relations can never be understood apart from Oedipal relations. For example, it was reliably reported that when Foulkes had a heart attack in his last group, several of the members of it cooperated with one another in an attempt to resuscitate him. However, shortly before he collapsed, these men were competing both with one another and with Foulkes himself. Both competition and cooperation characterised the relations among those who Foulkes called his "young lions". I was never sure that his British sons liked this somewhat Germanic epithet.

Since its inception, the Group Analytic Society International has been characterised by rivalry, the main patterns of which were apparent in the work with groups in Northfield. It is noteworthy that Tom Maine gave the first Foulkes Lecture, and that Pat de Maré had to wait a while before bringing the study of large groups to our attention. The main lines of rivalry were not so much between Foulkes and Bion but between Foulkes, Maine and de Maré. These rivalries have been continued and elaborated upon by their intellectual and clinical heirs. This can be seen in the development of group relations, therapeutic communities, organisational consultation, family therapy and group analysis itself. The development of Reflective Citizens events, which are comprised of an amalgam of these sub-disciplines, in the context of small and large groups, and drawing staff from several countries, is surely a creative response to this pattern of rivalry, which is not to say that the total is not greater than the sum of its parts (Mojovic, 2019).

***

I have no doubt that this work will be useful to students and colleagues alike, not only in group analysis but also in its sibling profession and training. I hope that this book will be widely translated into the languages of Europe from which we are likely to become increasingly alienated by the consequences of Brexit, and into Japanese and Mandarin with which we will become only slowly fluent. It is impossible to overstate the importance of the horizontal axis in any aspect of our work with groups and groupings. As the authors of the valuable chapters of this book make clear: the horizontal axis is the location not only of conscious and harmonious processes but also of deeply unconscious and contradictory phenomena. I have enjoyed working with my colleagues.

Earl Hopper
Series Editor

References

Freud, S. (1913). *Totem and Taboo*. Standard Edition XIII. London: The Hogarth Press.

Hopper, E. (1981). *Social Mobility: A Study of Social Control and Insatiability*. Oxford: Blackwell. Excerpts reprinted in Hopper, E. (2003). *The Social Unconscious: Selected Papers*. London: Jessica Kingsley Publishers.

Hopper, E. (1991). Encapsulation as a Defence Against the Fear of Annihilation. *The International Journal of Psychoanalysis*, 72 (4): 607–624.

Hopper, E. (1995). A Psychoanalytical Theory of Drug Addiction: Unconscious Fantasies of Homosexuality, Compulsions and Masturbation Within the Context of Traumatogenic Processes. *International Journal of Psycho-Analysis*, 76 (6): 1121–1143.

Hopper, E. (Ed.). (2012). *Trauma and Organizations*. London: Karnac.

Hopper, E. (2021). *The Return of the Scapegoat: The Covid Syndemic in the Unconscious Life of Groups*. Online Lecture for II Cerchio – Italian Association of Group Analysis, March.

Hopper, E. (2022a). From Remorse to Relational Reparation: Mature Hope, Communication and Community in our Responses to Social Conflict and to the Virus as a Persecuting Object. *Contexts. Issue 95, March*.

Hopper, E. (2022b). Processes of Scapegoating and Sibling Rivalry in the Context of the Basic Assumption of Incohesion: Aggregation/Massification or (ba) I:A/M. In S. Ashuach & A. Berman (Eds.) *Sibling Relationships and the Horizontal Axis in Group Analysis*. London: Routledge.

Hopper, E. & Garland, C. (1980). Overview. In C. Garland (Ed.) *Proceedings of the Survivor Syndrome Workshop* (1979). Group Analysis, Special Edition, November. Reprinted in E. Hopper (2003) *The Social Unconscious: Selected Papers*. London: Jessica Kingsley Publishers.

Hopper, E. & Kreeger, L. (1980). Report on the Large Group. In C. Garland (Ed.) *Proceedings of the Survivor Syndrome Workshop* (1979). Group Analysis, Special Edition, November, 93–97. Reprinted in E. Hopper (2003) *The Social Unconscious: Selected Papers*. London: Jessica Kingsley Publishers.

Limentani, A. (1989). *Between Freud and Klein: The Psychoanalytic Quest for Knowledge and Truth*. London: Free Association Books.

Mojovic, M. (2019). Serbian Reflective-Citizens and the Art of Psychosocial Listening and Dialogue at the Caesura. *Journal of Psychosocial Studies*, 12 (1–2): 81–95.

Schindler, W. (1951). Family Pattern in Group Formation and Therapy. *International Journal of Group Psychotherapy*, 1 (2): 100–105.

Seglow, I. & Hopper, E. (1973). Some Observations on Gender Identity in Therapeutic Groups. In A. Uchtenhagen, R. Battegay & A. Friedman (Eds.) *Proceedings of the International Congress for Group Psychotherapy*. Zurich: Karger Publishers.

Shakespeare, W. (1598). *Henry IV*. A play.

Shakespeare, W. (1599). *Julius Caesar*. A play.

Shakespeare, W. (1601). *Hamlet*. A play.

Shakespeare, W. (1611). *The Tempest*. A play.

Shakespeare, W. (1623). *The Winter's Tale*. A play.

Wooster, G. (2019). Transgenerational Metamorphosis in Shakespeare's Winter's Tale – and the Eurozone. Crisis. *Newsletter of EATGA*, No 17, Series 9, 19–25.

Preface

When Smadar Ashuach from the Tel Aviv Psychoanalytic group practitioners came to talk with me in London in 2016 we both realised that what would be fruitful was the complementarity of our different approaches to the importance of siblings in psychosocial life. In common we had not only our subject and our discipline, or "knowledge", but the fact that we were both clinicians and academics with the particular approach this combination produces. As clinicians we think upwards from the material with which we engage, as academics we look downwards at this: the result is a somewhat messy but hopefully creative melee of the two intellectual strategies. This is marked when, as here, the theme – siblings – is everywhere but un-cohered. An instance of this complementary distinction for me would my insistence (which could grow or diminish) on a "law of the mother".

If there is illicit desire among siblings – something tries to prevent its realisation. We look up from the ground of our clinical material, which is replete with the protesting toddler and the urgently authoritative mother; the mother persistently introduces "reality" – what is the feel, the sight, sound and touch of this combat? Yet the toddler's engagement with reality and with a prohibition seem different. We look down, as academicians – is this mother's demand for reality a "principle" (in alliance with, and opposition to, a "pleasure principle") whereas the threat of punishment might be a "law" like the "castration complex"? Does Freud's introduction from anthropology (already passé when he wrote) of a matriarchy in *Totem and Taboo* offer a space in which both principle and punishment can be contained? Jacques Lacan's "law of the (castrating) father" does not allow the possibility. . . . So we bring our own different clinical and academic trainings to the work in hand but we share the mixture as was so evident in lectures, discussions, talks and seminars when the group led by Avi Berman invited me to Tel Aviv in 2018. This most welcome book is the result of the Tel Aviv group's pursuit of the coming together of our complementary differences.

I have been asked in this brief preface to describe the diversity of my particular contribution. First and foremost I am a psychoanalyst working with *individuals*; siblings are very present in individual casework but they are not part of our focus on the vertical relations of a child to its parents. Group psychoanalysis to the contrary has always recognised their importance for what Earl Hopper very early on so importantly designated "the social unconscious". Earl and I trained together as individual "middle-group" or "independent" psychoanalysts in the British School. Neither of us had been medically trained, as was common at the time – my own background was English literature. For me, my psychoanalytic training and practise followed the publication of my book *Psychoanalysis and Feminism* – I was asking: where did these ideas about which I had read and written come from?

Apart from my debt to Earl's work and our collegial friendship, my knowledge of group work is from quite wide reading and a one-year small, median and large group training I undertook following the publication of my book *Siblings, Sex and Violence* in 2003. Although I have learnt from, been taught by and myself taught group psychoanalysts, I have not practised it as a clinician.

I have used my excellent but very British tuition in "infant observation" to study twins as siblings. The focus of this shifted because spot on for my developing thesis the twins unexpectedly received a sister when they were 16 months old. The girl twin lashed out at the baby whenever the opportunity arose; the boy retreated into a withdrawn depression. Today all three enjoy together a very sociable and intellectually successful late adolescence – they are, and always were, a delight as well as an important learning experience; they are a checkpoint in my forthcoming book, provisionally entitled *From Toddlers to Fratriarchy: The Sibling Trauma and the Law of the Mother.*

The twins' response to their baby sister confirmed the observational-theoretical shift I had made between *Mad Men and Medusas* in 2000 and *Sibling, Sex and Violence* three years later. It is not, as suggested in *Mad Men* that siblings are per se a traumatic experience inter alia – the significant trauma is the advent (or potential advent) of the baby who steals the toddlers' precarious identity. What led to my shift of argument? The question takes us backwards and forward. It starts with hysteria. Male hysteria is the foundational condition of psychoanalysis – in the midst of hysteria's abiding definition as female, it is the acclaimed presence of male hysteria which establishes the universality of unconscious processes.

Following the publication of *Psychoanalysis and Feminism* in 1974, I had discussed with my American publisher a book on male hysteria. It was on this gnarled and knotty subject that I had been stuck for many years when one day siblings arrived magically as though from nowhere. I was living in a very familiar village, staring at the sea and deciding finally I would have to abandon the subject of male hysteria unless in this idyllic setting some unlocking thought arrived. Siblings answered the call; offering themselves, clamouring for attention.

Almost as soon as male hysteria is discovered (more accurately "rediscovered"), although always known to be present in clinical and personal settings, it disappears from intellectual recognition. My interest in it revolved around its presentation as traumatic exactly at the crucial moment when trauma as psychosocially causative in the foundational thinking of psychoanalysis was being replaced by the notion of forbidden desire. Intrinsic to this shift to desire was the formulation of the Oedipus complex – incest with the mother – and subsequently, its prohibition from the position of the father – the castration complex.

The regular disappearance of male hysteria from analysis took with it the trauma that had previously enjoyed the limelight. Siblings restored trauma – but they also make its psychic role more complex in a way that is still today often missed in the obsessive preoccupation with trauma in more general psychological accounts. In the first instance, siblings demanded that hysteria be re-thought as a social malady: there is little point in being hysterical entirely on one's own. Siblings are definitionally social. *Mad Men and Medusas* (2000), the outcome of a contract for a book on male hysteria, tumbles over itself through having had shouting siblings added to it late in the day. Commentators split, for instance Rachel Bowlby heralded their presence as a major breakthrough while, then publisher's reader Lisa Appignanesi recommended their exclusion in the interests of clarity. They remained and, developing, being revised, re-thought, extended, shifting, they have stayed in a centre-stage position ever since.

In time siblings helped to change other observations of hysteria: it is indeed a universal but with a new gender divide. When anyone is hysterical the claim is to be the one and only subject, for women such a claim is pathological; for men this one and only status is ego-syntonic. For the position of women to be Object and Other is definitional as it is for other oppressed groups who thereby often are treated as feminine. But siblings also debouch onto other gender and feminist questions within a psychoanalytic framework. These issues may seem tangential. However the implications of ever-present existence of siblings still have to be discovered and in such a wide-open context any part of one's thinking can come into play. For me this is bound to include both feminism and literature.

Freud rightly noted that a psychic distinction between the individual and the social is spurious – individuals obviously internalise social relations. They do – but what of the other direction? How does the definitionally social sibling and its heir in friends and foe internalise the individual? How does the social take in the sameness and difference of the individual (female and male)? A feminist aspiration with a different concern touches on the same question.

Second wave feminism in the late 1960s had a crucial demand: "politicise the personal" – make the emotional, personal world of women the site of political analysis and strategy. It has just struck me that "the law of the mother" could develop in this direction – but more often what is achieved is not to politicise the personal but to personalise the political; to tell stories of individual sufferers rather than an analysis of the generic suffering. This is the missing perspective in Freud's contention about the individual and the social. The feminist perspective is: how do you analyse in a way that thereby gives autonomy and therein power and potency to the *social group* that is the Object or Other?

Freud gestured in this direction of the social and the individual when he offered a political analysis of brothers in *Totem and Taboo* – brothers sublimate their incestuous desire for each other relying on a contract not a prohibition to do so. But brothers are not Others. Sisters who receive an identical prohibition against murder and incest with the sibling baby appear as wives – wives make no contract. Freud's proposition of fraternal sublimation has led to there being more interest in male homosexuality than in siblings.

The law of the mother prohibits her traumatised toddlers – girl and boy – from getting rid of the baby or loving it in an embrace that assumes it is just more of itself: these are the roots of social murder and incest. This being the case, the sibling trauma in the context of the mother's law can rank alongside the Oedipus-castration complexes as an earlier foundational and psychosocial structural experience that will be repeated throughout life. This thought can go in many directions, one of which is the psychoanalytic understanding of trauma.

In a "foundational" trauma an absolute prohibition together with the desire which has been prohibited rise up from within the sufferer to meet the violence of the blow coming from outside which has broken through the protective psychic barrier. In the very many "ordinary" traumas of life, this historic internal trauma does not feature, or at least not prominently. The sibling trauma can use Freud's presentation of the case of Emmy von N – a text which tips between before and after psychoanalysis. Emmy insists Freud listen to one after another instance of her nightmarish experiences of death – her father does not feature though finding her mother dead does. Mainly her hysterical response to finding small animals traumatic can be taken to refer to her intimacy with her numerous dead brothers and a sister. She also tells Freud she has read about some boys thrusting a dead mouse into the mouth of one of them. Freud reads the article – there is no mouse. Where terror of the large animals that represent Oedipal parents will be overcome, a terror of small animals as siblings can persist throughout life.

Where castration *represents* death, Frau Emmy's hysteria *presents* death. This is the response of the sibling with the new baby. However, after the mother's law if it is successful we have not the presentation or representation but the socialising of illicit desires – the desires become instead the social requirement for war and marriage. If the law is unsuccessful, we have Frau Emmy's hysteria. Behind the invention of a dead mouse is the probable oral sexual engagement with a dead brother. Any trauma before the toddler's replacing baby would seem not to have a preceding history – the traumatised babies whom Winnicott describes respond not to the mother's prohibition of murder and incest but to the extreme life-threatening dependence of human prematurity.

The place of siblings and theories of trauma would seem to be on the same railway tracks. After this book's most welcome contribution there is still much work to be done by all of us.

Juliet Mitchell 18.07.2021

Introduction

Smadar Ashuach and Avi Berman

We were inspired to write this book several years ago, after noticing the lack of reference to sibling relationships in the psychoanalytic and the analytical group literature. The dominance of the Oedipal complex derivatives in the psychoanalytic literature seems to have overshadowed and marginalized the study of sibling relationships. The shift in analytic relationships from having an exclusively hierarchical nature to also include a mutual dimension has led, in our view, to increasing interest in the position of siblings in psychoanalysis.

In traditional psychoanalysis, basic concepts are either Oedipal or dyadic. We can describe belonging in the Oedipal thinking as a triangle of mother, father and child, in which the child belongs to his parents in passion or competition. The dyad approach offers mother–child relationships exclusively. Freud (1912, 1921) wrote about the masses and the primitive band that was born out of the son–brother relationships, that was oppressed by the ancestor, rebelled against him, tormented by guilt over the murder of the father, and established a legacy for him out of identification. But the Oedipal conception places the father as the creator of the primitive band and therefore eternally in the minds of the siblings.

The first human connection is established between child and mother, and the triangle of a child and parents is usually the first human environment the child experiences. However, sibling relationships are largely primary as well. The child's encounter with peers in terms of age and shared experiences may empower and evoke innate core emotions. This closeness may continue throughout the lives of those involved even after the aging and death of the parents. Siblings can be secretive and understanding, intimate and empowering, excluding parents from their conversations, but sibling relationships may also include experiences of comparisons between personalities, feelings of discrimination and a need that never ceases to preserve their rights and fight for their place.

Our basic assumption is that sibling relationships and parent–child relationships are areas that stem from distinct and independent mental sources, even when there is a reciprocal relationship between them. The attempt to base our psychoanalytic understanding solely on parent–child relationships ignores, or even denies, that sibling relationships exist in their own right.

DOI: 10.4324/9781003220060-1

This book is based on an approach according to which siblings are always represented in the mind, whether they exist in reality or not. Therefore, just as an infant expects there to be a mother and father, so will the infant expect there to be a sibling. Similarly, sibling representations exist in the inner world of the child as do parental representations. These internal siblings are also expressed in transference relationships in psychoanalytic work.

Siblings, real or imaginary, form complex and important relationships. Formative and fateful processes take place between them. These processes occur in the nursery, without parental supervision, as well as in settings outside the home, where there is no authoritative framework at all. In these spaces sibling relationships are most dominant, affecting deep-seated mental states independent of, and sometimes more than, parent–child relationships. Sibling relationships have an important and significant place both in the inner world and in the social, cultural reality.

The dyadic and Oedipal conceptions are inconsistent with the idea of parallel transpersonal connections. The sibling relationship is the psychoanalytic model whose duplication creates the social phenomena. According to our theory, they are independent and different from the idealized triangle that created them.

In this book we refer to parent–child relationships and sibling relationships as two distinct developmental axes: the vertical axis represents parent–child relationships and is an abstraction of hierarchical relationships of any kind; the horizontal axis represents sibling relationships and is an abstraction of reciprocal and non-hierarchical relationships. These axes span the entire space of influences, mental processes, emotions and thoughts.

In recent years, there has been a professional awakening, both in analytics and group analytics, around sibling relationships. An awakening that we believe stems from the rise of the relational approach and field theory.

Relational psychoanalysis emphasized the effect of the relationship between the therapist and the patient. This attitude of "two persons' psychology" thus shifted the relationship to a more reciprocal, mutual and less hierarchical one. The therapeutic relationship is between two subjects. The concepts that have emerged from the theory, like mutual recognition, enactment and resonance, are more suited to the horizontal axis.

Steven Mitchell, the founder of the relational approach, is among the leading voices of observing the human mind as transpersonal. In his words:

> What are the various reasons we are drawn to each other? Picture an oak leaf on a branch, asking the question, "Why am I hanging around with these other leaves?" . . . We are increasingly appreciating the implication of the fact that humans, like oak leaves, are not found in isolation, not possible in isolation. Human minds are fundamentally social phenomena that become focalized and, secondarily, elaborated by individuals.
>
> (Mitchell, preface, 2000)

Another approach in psychoanalysis that connects to the horizontal axis is "field theory", founded by Baranger and Baranger (2009) and inspired by

Bion. The field is a common matrix created by the joining of two people or more. The interpersonal field changes and emerges. From the moment they are formed and throughout each individual session, the separate existence of each participant becomes secondary to the existence of the field. The field is created jointly and affects each of the participants in it. It does not include a hierarchy and the vertical axis is not present within it.

The Berangers attribute therapeutic power to the field. The change in the field is responsible for the change within the patient. The shifting formation is the one that frees the patient from the fixations imposed on them in their life when they were subjected to the influences of other fields in his past. The therapist's function is to allow the field to form and be able to derive new meanings from the common decoding. In both relational approach and the field theory, the therapist is a partner in the formation of the field but has no authority or priority within it. The difference between the therapist and the patient has to do with responsibility, but not authority.

The role of the therapist also changes in this approach. The therapist does not decipher the patient and does not interpret them. The therapist is responsible for the degree of freedom that the field allows. The greater the degree of freedom, the greater the ability of the participants to feel and think without inhibitions, distortions or restraints. The therapist's position must recognize their own inevitable participation in the field and be able to switch between a participant and observer self-states.

We found the practice of the vertical and horizontal axes exists in other fields as well. For example, Deleuze and Guattari (1972), a philosopher and psychoanalyst, created a paradigm which enables two forms of cognition (epistemology) by means of two metaphoric concepts: the tree and the rhizome. These are two possible ways of thinking, observing and experiencing, which may address both internal reality (as a reflection on how one thinks and experiences things) and external reality.

The tree is a metaphor for clearly stratified, hierarchical structures; and the rhizome (French for botanic matrix of roots or grass), a metaphor for omnidirectional, flat structures. The tree has a rigid structure with distinct parts and clear directional relationships between them: roots, trunk, branches, fruits; the relationships are naturally asymmetric and easily described. The tree model corresponds to the vertical axis, used to describe modernist philosophies that attempted to define a single empirical truth, composed of distinct entities and causal relationships. In contrast, the rhizome is characterized by lateral growth, lacking a clear directionality or a single determining authority, where all parts interact with and affect all other parts, in a network of mutual and non-hierarchical relationships. The rhizome model corresponds to our horizontal axis.

Similarly, in the world of information and communication, authoritative sources of information in the forms of print and broadcast media are hierarchical mechanisms for methodically investigating and reporting the news. Social media, the epitome of internet-based human interaction, is inherently horizontal, composed of a vast network of sibling relationships. Moreover, the independence of social networks also illustrates their separation from the authority of the vertical axis. Social networks do not ask for permission from authority figure. Sometimes they rebel at something but they are mostly preoccupied with the relationships within them.

Local and global politics offer additional examples of vertical and horizontal axes and the corresponding parental and sibling relations. The internal political structure within each government is composed of clearly defined hierarchical roles and can be viewed from the prism of the vertical axis, while relationships between different subgroups under that government lack an inherent hierarchy or directionality, thus different municipalities, ethnicities and social classes form a network of sibling relationships. On the global scale, countries can be viewed as siblings operating in the absence of a parental figure, where initiatives such as the European Union are attempts to insert a vertical axis to a system otherwise operating solely on the horizontal axis.

Many of the leaders seem to be interested, politically, in the subgroup of their supporters only while differentiating themselves from the others and thus may produce a split in the societies. Leaders' response to these pressured tendencies tends to be nationalist isolation rather than encouragement of horizontal discourse.

During the production of this book the coronavirus pandemic started spreading all over the world, an example of an inherently horizontal event: disrupting the normal lives of people from all nations, social statuses, ethnicities and ideologies. We propose examining the response to this event from the view of sibling relations: the positive horizontal coping exemplified by the unprecedented cooperation and coordination in the pursuit of treatment and vaccination, along with the negative competition, envy, segregation and deprivation of certain groups. Both within and between different nations, examples of exclusion, discrimination and scapegoating are abundant.

In this book we emphasize the role of Juliet Mitchell's law of the mother in understanding sibling relations, as a comprehensive theoretical framework for psychoanalytic thinking.

In her writings, Mitchell (2003, 2006, 2018) discusses sibling trauma as the traumatic threat of annihilation experienced by the child upon the arrival of a sibling. This loss of one's dyadic bond with the mother and the expulsion of the child to the company of his peers out of home is a universal trauma, experienced by all, whether they are the eldest, middle, youngest or only children. The law of the mother then prohibits the child from processing this trauma by either getting rid of the sibling (murder) or by denying the sibling's independent existence and making them one and the same (incest). Thus the law of the mother defines the permitted space in which the child is to resolve the trauma, and threatens to withhold love, care and protection from the child if those boundaries are violated. This threat, in and of itself, is traumatic, equivalent in a way to the later castration threat of the Oedipal child. The successful resolution of the sibling trauma and the maintenance of the law of the mother force the child to develop positive coping skills for operating on the horizontal axis and push the child into peer groups and society at large.

Yet, contrary to Mitchell's assumption about the mother's all-present love, it seems that the law of the mother is also violated by the mothers themselves in the same way as mother's failure to provide good enough mothering to their children.

The mother who looks away when her son abuses his sister – and accuses her of lying when she complains – violates the law of the mother. A mother who constantly favors and/or discriminates against one of her children violates the law of the mother. Moreover, the mother who is not good enough might not be able to keep her alleged promise to love her children in a way that fulfils her part in the deal. She might be incapable to love them for keeping her law. These failures of protection and harmful behaviors are being focused upon and spoken about thanks to the wording of the law. When they are, they can be defined as violations of the law. The wording of the law of the mother enables the detection of its violations. In this book, we have chosen to give voice to the description of these violations and their price.

We include Mitchell's law of the mother unto the psychoanalytic tradition as an additional aspect of a mother's primary relationship to her children, and we propose to refer to it as a universal human point of reference in the spirit of psychoanalysis. It offers pre-conditions for sibling relationships in the broadest sense of the word that can be created and maintained as a safe and beneficial space.

Just as women can strictly adhere to the law of the father when they enlist to keep the vertical axis around them, so can men fulfil the law of the mother. When the law of the mother is internalized and implemented, even the siblings themselves – when they grow up – can exercise it and adhere to both laws. Individual therapy may benefit by the insights that derive from the additional perspective of the law and its implementation by the therapist. In group analysis the group facilitator, together with the group participants, can conform to the law of the mother.

We suggest that the law of the mother as a possible infrastructure for interpersonal and social coexistence. Violations of the law of the mother, or its absence in human relations, may cause deep-seated wounds and long-lasting harm to one's well-being. This results in peer relations as physical and sexual abuse, dehumanization, violations of rights and sabotage, among others. On the social scale it is possible that violation of the law of the mother might result in civil wars and revolution and counter oppression by vertical reactions. Many governments successfully and effectively enforce the law of the father, which maintains structure and order in the society, but fail to maintain the law of the mother. Favoring a political base over the opposition, attacking the well-being and validity of minority groups, and allowing bigoted and discriminatory policies and practices are all examples of violations of the law of the mother and result in polarized societies with hostile and unproductive relationships between different subgroups.

We propose that an understanding of sibling relationships allows for a new and important re-examination of individual and group dynamics, organizational vision and social processes, which would deepen and enhance the individual and group psychotherapy. As psychoanalysts and group analysts, we emphasize the re-enactment of sibling relationships in groups and in individual therapeutic relations that enables understanding, processing and treatment of the effects of sibling trauma and the law of the mother.

We curated this book emphasizing the perspective of the horizontal axis, by inviting authors with a variety of unique perspectives. The coexistence of ideas discussed here is itself a metaphor for sibling relationships: where ideas unfold in different directions, converge, complement, sometimes compete with each other, and by interacting in this way create a fertility of thought and inspiration for the reader to develop further.

While Mitchell's law of the mother plays a crucial role in both inspiring the creation of this book and in the ideas discussed in the book, it is not the only theory for the origins of sibling relations explored and discussed. *Hinshelwood* returns to the Oedipal complex and argues that it is the father, in violating the mother–child dyad, which produces a place for the third in the child's life. It is therefore the relationship between the parents that changes the child's experience from exclusivity to substitutability, and additionally places the child as an observer, resulting in the child's ability to contain exchanges between observer and observed. *Dudai* examines the transgressing relations between fatherhood and brotherhood as viewed in Zvyaginstev's movie *The Return*. *Billow* links the law of the mother to Lacan's concept of Enigma.

Gudmundsson and *Wilke* consider the concept of the matrix, one of the basic concepts of group analysis, to include horizontality regardless of the law of the mother. *Skowronska* and *Blanco* write about the concepts of transference between participants according to Foulkes, which create the reference to equals and peers. *Rappaport* and *Shoshani* write about the matrix of fraternity within a group of old friends-psychotherapists.

The book also discusses the historical, social and economic appearances of the horizontal axis. *Wilke* refers to the idea of equality, which underlies the horizontal axis, through one of its historical origins in the social occurrence of the French Revolution. *Rapoport* and *Kiper* refer to capitalism as a vertical expression with an aim that is disturbed, weakened and controlling the horizontal axis. This contains a critical statement about the therapeutic professions that participate, consciously or unconsciously, in calming individual tension, and especially by the psychoanalysis-based approaches that rely on the Oedipal conceptualization. This individual sedation is claimed to prevent these unified tensions from being directed towards challenging the existing vertical arrangement.

Berman and *Avrahami-Reshef* refer to the ideas of Deleuze and Guattari's about the tree and rhizome that resemble concepts of the vertical and horizontal axis. The tree and the rhizome may be characteristics of both epistemology and human relations.

In the book we strive to emphasize the applied benefit of deepening our understanding of sibling relationships and derivatives of understanding the horizontal axis. It seems to us that psychotherapy, family and organizational counseling may greatly benefit from the application of these ideas. *Ashuach* and *Talmi* show how the law of the mother contributes and furthers the understanding of the processes that take place in group relations conferences, organizations and society at large.

The family that upholds the law of the mother not only determines the fate of its children but also affects the establishment of the democratic psyche in our world; *Coles* refers to this through the Bronte family.

We argue in this book that the dominance of the Oedipus complex and its derivatives as well as dyad-based psychoanalytic therapy (mother–child, therapist–patient) may miss the significance and contribution of sibling relationship analysis. The individual therapist, aware of the contribution of the law of the mother and sibling trauma will include the meanings and processing of this trauma in their work and will include the violations of the law of the mother in the analysis of the transference relationship.

A number of authors in the book deal with the law of the mother through a discussion of its violations, the human suffering caused by these violations and the psychotherapy derived in order to alleviate this suffering. *Ofer* writes about the collapse of the law of the mother, *Breiner* writes about Ogden's novels in which he described the human injury in a sibling relationship abandoned by their parents and left unlawful. The gossip that endangers the existence of brothers is described by *Warhaftig-Aran* and *Mahler*. Some of the examples come from the events of the communist regime in Czechoslovakia. *Berman* refers to the phenomenon of discrimination that is so common in the relationship between mothers and their children. *Friedman* describes the failure of the law of the mother as we can see in the biblical story of Joseph and his brother.

The group analysis seems particularly close to the assimilation of thinking about sibling relationships and the horizontal axis. Some of the authors emphasize the focus of the group analysis' contribution in rehabilitating the sibling trauma of each of the participants. The trauma of the siblings produces distress from its very existence. *Ashuach* refers to exclusion from both the vertical axis (parent–child relationship) and the horizontal axis (sibling relationship) as one of its immanent derivatives. The developmental task on both axes is to accept this exclusion. Ashuach emphasizes group analysis as a place where the trauma of others can recover and gain an opportunity for repair. In the group, the past re-enact in the present. *Hopper* considers some aspects of scapegoating and sibling rivalry in the context of the fourth basic assumption of Incohesion, in the unconscious life of groups and group-like social systems. *Urlic* writes about adherence to the law of the mother in the group, by the facilitator and the participants, that makes it possible to process past traumas, renew mourning processes and direct them to creativity. *Stolper* refers to "sibling witnessing" that validates and acknowledges injuries and injustices both past and present in the group's "here and now". Witness participants express recognition and concern. It is characterized by being public, and being accompanied by "done" injunctions in violation of the law of the mother.

The group analysis also brings us closer to the idea that the vertical axis, represented by the facilitator, and the horizontal axis, represented by the participants, can have a conscious and goal-oriented cooperation between them (*Berman* and *Avrahami-Reshef*). It seems to us that precisely the recognition of the independence of these two axes promotes the characterization of such cooperation. In the group analysis, the facilitator, who recognizes the fertility of the horizontal axis, can be aimed at strengthening the participants' sibling relationships to deepen the therapeutic benefit of each of them. The fit and difference, the support and the challenge – all these are occurrences in the horizontal axis that generate a therapeutic benefit under the facilitator's ability and support on the one hand, and the lack of intervention – on the other.

References

Baranger, M. and Baranger, W. (2009). *The Work of Confluence: Listening and Working and Interpreting in the Analytic Field*. London: Karnac.

Deleuze, G. and Guattari, F. (1983/1972). *Anti-Oedipus: Capitalism and Schizophrenia*. Minneapolis: University of Minnesota Press.

Freud, S. (1912). The dynamics of transference. In *Standard Edition*. Vol. 12, pp. 97–108. London: Hogarth Press.

Freud, S. (1921). Group psychology and the analysis of the ego. In J. Strachey (Ed.), *The Standard Edition of the Complete Psychological Works of Sigmund Freud*, Vol. XVIII (1920–1922). London: Hogarth Press.

Mitchell, J. (2003). *Siblings: Sex and Violence*. Cambridge: Polity.

Mitchell, J. (2006). Sibling trauma: A theoretical consideration. In P. Coles (Ed.), *Sibling Relationships* (pp. 155–174). London: Karnac.

Mitchell, J. (2018, February 16). *Core Concepts: From Sibling Trauma to the Law of the Mother* [Paper presentation]. Group Psychotherapy Conference on Sibling Relationships, Tel Aviv University, Tel Aviv, Israel.

Mitchell, S. A. (2000). *Relationality: From Attachment to Intersubjectivity*. Hillsdale, NJ: The Analytic Press.

Sibling Relations

1.1 Group Encounters at the Boundaries of Developmental Epochs

Richard M. Billow

> I am working on the assumption that our psychic mechanism has come into being by a process of stratification: the material present in the form of memory traces being subjected from time to time to a *rearrangement* in accordance with fresh circumstances – to a *retranscription*.
>
> The successive registrations represent the psychic achievement of successive epochs of life. At the boundary between two such epochs a translation of the psychic material must take place.
>
> [Freud, 1896, p. 233, his emphasis]

Freud's (1896, p. 233) letter to Fliess introducing the concept of "nachtraglichkeit" (or afterwardness) shines a light on group process. In Freud's formulation, psychic growth could be achieved by the revisiting and amending of established developmental narratives ("registrations") amidst the fresh circumstance of analytic experience. The encounter is dyadic, yet remains intrapsychic, the "retransciption" being an accomplishment of the patient's insight, encouraged by the analyst's neutral presence, the associational sway of transference, and the accuracy of interpretation.

In group, the "re-arrangements" of developmental events delineate an individual, dyadic, and collective activity. The boundaries of the encounter are not only internal and symbolic but actual, interpersonal, and multi-personal. Each session is marked by intense, multiple, and often contentious interactions, in contrast to dyadic collaboration. The forward thrust of the session remains in the "here and now," and only sometimes does the group move to historical narratives of "there and then." "Retranscription of psychic material" is not a simple matter of member to member transmission. Ferenczi's "confusion of tongues" is typical, and likely. No one listens and resounds to the group events in the same way. What is epochal and traumatic for one member may represent a normative developmental experience for another. Multiple retranslations go on simultaneously, subjectified by each member, by the dynamic intensity of the group, and one's roles within it.

We are born in a social network (Freud, 1921), and it is the nature of human cognition to form assemblages (Piaget, 1969). An innate "groupality" creates

DOI: 10.4324/9781003220060-3

dynamic "internal groups" (Kaes, 2007) that, accordingly, structures the unconscious and forms the basis of object and social relations. The psychotherapy group is similarly structured. Individuals continually associate, combine, organize, and transform ensembles of psychic elements. Family members serve as prototypes, and in the course of development, other individuals acquire symbolic functions as mothers, fathers, sisters, and brothers, representing psychic qualities (e.g., warm, cold, sexual, aggressive, good, bad, nurturing, informing, etc.). Unconscious pre-Oedipal, Oedipal, and fraternal complexes are variously stimulated and underscore whatever is taking place.

In this chapter I describe my efforts to decipher and mediate among ongoing "translations" of psychic material that relate especially to fraternal relationships. For, in group, everyone possesses a sibling and serves as a sibling to others, all in the presence of the abandoning symbolic parent. The goal is analytic: to utilize opportune moments to understand, negotiate, and integrate developmental experience to propel psychic growth.

Case Example 1: Who Is My Brother?

The group received frequent updates from Jocelyn regarding litigation with her older brother – the hirings and firings of lawyers, court dates, the latest effronteries – reported with little emotion other than delectable pleasure in seeking retribution.

> I was the female lamb in a pack of male wolves. And my mother whelped them all, my brothers and even my father. My older brother was the only one who ever protected me, and now he's one of them, like my father, even worse. A devil, he's evil.

The uncompromising delivery of this usually reticent member gave us a sense of the fierce culture of Jocelyn's family of origin. "Yes, I learned their vocabulary," she acknowledged.

She entered one group in emotional turmoil unfamiliar to us. "I just received an invitation to my niece's wedding; I didn't expect one and don't know what to do." A panoply of tears, worry, and hatred followed.

> I'm really afraid to go. Did he invite me to humiliate? He's done that before at another affair. But I still want to go. My husband thinks I'm crazy, but I loved my niece. I haven't slept in three days. I had a couple of dreams about my brother dying, maybe that I killed him, and they were the best part of the week. I can be evil too.

Ignoring Jocelyn's confession, the group went to work, offering solutions to how she could go while saving face and maintaining dignity no matter how her brother behaved. Or maybe she should not go? This really wasn't about the niece, who should be mature enough to understand, everyone agreed.

Over many years in our group, Jocelyn played out her fear of undefined danger by "living under the radar," as she put it. Her timidity did not match her position in her adult family as a matriarch and successful career woman. "Who are you afraid of here?" we would ask.

> It's no one in particular, except Rich of course. I don't like it when he calls me concrete or disconnected. I have a long list [of slights]. I know he can be a nasty s.o.b. and I'm actually okay with that and I tell him off when I have to.

I was okay with that too, but not with her unwillingness to extend her self-understanding. I found myself inviting her to speak in every session – not always nicely, granted – and nursing her along when she did. Sometimes the group complimented her efforts. Their positive feedback and encouragement got us nowhere. I found her paranoia suspect and felt her resolute victimhood was as a cover-up and not a true emotional reveal. She stubbornly refused to take responsibility for her unconscious and its group derivatives. Like all of us, she had access to "radar" and unshared information. At times, it can be therapeutic to disrupt narratives of established patterns of victimhood, even when they represent significant trauma. My counterforce of skepticism and unwillingness to sooth her surrender to her wordless terror seemed to offer possibilities, whereas encouragement, explanations, and profusions of caring did not. I dramatized my impatience or satirized her excuses for not participating. What surprised me was that the group found me to be unusually patient and welcoming, even when being an "s.o.b." I suspected that she did too. Lacan (1977) advised establishing a "controlled paranoia" (p. 15) with certain individuals: "We must bring into play the subject's aggressivity towards us, because, as we know, these intentions form the negative transference that is the initial knot of the analytic drama" (p. 14). In being a s.o.b. and someone she could "tell off," I was the most knowable and safest member of our group.

I was heartened by Jocelyn's miseries. At last a view into Jocelyn's psychic interior: feelings of love and hate that I did not wish to disturb or close off. I wondered whether my pleasure in her distress symptomatized spiteful retaliation for "forcing me" to do the kind of supportive work that I did not want to do and hadn't been very successful in doing. Apparently, in being an "s.o.b." I filled the role of the spite-filled father/brother and gave Jocelyn some freedom to play safely with their split-off representations.

Her facile paranoia relied on a manic defense: a refusal to feel and work through what she was capable of knowing. In a maturational working through process different developmental epochs align, often painfully so. To reach an integrating "depressive position" Jocelyn would have to surrender the fraternal idealization and "situate herself in relation to different moments of her history" (Faimberg, 2005, p. 29). He who had been an amalgamation of the loyal big brother and the best qualities of what was mostly missing from her father (and mother) had become successively someone else: a distancing college student; a striving business partner to an unethical father, a bully, and a greedy heir.

In this significant session, Jocelyn acknowledged the true target of her fear, displaced from father to brother to our group:

> I thought I worked out my relationship with my father years ago. I remember the verbal bullying and put-downs, the threats to disinherit us [misbehaving sibs]. That's just what my brother is trying to do. I feel it in my body, some terror, I am so scared that he is going to hit me during the wedding. My father did hit us at family affairs.

Each group session had been a family affair. Were she to emerge from a protective internal grouping "frozen in a developmental time" (Bollas, 1984, p. 210), something "evil" could materialize. Would it emerge from her father, brother, a member, herself?

Discussion: Internal Groups Play Out in the Psychoanalytic Group

Layered with successive developmental "epochs" in which the brother transformed from guardian to persecutor, Jocelyn's fraternal dynamics spurred attraction and desire while simultaneously activating anticipatory fear. Mobilizing historical defense mechanisms involving psychic withdrawal and omnipotent control, allowed Jocelyn to participate "under the radar." While this strategy provided precarious safety during successive childhood epochs, they impeded her growth and development in our group and elsewhere.

Developmental Messages Populate Groups

We are born into "a network of desires and thoughts preceding each of us" (Kaes, 2002, p. 20, in Kirshner, 2006, p. 1010) and transferred through intergenerational "messages" (Laplanche, 1979). Jocelyn's father did not originate the threat and actuality of physical and verbal abuse but witnessed such behavior, lived within a patriarchal culture that allowed it, acted it out, and passed it on to his male heir. The deepest and most powerful messages originate in early periods beyond the developing child's intellectual, corporeal, and emotional equipment to understand. Further, they are transmitted without awareness by those who are themselves subjugated by such messages, and who would be horrified to know of their primitive affect and unconscious meaning.[1] In the following example, a maternal voice muffled and dominated a member's encounters with his group cohorts.

Case Example 2: A Manchurian Candidate

George was the oldest of seven "Navy brats," as he called his sibling clan, serving as an exemplary model to his younger brothers and sisters. Any child who stepped out of line could bring the threat of the father's wrath. His beloved mother never challenged her husband, even during his frequent absences at sea, but George was convinced that she did not always approve. He entered group in his early thirties, perplexed by his wife's insistence on divorce after a brief marriage. "She just lost interest and couldn't explain it more than that" was the best he could do. I soon came to understand what she meant. George was a handsome, modest fellow, happily ensconced as an associate professor of English literature at a local college. While possessed with a wide knowledge base, a prodigious vocabulary, and quick wit, he had surprising difficulty functioning with psychological depth.

When I asked for his feelings or responses to group happenings, he spoke in abstruse, metaphorical language, reflecting ironically on the players and proceedings. The group's considerations about his own psychology held greater weight than his own. "That captures how I feel, but I can't quite put it into words the way you do so well." He deferred to others to represent himself to himself. Over time we discovered that the tightly bound fabric of George's communication could rip apart when members ventured beyond certain interpersonal boundaries. More than once, members tried to link his unthinking "go along" attitude to his marital and later romantic difficulties. When they tried to dig deeper into his conformist behavior other than the obvious childhood ties to a domineering father, he became self-righteous, accusing the group of "piling on," or "not listening to what I'm saying, taking it way too far." While others tried to explain or reassure him of positive intentions, he relied on me to confirm them.

There were grave limits to what could be said and who could say it. As titular leader of an idealized internal group, only I could disturb it. Slowly and gingerly, I translated what others meant by their exploratory confrontations and why they might be frustrated, hurt, or angered by George's reactions. "It doesn't mean that they are right, but it's where they're at. Your wife didn't tell you what she was thinking – why remain perplexed?" I made it a point to call attention to our small victories, as when he brought an occasional dream or conveyed a feeling or emotional thought with conviction. He gradually developed some capacity to engage in disagreements and allow others to revisit them.

A greater victory occurred in a session when several members protested that he was being patronizing in how he offered opinions and advice. "You're acting like your father!" someone called out. I was surprised that George tolerated the intervention; moreover, he was amused. "Oh my god, that's just how I don't want to be!" "Welcome to the club," another member said, "we all struggle with that." But truly, he was not yet a full-fledged club member. Other than the few lively flare-ups (which I treasured and attempted to hold him to), he retreated into his characteristic bland friendliness.

The introjected father had entered our group space, and yet little had changed. During one recollection relayed with fondness, George told us something about his mother:

> You knew when you displeased her. She would put aside whatever she was reading and say "your father will hear about this"; that was scary enough, but she didn't have to say anything. She got an expression on her face that

could freeze you. All the sun went out of her. I was much more afraid of displeasing her than my father.

George had unwittingly revealed a violently inscribed parental message from George's superficially sweet mother. Maternal castigations – mostly nonverbal facial and tonal signifiers for transgressions – had terrorized George into meek submission. In group, even when verbally acting like a modified version of his father, he conveyed his mother's intentions, adopting some of her nonverbal skills to terminate what he considered improper sibling behavior. There were dangers in pushing boundaries of maternal introspections. Now I knew why.

Discussion: Assassinating the Minds of Disloyal Peers

The Manchurian Candidate (Condon, 1959) was a political thriller (made into two American movies) about a United States senator's son unknowingly hypnotized into becoming an assassin for a Communist conspiracy. A coded message (the Queen of Diamonds playing card) prompted the son to kill those standing in the way of his Russian-sympathizing mother's presidential ambitions for her husband. The novel resolves when the son, realizing maternal betrayal, shifts the intended target to his parents, and turns the gun on himself.

The young George intuited his mother's pervasive message to keep "in line," without the cognitive tools to understand why. To protect sustaining maternal idealizations, George shifted all developmental cruelties to his father. His mother, however, held the Queen of Diamonds. "All the sun went out of her face." George declaimed. An unbearably dark maternal "shadow" had hypnotic influence. Any member who intruded into George's maternally orchestrated psychology triggered an attack on their thinking.

An "interpolating signifier" (Laplanche, 1979) of maternal gestures governed George's mind and social behavior. We are all brainwashed, however, for every child wants to execute their parents' desires (Lacan, 1977). The protagonist of *Manchurian Candidate* turned the gun on himself to escape capture. If we are fortunate, sharing a murderous pact with siblings (Freud, 1913) makes that unnecessary. Traversing developmental epochs with sufficiently irreverent fraternal figures provides multiple opportunities to translate parental messages, partially freeing the next generation from their control.

While surrounded by siblings, but blindly playing out their mother's "card," George had suffered through developmental epochs without their support. Entering our group with difficulty maintaining his own point of view, he came to trust other members as needed siblings who could complete his thoughts and validate his feelings. Except when the topic turned to mothers. Until now. A group discussion provided a fortuitous moment to address him while unarmed and mentally available. With new understanding that his description of his mother provided, we took opportunity to sabotage the plot.

Case Example 3: The Therapist's Fraternal Dynamics Play Out in Group[2]

"Stop, you're spinning." "You're ranting, we got it!" The members reasoned and remonstrated as an unstoppable Marcia continued: "You don't understand; let me explain what I mean." "Sorry to cut you off. I didn't realize." "I just needed to get this out; I don't need feedback." Even when yielding to interruptions (often to her interruptions!), Marcia negotiated the terms: "I'll try to hear you, but don't tell me I'm 'spinning.' Think of another word. Not 'ranting,' that's worse. I know I do this sometimes; that's why my [ex-]husband hated me, but he criticized me no matter what."

Marcia rested comfortably with the knowledge that she was not hated but rather enjoyed and valued for her lively presence. She affably rebutted confrontations and criticisms with frank acknowledgment: "I don't want to do group your way. "I know, I know, it's my mother, I fight back and don't let anyone pressure me to be or to do."

Defending against an internalized mother, Marcia fought to live within a protected zone of entitlement. While careful with the other female members, she acted with impunity towards men. A source of energy and delight to her father and brothers, she did not expect or enjoy being challenged by their group representatives. Humorously recognizing their limits, members turned to me to "do something"; "she listens to you, sometimes." While making efforts not to embarrass her, I called attention to how she shuts others out and halts exchanges. "[Marcia:] Okay I get it, let's move on."

My work seemed tolerable to Marcia and good enough for the group, but Hank complained that I was charmed and seduced. There was truth in the accusation, although Marcia claimed that Hank was the true favorite since he often talked like me. There was truth in her rebuttal too, for I admired his insights and how well he expressed them. As the most educated member of his family, Hank was groomed to be the "messiah" (his word). Not surprisingly, such parental favoritism did not sit well with his younger sisters, who took many opportunities to relay his every infraction real, exaggerated, or fabricated. Hank repeatedly tried to educate Marcia on her disconcerting effects on his concentration only to set off Marcia's defensive wall of words.

On one occasion, with an uncharacteristic loss of patience, he called out "shut up already" and held his ears. Marcia did not take this remark with the warm humor intended. "It's one thing for Rich to say this to me, but not you." Hank tried to repair: "I thought we were friends." "Not that kind," Marcia retorted steamily. Other group members tried to adjudicate. Hank could have said it better, but his frustration was understandable, and maybe I as the leader should have done more. "He was trying to talk" someone explained, to which Marcia countered coolly, "go ahead, I'm not stopping you."

Hank blanched and said little for the session's remainder. He did not appear for the next two weeks, and when I asked him about his absences in an individual session, he said he was thinking of dropping out. "Something went horribly wrong." There was no repair, given the fearsome "intensity" of Marcia's anger. What intensity? I inquired skeptically, adding truthfully that I did not notice anything different from Marcia's animated piques that I, along with the other male members, were regularly subjected. "Talk it out with Marcia," I suggested. "No," he replied without rancor, "I don't think you can protect me from Marica, not sure that you would even try."

Hank took several months after returning before addressing Marcia. He haltingly described the deep fissure in their relationship and expectation of group denunciation. Marcia reassured Hank that she hardly thought about it, maybe not at all. Hearing from the group that her reply did the opposite of reassure and might have hurt, she clarified:

> I'm not saying I don't think about you. You're very important to me and I hated it when you didn't come to group. I just don't like it when you act superior like a professor and tell me what to do. That's Rich's job.

Hank's air of superiority, purified in an atmosphere of parental favoritism, did not sit well with Marcia, who would not tolerate a symbolic sibling putting limits on her. Neither was an innocent "done to" in their internal sibling groupings, nor in their replications here and elsewhere. I was confident that they would work it out to the advantage of both. Taking efforts to revamp his relationship to Marcia, Hank became less the professor and more the peer to his group cohorts. For Marcia, Hank provided a persuasive learning experience regarding her effect on others – a thoughtlessness that could cut deeply (and which likely contributed to her failed marriage).

Discussion: The Analyst Meets Peers of an Earlier Self

I had agreed with Hank that something had gone wrong but not "horribly" so. What had he been expecting? I considered the question too: who were these antagonists to each other, and who were they to me? Hank's "shut up" fleetingly disrupted Marcia, who shrugged him off with the confidence of a lifetime of male adoration. The group had no zone of safety for Hank, no trustworthy parent or sib to witness, partner, and counter unfair treatment. "I'm so disappointed, I expect better of you" haunted Hank's inner groupings, a stereophonic familial message he had transmitted to Marcia (and to me), and which he had heard returned in her harsh rebuke.

Whereas I registered Marcia's anger at Hank, I assessed hers as not severe, and not entirely believable. While Hank (and I) had assumed his "shut up" and gesture of covering his ears were brotherly communications and typical, Marcia heard an unprivileged paternal injunction. "I just don't like it when you act superior like a professor and tell me what to do. That's Rich's job." Other members had entrusted that job to me as well: "Do something, you deal with her [Marcia]." For Hank, my voice proved unreliable, and he risked his own. No one had shamed him or gullibly denied Marcia's share of responsibility.

Yet, despite contrary evidence of support, Hank found himself once again in an internal group, keeping himself at emotional distance from distrusted family members.

Each of us heard words and viewed that which passed in the group space in terms of our own developmentally influenced relational complexes. Other than my own sporadic behavior, I could not conjure reveries of mean childhood play with siblings. My grudges are mostly vertical and relate to successive developmental periods revolving around authority figures – they continue today. Like Marcia, I had a parent who talked over and at me, and like Hank, one who was disappointed that I didn't do better (Billow, 2019b). At one time, Marcia or Hank could have become that parent to me. I complimented myself for having matured and relating to both with such warm aplomb.

"Shut up," "no you shut up, you're not my boss" – such momentary sib flare-ups extend to adolescent courtship rituals and were enjoyably familiar. Informed by nostalgic romantic reveries of my adolescent epoch, I heard and saw nothing worrisome or undeserved in Hank's "shut up" and pantomime of covering his ears, and I was surprised but not troubled by the intensity of Marcia's feisty retort. Both were troubled by their interaction, however. While short-lived for Marcia (or so it seemed), and left unresolved, it persisted for Hank. Failing to be troubled, I did not anticipate the depth of Hank's psychic pain that existed out of the range of my sibling experience, and I unwittingly confirmed Hank's contentions regarding me as a failed father figure. To do better, I had to meet both at the boundaries of their developmental epochs.

I found myself breaking in more often, saying kindly but forcibly: "Marcia, hold back, give others a chance"; "you're getting off subject"; "you said your opinion well, you don't need to repeat it"; "you're not hearing what people are saying to you." These types of comments were not easy for me and I hated making them, remembering how often I was on their receiving end from my parents. In subjecting my behavior to developmental "re-arrangements," I become more the boundary-enforcing parent (pleasing Hank) and less a sibling. and was not always judicious. I had limits to my patience (as did my parents, I sympathized), which varied according to whatever else was going on in the group and me personally. However, learning from what my parents did not do, I expressed regret and adjusted. Even a warm smile could repair, but when Marcia occasionally left a session feeling hurt, I did too. That felt more mature, better than just feeling good about myself.

In critical group encounters, vestigial remains of fixed identities and frozen roles reappear, and with so many internal as well as actual group voices resonating in the analyst's "third ear," we cannot immediately (and rarely, conclusively) resolve who is doing what to whom. Mitchell (2003, p. 11) asserted that before siblings "are equal in their sameness to each other for their father, children must be equal in their difference from each other for their mother. This will be the first vertical relation for siblings." In actuality, children are not equal to parents, whose unconscious complexes are variously stimulated (Magagna, 2014). Likewise, group analysts do not relate to each member equally. Each member takes shifting roles in our internal groupings, many of which connect to developmental experiences of being with siblings and serving as one. While we speak through the voices of our own development, others receive us according to theirs.

Psychotherapy Groups Provoke Fraternal Trauma

Groups are busy, even when silent, for the participants are coping with profound fraternal trauma: "*Then came another baby and brought you grave disillusionment*" (Freud, 1937, p. 261). Confronted with the group, the unconscious experiences massive loss (Debbane et al., 1986, p. 523). Members (re)discover an interpersonal world of "like me's," confirming fears of no longer being exclusively "cared for and loved" (Freud, 1905, p. 194ff). The infant fascinates on peers; likewise, the group member, who greets peers as extensions of ourselves and hates them as our replacements (Mitchell, 2003).

Freud (1921, p. 120) described how

> the fact that the younger child is loved by the parents as much as he himself is . . . he is forced into identifying himself with the older children. . . . What appears later on in society in the shape of . . . "group spirit" does not belie its derivation from what was originally envy. . . . Thus social feeling is based upon the reversal of what was a hostile feeling into a positive-toned tie in the nature of an identification.

Groups camouflage a collective loss of identity, a loss I also feel and must cope with as leader (Billow, 2021a, 2019b).

Whenever a group convenes, the leader should be warm and hospitable without overstaying the welcoming process by being too friendly, too sensitive, or too empathic, all of which may pressure on people to behave similarly. Therapists must possess "a certain amount of cruelty" and not be "too nice," Carl Jung declared (Atlas & Aron, 2018, p. 117), which fits the developmental role of siblings, too. To be necessarily cruel, the analyst must be willing and able to adopt a challenging fraternal *presence* (Billow, 2019a). Interpretation alone does not sufficiently disturb a mutually protective fantasy of how groups and members are supposed to be (Caper, 1997). In upholding am exclusively vertical relationship to the group, the leader unintentionally reinforces an idealized *family* fantasy involving the analyst-parent as "pillar of the faith" (Lacan, 1977, p. 219), an unwavering model and enforcer of appropriate thought and behavior. In every group, painful fraternal traumas fester; left unaddressed, we risk burdening members with needless suffering. To set up the grounds for "translation of psychic material," it is important to disrupt ritualized roles behavior, fraternal as well as parental, mine as well as other members.

A group is not so different from the immature child who, through successive developmental stages, needs adults to follow and also to separate from and engage with peers. For some members it may be important for the analyst to serve as a symbolic sibling; for others it is imperative not to be one. Members may implore us to "do something" and assert parental weight; they turn to us for safety and clarity in the midst of sibling conflicts. Like a parent, we cannot protect a group from growing pains and inevitable fraternal struggles. Some becoming braver and more spontaneous, others more circumspect and self-conscious.

Re-transcribing the *Container-Contained*

Bion (1965) formulated an essential relationship between socialization and emotional development in terms of the container-contained:

> The individual cannot contain the impulses proper to a pair and the pair cannot contain the impulses proper to a group. The psycho-analytic problem is the problem of growth and its harmonious resolution in the relationship between the container and the contained, repeated in individual, pair, and finally group (intra and extra psychically).
>
> [Bion, 1970, pp. 15–16]

Bion's symbolic representation [♀♂] ideographically represents *multiple* interacting elements, encompassing internal, dyadic, triadic, and group relationships.

To pass through "successive epochs of life" (Freud, 1896, p. 233) the developing individual needs containment by self, dyadic partners (vertical and horizontal) and groups: small (the family) and large (the sociopolitical world). In some encounters we aim to function as the benevolent maternal figure who *holds* the group and establishes nonverbal bonding. In others, we aim to *bind* the group to language, being the emblematic father who enters with thought and imposes the use of words (Billow 2013; Lacan, 1977). And as a sib, we want to be available to *play* and joyfully let ourselves to be played with. After all, the analyst functions in a setting amid "like me's" and should feel and be treated as one. In reducing traditional asymmetry in psychotherapeutic relationships, the analyst relates as one "more simply human than otherwise" (Sullivan, 1947, p. 7), down to earth and on our toes. The elaborated version of the container-contained grounds and expands our technical options, clarifying how we may shift our symbolic boundaries. Bringing these functions into conceptual focus frees up the analyst to meet others at various developmental levels and traverse them experimentally.

Conclusion: Penetrating Epochs of Development

Approaching the analytic patient, Bion (1977, pp. 48–49) advised formulating a method that can "penetrate the barrier" between different layers of the personality. Supporting a pluralistic rather than a one or two-person psychology model, analytic group psychotherapy presents a methodology particularly suitable to reveal these layers, since a broad developmental range of their derivatives display themselves in vivo. All members have opportunities to call forth, mentally rehearse, and publicly revise relationships in which maternal, paternal, and fraternal figures from different developmental epochs play their parts. In making one's own translations – from then and "them" to now and "us," each member establishes integrating links between one's own psychic growth and the growth of others. The group penetrates the core of identity; we mature and are gradually transformed.

Notes

1 From Freud (1905): "A mother would probably be horrified if she were made aware that all her marks of caring [derived from her own sexual life]? were rousing her child's sexual instinct and preparing for its later intensity. . . . She is only fulfilling her task in teaching the child to love" (p. 223).
2 I discussed aspects of this case in Billow (2021b).

References

Atlas, G., & Aron, L. (2018). *Dramatic Dialogs*. New York: Routledge.
Billow, R. M. (2013). Appreciating 'Le Non/Nom'. *Group Anal.*, *46*:33–47.
Billow, R. M. (2019a). Doing our work: Words, deeds, and presence. *Int. J. Group Psychother.*, *69*:77–98.
Billow, R. M. (2019b). Attention-getting mechanisms (AGMs): A personal journey. *Int. J. Group Psychother.*, *69*:408–433.
Billow, R. M. (2021a). *Richard M. Billow's Selected Papers on Psychoanalysis and Group Process: Changing Our Minds* (T. Slonim, Ed.). London: Routledge.
Billow, R. M. (2021b). Opening Laplanche's window: Transference-countertransference in psychoanalytic group psychotherapy. *Psychoanal. Q.*, *90*:1.
Bion, W. R. (1965). *Transformations*. London: Heinemann.
Bion, W. R. (1970). *Attention and Interpretation*. London: Tavistock.
Bion, W. R. (1977). *Two Papers: The Grid and Caesura*. Rio de Janeiro: Imago Editora Ltd.
Bollas, C. (1984). Moods and the conservative process. *Int. J. Psychoanal.*, *65*:203–212.
Caper, R. (1997). A mind of one's own. *Int. J. Psychoanal.*, *78*:265–278.
Condon, R. (1959). *The Manchurian Candidate*. New York: McGraw-Hill.
Debbane, E., deCarufel, F., Bienvenu, J., & Piper, W. (1986). Structures in interpretations: A group psychoanalytic perspective. *Int. J. Group Psychother.*, *36*:517–532.
Faimberg, H. (2005). *The Telescoping of Generations: Listening to the Narcissistic Links Between Generations*. London: Routledge.
Freud, S. (1896). Letter 52 from the extracts from the Fliess Papers. In *S.E.* 1:233–239.
Freud, S. (1905). Three essays on the theory of sexuality. In *S.E.* 7:123–244.
Freud, S. (1913). Totem and Taboo. In *S.E.* 13:1–161.
Freud, S. (1921). Group psychology and the analysis of the ego. In *S.E.* 18:70–92.
Freud, S. (1937). Constructions in analysis. In *S.E.* 32:255–270.
Kaes, R. (2002). *La Polyphonie du Reve*. Paris: Dunod.
Kaes, R. (2007). *Linking, Alliances and Shared Spaces: Groups and the Psychoanalyst*. London: International Psychoanalysis Library.
Kirshner, L. (2006). The work of Rene Kaes: Intersubjective transmission in families, groups, and culture. *J. Amer. Psychoanal. Assoc.*, *54*:1005–1013.

Lacan, J. (1977). *Ecrits* (A. Sheridan, Trans.). New York: Norton.

Laplanche, J. (1979). *New Foundations for Psychoanalysis* (D. Marcey, Trans.). Oxford: Basil Blackwell.

Magagna, J. (2014). Envy, jealousy, love, and generosity in sibling relations: The impact of sibling relations on future family relations. In *Siblings: Envy and Rivalry, Coexistence and Concern*, ed. K. Skrzypek, B. Maciejewska-Sobczak, & Z. Stadnicka-Dmitriew. London: Karnac, pp. 195–217.

Mitchell, J. (2003). *Siblings*. Oxford: Polity Press.

Piaget, J. (1969). *The Language and Thought of the Child*. Cleveland: Meridian Books.

Sullivan, H. S. (1947). *Conceptions of Modern Psychiatry*. Washington, DC: William Alanson White Psychiatric Foundation.

1.2 Siblings and Groups. Groups of Siblings?

Maria-José Blanco

Introduction

Transference and the Transference Level: 'Making the Unconscious Conscious' (C.G. Jung)

Kreeger defines transference as 'the psychological process by which feelings, attitudes and wishes, originally linked with important figures in one's life, are projected onto others who have come to represent them in current life' (1991). Schlapobersky, defines it as 'a feature in all our relationships in which behaviour, relationship patterns, emotions, fantasies or all these psychological attributes arising from childhood experience are lived out in later relationships – in this case the group – *as if* they belonged there' (2016, p. 374). As Foulkes explains, transference is a term taken from individual psychoanalysis (Foulkes and Anthony 1957, p. 17). 'The psychoanalytic situation is known as . . . a "transference situation"' (60). Foulkes sees the transference level as 'the level most often envisaged by group psychotherapists of analytic orientation, for whom the group represents the family, the conductor father or mother and the other members siblings' (1964, p. 115). He saw the 'transference situation' as the place 'where past and present meet' (Foulkes and Anthony 1957, p. 50) and referred to the group-analytic group as a 'transference group' (Foulkes 1964, p. 74). He believed that if the patient is able to see the link between present experiences in the group and their past relationship with their parents and siblings, this 'recognition of the historical Transference significance often follows change' (Foulkes 1975, pp. 127–128). Anthony highlights the importance of the therapist's own feelings and the need to deploy them in benefit of the group (Foulkes and Anthony 1957, p. 144), and Hopper sees the conductor countertransference, or what he calls 'co-transference',[1] as 'a useful communication tool' (2006, p. 555).

Groups of Siblings, the Horizontal Line

Whenever Foulkes wrote about siblings, he linked it to transference and the transference level (Foulkes 1975, p. 127, 1964, p. 64 and p. 115; and Foulkes and Anthony, p. 101). He did not develop the idea of sibling relationships in

DOI: 10.4324/9781003220060-4

groups, although he gave importance to the sibling transference and compared the dynamics of the group to family dynamics (Foulkes and Anthony 1957, p. 50). Foulkes called the family the 'root group' (Foulkes and Anthony 1957, p. 31, p. 113, p. 266). This is the first group where disturbances arise (266) and the therapy group becomes the place where the disturbance is expressed (266). 'To be a member of a group-analytic group is ultimately, at least, a regression to the nursery group stage' (Foulkes 1990, p. 241) or, in other words, to the sibling group.

Mitchell argues that the development of group psychology is impossible without looking at sibling relationships (2003, pp. 12–13). Mitchell also develops the idea that the differences between psychoanalysis and group analysis lie on the axis of the relationships, the psychoanalytical being vertical, between the psychoanalyst and the patient/client, and the group analytic being horizontal, between all the members of the group including the conductor (11). Foulkes referred to group analysis as 'horizontal analysis' (Foulkes and Anthony 1957, p. 42, p. 53). Sibling relationships have a horizontal character, which does not preclude their also containing vertical elements.

In the classical psychoanalytic context, transference occurs between the patient and the analyst. I will argue, following others, that, in the group situation, transference occurs between patients, both 'in the horizontal level (to peers) and at the vertical level (to the conductor)' (Prodgers 1991, p. 393). I will add, as others have also done before (Mitchell 2003, p. 14; Papiasvili 2011, p. 292; Philips 2014), that the horizontal level of the transference could include both the conductor and the members of the group. 'The group situation provides an indispensable means of bringing essential patterns into focus . . . a whole spectrum of relationships in active operation before our eyes' (Foulkes and Anthony 1957, p. 50). Transference arises out of past relationships to significant figures, siblings have been, in most cases amongst those figures (Grant and Crawley 2002, pp. 1–7). The conductor's own patterns in early life inevitably influence the way he or she takes up the conductor role. As Anthony says 'he has to watch his own reactions' (Foulkes and Anthony 1957, p. 145).

Shapiro and Ginzberg see a logical link between sibling relationships in the members' families and the transference amongst the members of the group; they wonder why clinicians don't use such transferential phenomena when giving interpretations in their groups (2001, p. 328). Rabin sees how the study of sibling and peer transference can 'enrich the therapist understanding of the group dynamics' (in Shapiro and Ginzberg 2001, p. 328). While Parker wonders whether the seeming reluctance to write about sibling relationships in groups derives from 'our own sibling difficulties' or whether we are 'daunted by their complexity' (2016, p. 5).

We can see that sibling rivalry has been a focus of study in relation to groups, but there are relatively few studies dealing more broadly with sibling relationships in groups. Even though rivalry is inevitable in the group's life, the relationship between the different members of the group can present many other characteristics of sibling relationships which contribute to the therapeutic process and to change.

Why Is Sibling Transference Important?

Given, not chosen, siblings are the first peers and companions, the first people to play, argue, share with, to compete against. Siblings play an important role in the development of our personality and, as Coles explains, they 'play a crucial part in the development of our mind' (2006, p. 3).

Being the first born, the first male, the first female, may contribute to having a more powerful role or carrying more responsibilities. In a therapy group, older members (not in age but in group chronology) may also feel a sense of power, or responsibility, while younger ones may feel rejected by the older ones. These roles, in a family, change over time, in the same way that the roles of the conductor and the other group members change as the group develops (Foulkes 1964, p. 63).

Despite its limitations, Adler's theory of the significance of birth order in shaping people's characters help us to think about individual histories and how these characteristics are recreated in patients' relationships to each other, in the group. Foulkes stated that we are shaped by the family group (1990, p. 231) and Elias explains how the development of an individual would depend 'on the structure of the group in which he grows up, and finally on his position in this group and the formative process it entails' (1991, pp. 21–22). Greif and Woolley look at adult siblings' relationships and outline some of the characteristics of these. They also talk about positive aspects of sibling relationships, such as support and social network and the learning of basic interactions such as: 'cooperate and deal with competition'; 'opposite sex interaction'; 'negotiate differences'; 'deal with loss' and so on. Such factors relate closely to the development of a therapy group, where members come to accept each for who they are, share resilience and hope, and want things to work out for everyone (2016, p. 7). Bonds strengthen over time and their influence can bring change. Hope-Price writes about hostility in families and therapy groups and the importance of being open about the hostility and its resolution as 'crucial to the therapeutic change' (1982, p. 1). 'Working through' the sibling transference (Kreeger 1991; Hopper 2006, p. 554) is the way to understand feelings from the past and to 'free [one]self from the grip of mechanisms of repetition' (Kreeger 1991).

The Clinical Context

Group Dynamics: A Group of Siblings, Positive and Negative Interactions in the Group

I am going to use the training group I ran at an outpatients psychodynamic psychotherapy service in a NHS hospital, in London. It was a slow open, mixed group, which met once weekly for an hour and a half for just over three years. The local borough is very diverse in culture, ethnicity, and economic circumstances and this is reflected in the range of patients that the department treats. Most of the group members were in employment. Their main presenting problems were depression and anxiety and most were taking medication for depression. Sibling transference was a vital tool in helping me and the members of the group to understand our interactions and reactions to other members.

The Older Brother – Malignant Mirroring/ Negative Projective Identification

In the group's second session, Anthony had been very quiet, which made me uncomfortable; he had always spoken a lot, during our one-to-one sessions and in the first session of the group. Another member of the group, Ehsan, had monopolised the first session and was doing so, again, in the second. While in the first session Anthony had communicated with Ehsan about their common careers, mental health problems, and other circumstances of their lives, this time Anthony seemed annoyed with Ehsan. In Mitchell's words, the switch in attitude, between the sessions, was like 'the hugs that turn instantly to blows' (Mitchell 2003, p. 20). While their common backgrounds: sophisticated language, working as civil servants, having been bullied at school, and so on, had helped their bonding in the first session, their competitiveness and controlling nature clashed in the second one. Lucas, who had not spoken very much in either session said to Ehsan, 'you talk a lot but your words don't reach me'. That sentence was the catalyst for Anthony to tell Ehsan how he had taken lots of space in the session and how he was undermining other members of the group with his superiority and his arrogance. Anthony said to Ehsan 'you want to control the group'. Anthony was very aggressive towards Ehsan, accusing him of being arrogant and believing that he was cleverer than others. Ehsan left the group at the end of the session looking like a child having a tantrum; he slammed the door and never came back. Battegay writes about the 'Sacrifice of Isaac' and gives an example of a member of his group exposing his problems, while the rest of the group feel relieved that they don't have to talk. Ehsan became a sacrificial figure for the group and, as it was early days, I was not able to 'work through this tendency' (1983, p. 217).

Freud believed that 'Sibling identification occurs in response to sibling rivalry' (1921). This was a clear case of negative projective identification or of malignant mirroring with Anthony 'killing' Ehsan with his 'hatred', 'hated by the older child, hated to death' (Mitchell 2003, p. 43). Schlapobersky speaks of this kind of transference process and explains how, while this is happening between two people, the rest of the group, including the conductor, are witnesses of their exchange. He goes on to say: 'Their reparative dialogue can then become a nucleus for a widening discourse . . . that comes to include the group as a whole' (2016, p. 371). The 'reparative dialogue' between Anthony and Ehsan was not possible, but the subsequent discussions about what had happened did establish a discourse in the group matrix, which was then drawn upon, when another similar conflict happened, some months later, with the incorporation of new members into the group.

The Younger Siblings – Sibling Rivalries/Malignant Envy

SESSION 23

Teresa is very jealous of her younger sisters, as they both have husbands and a comfortable life, while she is a single mother of a 'difficult' daughter; she has not had a relationship since her daughter, now a teenager, was born. When two new members, Fiona and Noah, arrived in the group, Teresa found their presence very disturbing. In their second session, the new members had given a lot of support to Pam, while the rest of the members had been unusually quiet. Towards the end of the session, Teresa expressed annoyance with Shane and Tracy for 'teasing' the conductor. She told them of the 'older brother' (Anthony), who couldn't stop attacking me. Fiona defended Shane and Tracy and Teresa angrily informed her, 'You don't know how this works'. In this moment she seemed to be relating to me on both horizontal and vertical axes, both defending me as a sibling in the group, who was being teased, and, at the same time, wanting to be mummy's favourite, showing off that she knew better than the younger members how the group worked. Fiona then turned to Noah, and said, 'You see, this is what I was asking you about the other day, I don't know how this is going to work'. This further inflamed Teresa's anger; the idea of Fiona speaking with another member, outside the group, outraged her. 'So, you talk to him but you cannot talk to me? You cannot even look at me.' Fiona, touching Teresa on her arm, said, 'I am sorry'. Teresa pulled her arm away. Raising her voice, Fiona said 'I try to apologise and this is how you treat me'. Teresa declared that she couldn't cope with the group and needed to leave, but it was Fiona, who left the room. After the session had ended, Fiona came back to pick up her bag. She said, 'I left so that Teresa could say good bye to the group'. At that moment, her wish to get rid of Teresa was very strong.

A re-enactment of the first conflict seemed to be developing before my eyes, but experience of the first allowed me to understand that I needed to respond in a different way. In contrast to the first conflict, both women came back to the group the following week and the group was able to talk about the difficulties. I brought the focus of the anger towards myself, for having brought new members into the group, and they were able to speak about their feelings towards the birth of the younger sibling. 'The one who feels displaced refuses to recognize the new-found sibling – the other' (Mitchell 2003, p. 133). Teresa felt she did all the work in the group had the responsibilities, had to look after me while the younger 'siblings' broke the rules, the boundaries, by talking outside the group. I, on the other hand, felt annoyed with Teresa for not welcoming the new comers. As the youngest in my family I felt great empathy with Fiona and Noah who were trying to find their place in the group.

Sibling Support/Empathy

Tracy had lived in a foster home from an early age. When she was nine, she went back to live with her mother and her stepfather. Her mother was very aggressive and abusive. She made Tracy look after her younger brother, feed him, change his nappies, and take him to bed. If she did not do what she was told, she was beaten. Tracy was very protective of her brother, as she did not want him to receive the same abuse that she was getting from both mother and stepfather. She always made sure that he would be on time for school, even though that meant she was late herself. She was always late for the group.

When Noah and Fiona joined the group, Tracy who had been very quiet from the beginning, started talking more. She was specially drawn to talking to Noah and he seemed to understand her. He talked about her anger, when she was not there, and understood her feelings even though she never spoke of anger in the group. The rest of the members noticed the change and commented, when she was not there, on the fact that she seemed to relate to Noah better than to any of the older members of the group.

When the last new member, Cass, joined the group, Tracy began to arrive on time. The first session with Cass, Tracy spoked at length. The other members were very surprised.

It became clear that the birth of a new child in the group, someone she could look after and protect, allowed Tracy to find a place for herself in the group. Subsequently, by coming on time and speaking, she began to give others the opportunity of knowing and trusting her.

Sharing/Resonance/Exchange

SESSION 50

Teresa had been thinking about leaving the group. She came to see me in a one-to-one session. She said that she found the new members, especially Fiona, difficult to deal with. She worried about breaking of boundaries, and felt that Fiona did not understand the rules of the group, as the founding members did. I wondered whether she felt that I had not been as strict with the new members as I had been with the 'first born'? Had I become a more relaxed 'mother', who did not discipline her younger children?

After having the one-to-one session with me, she decided to come back to the group and try again. The talk turned to sharing and how she preferred to be on her own rather than with other people; she did not like groups. She spoke about playing shops on her own, when she was little, she would be both shopkeeper and customer. Pam also liked to be on her own, even though she knows that it is not good for her and that the best moments are when she is with others. She said that she had found it difficult to share, even though she liked playing with other children. When she was little, she had a kitchen that she never let her half-sister play with; it was hers and she did not want to share it. Pam told the group about going to a concert, with her oldest friend and her mother's friend; being there with them may have been the happiest she had felt in 15 years. I spoke of sharing the space with others in the group, linking it with the fact that Teresa and Pam were firstborn and that there was a big age difference between the two of them and their siblings. Teresa said, 'Yes, we were like only children'. Pam said, 'I sometimes remind myself that I am one of five, but I am the only child, for my father and mother as a couple'. Lucas spoke, then, to say that he had never had anything that he could call his own. Being the youngest of 11, everything had belonged to others. This led him to speak about his own body not being his. For the first time, he spoke about the sexual abuse he suffered when he was a child. He never talked about it at home and since the group had started he had in his mind that he needed to tell them. I wondered whether telling the group at that moment had to do with the theme of sharing. Was he sharing the only thing that he had never shared before? Would that make him part of the family of the group, where he had always seemed to be on the edge, since the beginning?

The idea of 'sharing' in therapy groups is in everybody's mind. Sharing the therapist and the time and sharing their thoughts with others, who sometimes would mistreat them. When Lucas talked about the bathroom being the only place where he could be on his own, I thought of him hiding in the group bathroom, with his silences. Meanwhile, Teresa and Pam knew how to share, but while Pam had learned to enjoy sharing, Teresa still would like to have me for herself and not accept new members who may interfere with her playing.

'Siblings and peers can care for or destroy but also they can mirror – the baby can begin to form some image of itself through others who are like it' (Mitchell 2003, p. 136). In this session the members of the group resonated with each other being able to reflect on what it means to share in the group.

Discussion

In the life of the group, there were two major conflicts, clear examples of malignant mirroring or negative projective identification. In the first case, the members of the group, myself included, were not ready to deal with the conflict and, consequently, two members left the group. In the second case, we were able to work with it, sometimes explicitly drawing on the earlier experiences. In hindsight I could see how the sibling dynamics were present from the birth of the group. My own feelings, as the youngest sibling in my family, the only sister, who in many cases felt undermined by older brothers, were important at the start of the group's life. Both Anthony and Ehsan had evoked in me feelings of being the youngest sister, who didn't know what she was doing. Both very intelligent and competitive, they seemed confident when speaking and had achieved well in their careers. At the same time, they both had been neglected as children and had found it difficult to develop good relationships, including good attachment to their own siblings. I was initially unable to grasp the significance of this dynamic. After bringing new members into the group, similar sibling dynamics emerged. In this case, I was better able to understand the rivalry and separate myself from the sibling dynamic, in order to provide a parental containment. As Philips explains: 'vertical relationships create the "secure base"' (Philips 2014, p. 4).

The therapy group can be the place 'to examine and change old roles' (Ashuach 2012, p. 160). Relationships and members' roles evolved as they spoke about their roles in their families and how they had felt unable to change these. The only way for such changes to occur, in family or group, is to bring the hostilities into the open and work with them (Hope-Price 1983). The conflicts and hostilities towards each other were talked about and, in most cases, resolved. There was also positive sibling transference between group members, who felt the support given by others. Some of these changes were reflected in the experience of bringing the last member, Cass, into the group. The attitude of the group towards her was more open and respectful and she was not driven into a role, prematurely. This suggests a move from rigid, constraining sibling relationships to more supportive and open forms.

Ehsan and Anthony's conflict seemed to contain what Nitsun describes as the anxiety of the early days in a group's life. He links it to what Winnicott called the 'unthinkable anxiety' (Nitsun 1989, p. 250) where fear of rejection and attacks are anticipated (251). In Teresa and Fiona's case, what they seemed to expect from each other was also rejection and attack. The verbal exchanges in both conflicts were so quick that no one else could intervene or understand what was happening. They were all anticipating it, nothing needed to be said – just as it had happened before in their families.

Once Teresa and Fiona had engaged in their conflict, they were able to bring more complex accounts of their family histories into the group. Both of them harboured strong feelings of unfairness – Teresa for the birth of her sisters and the loss of the space that was hers, Fiona for the time and space that her older disabled brother received from her mother. Previously, they presented simplified, idealised pictures of their early histories, but later they were able to uncover their relationships with their siblings much more fully. This, in turn, allowed them, and others, to confront difficulties within the group, rather than running away from them. Brown explains that 'destructive rivalry . . . has to be fully acknowledged and worked with in the group before it can be transformed and transcended' (1998, p. 323).

Conclusion

Transference is central to psychoanalytic and group analytic theory and practice, but sibling transference has not received the attention that the transference between patient and therapist has had, over the years. One feature that differentiates group analysis from psychoanalysis is the horizontality of the relationships. Reviewing the group analytic literature, it is clear that sibling transference and sibling relationships play an important part of the group dynamics. Even though, until recently, there had not been much written about it, the last few years has seen a resurgence of articles and essays on sibling relationships and sibling transference.

Since establishing the group, I started focusing on birth order and on how this influences the roles that were given, and taken, in families. In many cases, these roles needed to be transcended, in order to allow development. Frequently, this process entails conflict and its resolution, before changes can occur. Hostilities were present in the group, but the members were able to live through periods of intense conflict and resolution. They were part of, or witness to, these processes of change. By speaking about their sibling relationships and their place in the family, the members of the group were able to understand how the other felt. The older siblings, who found it difficult to share, were witnesses of the feelings of the younger, who felt he didn't have anything he could call his own. Through their encounters in the group, older and younger siblings are able to experience revelation of, and insight into, the experience and perception of the other.

My role in my own family, as the youngest sister, influenced the way I initially conducted the group. As youngest sister of older brothers, I was desperate for acceptance as a member of the sibling group. The uncertainty that I felt in the group, as an inexperienced group therapist, evoked in me the sense of exclusion, which the younger child feels. I needed to grow out of that role in order to be able to provide the group with a safe base. My own change and development allowed change in the other members of the group

Reflecting on sibling transference initially helped me to grasp the dynamics in the group and eventually to make sense of them. The members also started to consider transferential feelings towards each other and to relate them to family histories. The first conflict and dropouts forced me to confront elements of my own sibling transference, in order to take up the role of conductor/mother, which the group needed. The conductor's own sibling transferences are an integral part of the process of group development. Once a safe base was put into place, the members were able to relate to each other as siblings. Parker feels that, 'The distinction of sibling relationships – in whatever form – is the sharing of parents' (Parker 5), and the members of my group needed, first of all, to compete for my attention before they turned to each other. Gradually, I started being needed less and left more space to the individuals to relate to each other, like the good enough parent. Brown distinguishes between the immature and the mature group, where the members don't need the conductor as she has been internalised (Brown 325).

Note

1 Co-transference: 'The relationship between the client's unconscious and the therapist's unconscious' (Tomkins 2011).

References

Ashuach, Smadar (2012) 'Am I My Brother Keeper? The Analytic Group as a Space for Re-enacting and Treating Sibling Trauma', *Group Analysis*, 45 (2), pp. 155–167.

Battegay, Raymond (1983) 'The Phenomenon of the "Sacrifice of Isaac" in Therapeutic Groups', *Group Analysis*, 16 (3), pp. 217–227.

Brown, Dennis (1998) 'Fair Shares and mutual Concern: The Role of Sibling Relationships', *Group Analysis*, 31 (3), pp. 315–326.

Coles, Prophecy (2006) *The Importance of Sibling Relationships in Psychoanalysis* (Oxon: Routledge).

Elias, Norbert (1991) *The Society of Individuals* (London: Continuum).

Foulkes, S.H. (1964) *Therapeutic Group Analysis* (London: Allen and Unwin).

——— (1975) *Group-analytic Psychotherapy: Method and Principles* (London: Karnac).

——— (1990) *Selected Papers. Psychoanalysis and Group Analysis* (London: Karnac).

——— and E.J. Anthony (1984) [1957] *Group Psychotherapy: The Psychoanalytic Approach* (London: Maresfield Reprints).

Freud, Sigmund (1921) *Group Psychology and the Analysis of the Ego*. The Standard Edition of the Complete Psychological Works of Sigmund Freud, Volume XVIII (1920–1922): Beyond the Pleasure Principle, Group Psychology and Other Works, 65–144. http://freudians.org/wp-content/uploads/2014/09/Freud_Group_Psychology.pdf

Grant, Jan and Jim Crawley (2002) *Transference and Projection: Mirrors to the Self* (Buckingham: Open University Press).

Greif, Geoffrey L. and Michael E. Woolley (2016) *Adult Sibling Relationships* (New York: Columbia University Press).

Hope-Price, Gloria (1982) *Sibling Rivalry in the Therapy Group*. Unpublished Dissertation.

——— (1983) *Resolution of Sibling Rivalry in the Therapy Group*. Unpublished Clinical Paper.

Hopper, Earl (2006), 'Theoretical and Conceptual Notes Concerning Transference and Countertransference Processes in Groups and by Groups, and the Social Unconscious: Part I', *Group Analysis*, 39 (4), pp. 549–559.

Kreeger, Lionel (1991) *Transference and Countertransference in Group Psychotherapy*. Unpublished Paper.

Mitchell, Juliet (2003) *Siblings: Sex and Violence* (Oxford: Blackwell).

Nitsun, Morris (1989) 'Early Development: Linking the Individual and the Group', *Group Analysis*, 22(3), pp. 249–260.

Papiasvili, Eva D. (2011) 'Sibling Transference Phenomena in Experiential Process Groups', *Group*, 35 (4), Siblings and Groups, pp. 289–303.

Parker, Val (2016) *"The Sibling Blind Spot" Has Group Analysis Neglected the Complex Issue of Sibling Dynamics*? Unpublished Talk Given as Part of New Readings (London: IGA).

Philips, Caroline (2014) *The Influence of Sibling Relationships in the Development of the Group Including the Group Conductor*. Unpublished Clinical Paper.

Prodgers, Alan (1991) 'Countertransference: The Conductor's Emotional Response within the Group Setting', *Group Analysis*, 24 (4), pp. 389–407.

Schlapobersky, John (2016) *From the Couch to the Circle: Group Analytic Psychotherapy in Practice* (Oxon: Routledge).

Shapiro, Elizabeth L. and Raphael Ginzberg (2001) 'The Persistently Neglected Sibling Relationship and Its Applicability to Group Therapy', *International Journal of Group Psychotherapy*, 51 (3), pp 327–341.

Tomkins, Gary (2011) *Clarifying and Re-mystifying Transference, Counter-Transference and Co-Transference: A Guide to Avoiding Procrustean Psychotherapy*. Bristol C.G. Jung Public Lectures. www.individualpsychotherapy.co.uk/articles04.htm

1.3 Far away from home

A study of sibling relationships in Thomas Ogden's novels

Shoshi Breiner

My brother and I (introduction)

When I was four years old, I liked to daydream. As I walked down the street, I might walk into a pole or other treacherous object. Like Lewis Carol's capricious Queen of Hearts, I wanted to yell, "Off with their heads!"

It seemed to me, at the time, that the world was nothing other than a colorful backdrop, a stage built to adorn my life. Through my childish eyes, I was not only the center of the world. To me, the entire world had been created to contain me, and even my parents were actors in a singular role. In these moments, when I would sink into my reveries, a deep wonder would steal into my heart over this extraordinary arrangement, possibly a last vestige of humility, but for the most part I was overcome with great elation, which even the obstacles that came my way failed to subside.

I was an only child and grandchild, and even an only niece. The world was an oyster, that I alone was born from. And then, I was informed that my mother was with child, and a new brother or sister would soon be born. The Queen of Hearts still felt secure in her kingdom. Here was my mother, giving me a gift, a sort of doll to do with as my heart pleased. And then my brother was born. All at once, I lost all control over my mother's actions. It was clear that she was consumed with caring for the baby, not in order to give him to me, but in complete attentiveness to his needs, health and wholeness, without regard for me – or my fury and indignation. Beyond my panic of abandonment, beyond the jealousy, insult and rage, not to mention revenge fantasies, more than anything I felt the terrible grief over losing my ability to daydream. I understood that I had been wrong, that nothing had been created for me. Here was my mother, caring for my brother as a separate entity from me, focusing all her attention on him. [I will never forget her tears when he fell ill with severe diarrhea, and her words, "But this is the end of the world!"] Now that little fool could think the whole world was built for him. The kernels of doubt I had before about the meaning of reality now became painful certainties. My expulsion from Eden became the source of my sorrow, but also the source of a certain tenacity and creativity.

My mother, in all her wisdom, noticed my plans for revenge, and warned me, gently but firmly, that if I hurt my brother, I'd live to regret it. It was clear to me,

DOI: 10.4324/9781003220060-5

without any if-thens, that hurting my brother would destroy any last affections my mother held for me. And so, in her presence, my behavior was exemplary, but when she turned her all-seeing eyes, my brother might get a little pinch here or there. And when he was under my care, I might not stop drawing or building while he wailed bitterly beside me. His choked sobbing was a perfect backdrop for my artistic endeavors.

Along with this storm of feelings, I was surprised to discover that he was also cute, that I would melt in the light of his smile, or when he reached out for me. He adored me, and sometimes even preferred me to our parents. His first words were the distorted syllables of my name. I loved him and hated him and did not know what to do with all my conflicting feelings. Though my mother's warning was no longer pronounced in the house, it echoed inside me, in my own voice.

To use Winnicott's words, my false-self gained its full scope; my accommodating side grew stronger. I learned to give in, make do, share and delay gratification. The world transformed from a wide-open space to a crowded place where I sometimes had to elbow my way to the front, to pretend I was happy when a subdued rage boiled inside me.

According to Juliet Mitchell (2006) the eldest child must contend with an unexpected rival. At first, he excitedly awaits the baby, who will be another like him, a sort of twin or extension of his own self. But when the baby arrives, this narcissistic love shatters because the baby is "not me." That same "not me" baby becomes the object of hatred and jealousy.

In my adult life, my powers of imagination served me well. I became an artist and author, and I create worlds in which I do as I please, but the feeling of bitter disillusionment maintains its hold on me. In my novels, I have found myself writing time and again about sibling relations.

Ever since Freud, many authors have adopted psychology as the infrastructure upon which their characters' actions are organized. Others adhere to motivations such as fate or chance. Since I count myself among the first group, I naturally read the writings of many psychoanalysts, especially contemporary ones. A writer who particularly attracted my attention was Thomas Ogden. For me, as a writer, part of my fascination with psychology is through its writing. In my view, Ogden's academic articles stand out for their exceptional fluency and clarity. His clinical examples are short stories with structure and cadence that rivet the reader and make the imagery come alive. He himself declares, time and again, his love of writing: "Analytic writing has been one of life's pleasures for me," he writes, and goes on to describe how he must artistically create, in words, the analytic experience. However, although the psychoanalytic writer must treat the incident described as a fictional event, s/he must also, contrary to the author, remain true to the fundamental facts of what actually happened. Ogden also wrote several articles in which he psychoanalyzes literary works [and even co-wrote a book with his son, "The Analyst's Ear and the Critic's Eye," in which he linguistically analyzes his own literary analyses].

For the sake of transparency, I will admit that my literary reading differs from my reading of academic texts. In my field, or in the spirit of this paper – in my professional home, my critical eye doesn't miss much. The universal measures of writing (which have become more obscure nowadays), together with my individual tastes, influence my reading, and this will be reflected later in this chapter.

I will add another personal statement before what follows: this chapter can be read on its own; I endeavored to provide the reader with enough information to understand the context of my comments, but those who have read Ogden's two novels will reap a greater benefit.

It's all mother's fault [dysfunctional families]

We can say that literature takes a collection of events and groups them into a coherent sequence with meaning. What unifies them are the interpretations of our fevered minds.

In both of Ogden's novels, he describes dysfunctional families, families in which the children are under the authority of mothers who treat one of the (male) children with cruelty, while the father is a weak character. In one case, the father dies in an accident, and in the other the father is consumed by guilt and fails to defend his children from the mother's abusive tyranny. As a result, the home, which is supposed to be a safe space, becomes a trap with no emotional escape.

Ogden claims in his psychoanalytic writing, in the spirit of Winnicott, "The unique character of every infant involves certain aspects of the mother's emotional capacity and breathes life into them . . . Since the baby plays a role in the mother's creation, no two babies have the same mother." When Rose gives up her son Damien to her sister for adoption, she says, "Some children simply are not a fit with their parents. . . . From the moment his was born he didn't feel like my child. . . . No child is born unlovable, but a child may be born to parents incapable of loving him" (47).

Both of Ogden's novels are told from the point of view of an all-seeing narrator. The power he takes for himself as narrator is unlimited. On the contrary, as in the title of his first novel: he tells the story with details left out, which he slowly exposes. This manipulation [which I discuss at length later] creates suspense and surprise. In the end, the reader learns that Rose had been separated from her husband for a period of time and had had a love affair that left her pregnant with Damien. Although she was the only one who knew this, we learn that her husband Brian also never treated Damien as his own son. Damien became the unwanted, superfluous child – so unwanted that his mother felt she might harm him if he stayed at home. This is what leads her to give him up for adoption, to her childless sister. Her sister, who is incapable of intimacy, conditions the adoption on the fact that Damien will never see anyone from his family again. And so, overnight, the boy's mother and family disappear from his life. The transition is traumatic: "He was being asked to switch not only mothers, but also families." Abolishing the child's belonging to home and family is so dire that a child cannot even imagine it. This distancing, which is unfathomable to him, exposes him as vulnerable to infinite cruel outcomes, and therefore he must always be on the defensive and anticipate the worst.

A few years later, Damien returns home [after his aunt despaired of the adoption]. The many abandonments he experienced in his short life made him a stranger wherever he went. "Damien felt as if he had awoken, or maybe he was still dreaming, and found himself in a different world – a world in which he was a visitor, and he didn't know how long he'd be allowed to stay, no matter what anyone said" (120).

In Maslow's hierarchy of needs, the need for love and belonging is a person's third need, after the necessities of sustenance and security. Without love and belonging, people are vulnerable to loneliness, detachment and social anxiety. Clearly the home, and the mother, create the feeling of belonging that is so crucial to an infant. To Damien, who was denied this feeling of belonging, it becomes on the one hand the most desirable object and, on the other, a thing he has no natural ability to attain, and therefore he feels doomed to be an eternal outsider.

In *The Parts Left Out* (hereinafter Novel A), we meet a family whose mother experienced a psychotic episode during her pregnancy with her eldest daughter, Melody. With her grandmother's help (the father Earl's mother), Melody has a relatively harmonious childhood, but when her grandmother leaves and her brother Warren is born, her mother Marta quashes Melody's little rebellion by locking her in the closet. "Melody only needed to be latched in the closet a few times before she learned to behave, and she's been a very cooperative child ever since" (11). Here, the narrator's ironic tone is clear through the mother's thoughts.

Warren, on the other hand, does not give in to his mother, and in his case the closet is of no help. His thumb-sucking at age 11 drives Marta crazy: "He had ceased being her child, and she had ceased being his mother; he was an animal that she had to break, and she was a woman who could not rest until this task was done" (23). Marta, whose father sexually abused her as a child and teen, and later emotionally abused her, becomes a woman lacking introspection. She feels like a stranger among humans and prefers the restorative power of books over human relationships. She despises men, manages her life according to social appearances. Melody pleads to her father to "stop her mother from treating Warren so cruelly. 'She's insane, you know that. Why don't you stop her?'" And his answer is, "It's not that easy. Your mother's pride has been hurt by Warren. She suffers when Warren embarrasses himself and her at school and in front of neighbors" (24).

The struggle between Warren and his mother is interpreted by the narrator: "At stake were his will and her will. Neither of them had anything but their will to call their own" (17). Who knows how this struggle would have ended, if the mother had not attacked her son with a knife, threatening to chop off his offending hand, an act which finally enlists the father to protect his son. Earl tries to block his wife from the child, and the blow that lands on her is a death blow. A former baseball player, the intensive blow Earl deals his wife is too powerful for the small woman that stands before him.

It seems that beneath the narrative, a second, hidden story is playing out, which the reader partially understands independently, and the rest is revealed by the narrator in due time: Earl and Marta's relationship has been forced upon them. Marta did not want a family, and became attached to Earl due to an unwanted pregnancy [Melody]; Earl is in love with Marta's sister Anne, but as an honest man who was raised in a decent and loving family, he sacrificed himself to live with Marta – who should not be abandoned due to her pregnancy or unstable emotional state. Marta is willing to accept an obedient daughter [or apparently obedient, it should be noted], but not a son who, though he is devoted to her, rebels against her as well.

Warren's rebellion exposes to the world the severe deprivation he experienced from his mother, and although she is unaware of this interpretation [thumb sucking at a late age], he unconsciously treats her murderously. The absent father steps up suddenly when he apparently saves his son's life, but the excess force he uses against his wife is driven by an accumulation of rage and frustration, and no less by his will to remove the obstacle that stands in his way of his love for his sister-in-law.

As a psychoanalyst, Ogden probably encountered stories of destructive mothers like those he wrote about. In his second novel, he dedicates the book to his mother's memory. In interviews after the book's publication, Ogden emphasized the crucial role his mother played in shaping him as a person and psychoanalyst. It seems he is making a concerted effort to separate his mother from the destructive maternal characters of his novels.

The good brother

In both Ogden's novels, we find a variety of sibling relationships; both novels deal with children as the current generation and parents as the previous generation. In both generations, the protagonists' siblings play a significant role. In both novels, we are witness to the fact that in dysfunctional families, siblings replace parents.

> The disregard for sibling issues in the psychoanalytic literature arose mainly due to its attention to horizontal transference relationships – siblings and peers of the same age, as driven by the vertical transference relationship – between parent and child. The literature of family and group psychology tried to give sibling transference importance in and of itself, but it mostly emphasized that problems were an indication of a dysfunctional parental system.
>
> (Ashuach, 2012)

In Novel A, we meet the father Earl's brother and sister and see their influence on him. We also meet the mother's sister, Anne, and see their complex sibling relationship. As the [omitted] details unfold, we discover the fatefulness of this relationship. But at the forefront of the story are the relations between the children in the family: Melody and Warren.

In *The Hands of Gravity and Chance* (hereinafter Novel B), we meet Rose, the mother of the family, and her sister Margaret. In this story, the father was killed in an accident, and we have no information on his family. The children, Erin, Damien and Catherine, are the protagonists of the story and their complicated relationship shapes the drama of the story.

Both novels present a variety of parent–child relationships and show how these relationships may leave a deep and traumatic imprint on children. But for Ogden the psychoanalyst, this does not suffice. He points to the brothers as potential critical players in shaping the minds of the protagonists. Freud, for his part, was not concerned with examining sibling influence. He was interested in the vertical axis, which represents the relationship between the father (and mother) and their children, and thus he reflects a world of various hierarchal relationships.

Juliet Mitchell's contribution to psychoanalytic thought is the assumption that the horizontal axis is formed by sibling relationships (2006). In her view, the mother, as opposed to the father, is the one that generates the sibling relationships and their horizontal abstraction. In her writings on the law of the mother, she includes two basic principles that describe this. First, the mother is the one who distances her children from the dyad, but also from the triad, into the social world of his peers. Generally, the child's place is usurped by the baby born after him. The second principle is the dual prohibition she imposes on her children: they must not hurt each other, and they must not commit incest. She threatens to deny her love to anyone who breaks either of these rules. The horizontal axis exists within the law of the mother's partial and turbulent success.

Although I did not find that Ogden's academic writing explicitly addressed sibling roles, he gives them so much weight in his literary writing that it begs the question whether traditional vertical psychoanalysis can explain the human psyche without consideration of the siblings' horizontal influence.

The horizontal view envisages sibling relationships as nonhierarchal, as an experimentation in the home that anticipates our later social relationships. Freud saw the birth of a sibling as a great threat to the elder child, who gets pushed aside. However, he also believed that confronting the threat by forming a response, repetition and identification, leads to the development of a sense of social justice and solidarity (Freud, 1921).

And this is how he expands his education under the influence of his younger sister.

> Earl remembered Leslie reading him the opening pages of *Of Mice and Men*. . . . He remembered that he'd been choked with tears and he had to make a concerted effort not to let his voice crack. . . . All these years later, he remembered her saying that, and how astounded he was that she'd been able to put words to what he'd been feeling.
>
> (136–7)

The use that Ogden makes here of Steinbeck's story reveals a few parallels with his own novel: the two protagonists Lenny [who was mentally disabled] and George, who acts as his older brother, dream about buying a farm. Their dream shatters, as does Earl's dream to escape the farm – because of his wife. In *Of Mice and Men*, the female protagonist is killed by a man who misjudges his own strength, as is Marta in our story.

Marta's sister Anne appears suddenly in her life, bringing with her a youthful and refreshing spirit, based in her knowledge of contemporary music. Talking about music touches Marta's troubled soul and opens a door into an enchanted world. The influence of siblings in both novels is demonstrated through their musical and literary tastes. This repeated theme, aside from revealing Ogden's own preferences, illustrates the character of horizontal sibling relationships. This is distinct from parent–child relationships, in which children often distance themselves from their parent's tastes or even reject them completely out of youthful rebellion.

Damien, who was ejected from his family, learns, upon his return, all his social skills from his brother Erin. After they see *Rocky* at the cinema, the sensitive Erin suggests a role-playing game in which he plays Micky, the manager of Rocky's boxing club, who took him under his wing. Damien becomes Rocky, "It was never entirely clear to either boy whether they were speaking for themselves or for the characters they were imitating" (131).

In Rose's view, Erin took it upon himself to be a father figure for Damien: "Erin was the innocent – he really believed he could give Damien all that he'd never had from their father or anyone else" (132). Even in her thoughts, Rose doesn't believe that such a replacement is possible. Ogden uses words that warn of impending disappointment: "innocent" and "really believed."

Brotherly sins

However, these interactions contain more than loyalty, love, expanding knowledge and skills. There is also competition: Anne and Marta secretly compete for Earl's love, and even though Marta isn't really interested in him, she is insistent that he not meet her sister.

Catherine is jealous of the close bond that forms between Erin and Damien:

> The only thing that had bothered her when Damien showed up was the change in Erin that resulted. There was no room for a girl in the games he dreamt up for Damien. It was as if she didn't exist for the two of them. She hadn't *gained* a brother when Damien arrived, she'd *lost* one.
>
> (164)

These relationships have disappointments and abandonments, which might hint at the ambivalence below the surface in sibling relationships, even while only the protective and formative aspects of siblinghood are outwardly visible.

Earl is hurt and disappointed when his brother goes off to school and they grow apart: "But when Paul got married, I hardly ever heard from him. I thought he was a fraud, and that he had just been acting like a perfect older brother, and had never really liked me or enjoyed being with me" (63). This is exactly how Damien feels towards Erin when he goes off to university and disappears into his new life: "He had given his solemn word to Damien that he would stay in close contact with him during his freshmen year at university. . . . But everything changed the day he arrived at school" (245).

It seems that every time the elder siblings spread their wings and discover the world outside the family, they shed the heavy burden of responsibility they had carried, as parental children, and grow apart from their siblings. The law of the mother, as defined by Juliet Mitchel, does not include a prohibition on sibling abandonment.

In Novel A, it seems that Warren and Melody fill each other's worlds.

> Having little time for anything but school and farm work, they were one another's best and only friend. The deep tie between them was evident to anyone who saw them together, though the nature of that bond was known only to the two of them.
>
> (9)

The narrator leaves a space to be filled by the reader's imagination. As Randy, the local deputy Sherriff, puts it: "Melody and Warren had created a family of their own from which he and everybody else, including Earl, were barred" (38).

Melody loved talking with her brother. Despite his youth, she felt he was smarter than her: "Warren thought she was the prettiest girl in the school. He wished she could be his girlfriend, but he knew that wasn't allowed." Furthermore, "Warren and Melody had an unspoken agreement not to talk about anything related to sex. . . . He had begun to have wet dreams, which scared him, but he would never tell Melody about that."(p. 62) It seems that knowing that incest is forbidden is almost intuitive.

In Novel A, Ogden presents the full range of possible emotions and attitudes within a family: love, hate, neglect, cruelty, tenderness, betrayal and loyalty, devotion and murderousness. On the issue of incest, the brother and sister walk the thin line of the fantasy. Murderousness is present only between the mother and father; it seems to have no place among the children. However, examining the familial power structure following the mother's death reveals that her death violently tears open the protected and private space created by the siblings. A new player, the children's aunt Anne, gets thrown into the mix when she attends their mother's funeral. Melody is instantly dazzled by her beautiful and fashionable aunt, who radiates positivity and warmth. She wants a mother like this woman, and since clearly her father is equally charmed by the guest, the path to happiness seems assured.

Warren, on the other hand, is insulted by his sister and her enchantment with their aunt Anne. He is disappointed by Melody's impression of Anne, whom he finds to be phony. It seems that Warren, a sensitive child, feels that his exclusivity over his sister has been broken, since the two figures that populated his inner world are now gone: his mother died because of him, and now his sister has found a replacement for him, and he no longer has any reason to live.

Mitchell's law of the mother, maintained to varying degrees in families, may be violated in the mother's lifetime as well, as we see in Novel B, but after a mother's death, conflicts may erupt between siblings, as deep passions are exposed when the threat of the whip disappears [this may be another possible explanation for conflicts among siblings over inheritances, where material things are just a metaphor for competitiveness, jealousy and vengeance]. Warren writes a suicide letter addressed to his sister alone. In the letter, we find an explanation for his murderousness toward himself:

> I dread everything that will happen from here if I continue to live . . . You are the only good thing that happened to me in my whole life. I would hate to feel that I'm holding you back because you want to take care of me. I'm not made for this life and you are.
>
> (212)

A closer reading of the text reveals a hidden accusation: I'm afraid of what will happen when I'm not longer your favorite, I'm an obstacle on your path to a new life and so I'll leave [and we'll see what kind of a life you have now . . .]. Even if he is hasty, even if he doesn't completely understand what he is doing to those he is leaving behind, his actions intentionally hurt his sister. The violence is not only toward himself but toward her and his father as well.

In Novel B, Damien violates the first rule of the law of the mother in the beginning of the story: the novel opens with a scene in which Catherine suddenly leans forward and loses her balance, falling down the stairs until she hits the wall at the base of the stairs. Damien, who was standing behind her, later tells his brother Erin, "I pushed her. I tried to get my hand on her shoulder to pull her back, but I couldn't" (31). Erin, who was standing next to him and witnessed the fall, adamantly denies this, but Damien insists. Damien himself isn't quite sure whether he tried to pull her back or push her. This is testimony to the ambivalence he feels towards his sister, who was their mother's favorite. A whiff of unconscious revenge arises from Damien's feelings of guilt.

As for the law of the mother in the second story, here Ogden breaks down the barriers of fantasy and turns the attraction between the brother and sister into reality. To lay the groundwork for breaking the taboo, we learn that Damien was separated from his family and lived at his aunt's house for years, during which he had no contact with his siblings. On top of this, his mother didn't fulfill her motherly role when he was at home. But, above all else, we discover that the children did not have the same father. In this case, the siblinghood was entirely theoretical in terms of the protagonists' feelings. Lacking a common past makes their meeting, when they are teenagers, an event that has intimacy but also novelty and mystery.

In his book *Can Love Last?* Steven Mitchell (2002) claims that passion seeks submission, adventure, renewal and the unknown, while love seeks anchoring and connection. In passion, we seek what is missing in ourselves, that we have shunned, but also what lies beyond ourselves, outside the boundaries of self-knowledge, what in normal circumstances we protect tenaciously.

Thus, Damien finds in his sister both familial stability [love] and the mystery of alluring newness [passion]. For her part, Catherine finds features of the unknown and enticing stranger as well as the intimacy of a relative, who is ready to risk himself for her protection. Moreover, owing to her disability after the fall, the teenage Catherine feels repulsive and that no boy would be interested in her. The fact that her brother is interested in her makes him, in her mind, the only candidate for experiencing romance.

Damien's sense of detachment and transience produces in him an urgency to find stability and belonging. His first step was to create a deep bond with his brother. This is clearly within the boundaries of acceptable conduct. What the brothers want is to stop time. Guarding what they have becomes a life mission for those who are robbed of it time and again.

It is interesting to compare Damien's longing to freeze time with Warren's similar longing. Sucking his thumb at age 11 is described as a manifestation of the boy's iron will against his mother's iron desire that he stop. What we see is a timeless clash of wills. But a subversive reading might claim that of all possible demonstrations of will, thumb sucking has something infantile and regressive, a declaration of unwillingness to grow up by a child who tries again and again to re-enact the period of his life that left him unfulfilled. [Or, as Winnicott would say, he is trying to destroy the object/mother to encounter the object that survives destruction, but in Warren's unfortunate case, his mother lacks the ability to contain and therefore is a dead object.]

In reality, time cannot be frozen, and neither can the sense of security Damien established with Warren, so when Erin leaves, Damien grows closer to his sister. He enters her room like entering a temple of femininity, stimulated by curiosity and caution. When she shows him the clothing she makes but doesn't wear, to him the words "sounded as nonchalant as a fire alarm: You don't wear your clothes! You're completely naked" (182). Damien's courtship of Catherine is short and decisive. Her receptivity hastens their sexual connection. After their first kiss, Damien thinks,

> He knew that many people would find what they'd just done appalling, but at that moment, he didn't care. It didn't feel like a brother and sister kissing. He had never for a minute in his whole life felt that she was his sister. . . . He felt like a foundling who had been taken in and treated 'just like' a member of the family.
>
> (189)

It seems that Damien and Rose reflect each other's feelings of guilt and murderousness. Towards the end of her life, Rose thinks that her children's incest is "the most profound indictment of a mother that there could be" (248). She tells her sister that her pain is so great that death feels like her only escape, and thus she opts not to go ahead with the chemotherapy that would have prolonged her life. Like Warren's thumb-sucking, her children's incest is like a mark of Cain on the forehead of an abusive and neglectful mother, which cannot be concealed.

The incest, which at first seems like a decision they can live with, closes in on the brother and sister. To protect their secret, they both give up their careers to hide out in a new place where they hope to escape persecution. Damien understands that he would be perceived by the world as a pervert, and thinks to himself, "Damien would forever be . . . the sick kid who was having sex with his sister" (216).

Why were parts left out? On literary manipulation

As in life, the end of the story is unlike the beginning of the story. Margaret suffers terrible loneliness when her sister Rose shuts herself up in her house and surrenders to her disease, lacking the will to fight. Margaret, the woman who didn't know how to love, who failed to connect with Damien when he was a dejected young child, forges a brave bond with Damien and Catherine as adults, supported them both emotionally and financially and in a way becoming the closest person to them. This is the gift of total love she grants her sister on her deathbed. The empathy Margaret shows her niece and nephew does not blind her to the world's moral judgment of them. In fact, Margaret's point of view, through literary manipulation, becomes the reader's point of view, who is swept into this tragic and fateful story, as hinted in the title. In the closed world of the story, it seems the siblings have no choice but to feel act and they do. The reader may ask, how is it that I understand and identify with them and their suffering even though I know that they violated the most sacred taboo, and such a violation cannot be justified?

One of the things that stands out in Ogden's novels is the infinite power he takes as an omniscient narrator. In his book *Death of the Author*, Roland Barthes asserts that the hegemonic position that author once enjoyed is no longer credible in contemporary times, rather it is the reader who must unleash the subversive potential of the text. This statement refers to the fact that contemporary readers expect writers to explain their absolute knowledge. A writer must choose a single point of view, or two at most, to which he remains loyal and all other information must be supported by evidence such as letters, conversations or hearing other characters without their knowledge. The author's hegemony is no longer credible if he is free to wander arbitrarily between the viewpoints of his characters. Catherine says to Damien: "I like books that are convincing because the book works, and the author trusts the reader to do their part of the work" (137). In an interview published in Haaretz in 2017, Ogden himself says, "Leaving out parts shows respect for the reader's ability to respond not only to what they read, but to participate in writing the novel." As an author, Ogden does not always follow his own advice. In Novel A, this is especially noticeable when the narrator takes on Earl's viewpoint. Is it acceptable to us as readers that only after his death does Earl "remember" that he has been having an intense telephone affair with his sister-in-law for the past year?

Leaving out details from the protagonist's consciousness to create tension in the story is not at all credible. He cannot even claim, as a psychoanalyst, that such incriminating details were suppressed. They were clear to the protagonist all along and were left out of his narration in a way that feels unnatural and manipulative. As for his alternating points of view, it is possible that his experience as a therapist, who is brought into a people's psyches on a regular basis, tempts him here as a writer – to recreate the pattern of constant migration from one personal story to another. It seems he is tempted to explain and interpret his each and every character. Thus, he deprives the reader some of his right to read between the lines.

The way in which the omniscient narrator moves in and out of the story's details also seems arbitrary, practically dependent on the author's mood, regarding the rate at which he reveals details, and especially information given to the reader. For example, the fact that Damien was sexually abused by the driver his aunt hired is mentioned in a single short, obscure sentence. "He was a quiet man, well acquainted with the world, who molested Damien" (63). The event is never touched on again, nor is its effect on Damien, until the end of the book. Did Ogden trust his readers to draw conclusions themselves, while he spends pages detailing Damien's work as a literary editor and Damien and Catherine's seclusion? In the case of sexual harassment, the author seems to believe that the reader has enough information to understand Damien's complex emotional upheaval, making it unnecessary to get into the gory details.

In the same interview in Haaretz, Ogden says:

> When I was three, my mother started psychoanalysis, and even though she never spoke to me about it, I was always aware of her appointments. As a three- and four-year-old child, I didn't know what "appointments" were, but I knew she left the house to go to them and that there was a new presence in our family. We were me, my brother who was 2 years younger than me, my father and mother, and there was always a fifth person at the table.

This is the only mention of Ogden's brother that I found. [In general, it is a touching story, on the roots of Ogden's connection to psychoanalysis and even the presence of the analytic third, or as it appears here, an abstract but arbitrary fifth presence.] As earlier noted, I did not find any writings on siblinghood in Ogden's professional writings, and his engagement with the topic in his novels aroused my curiosity. Both novels feature a brave bond between a younger and older brother. In both cases, the relationship and its shattering are described from the younger brother's point of view, and therefore I assumed that, as writers often do, Ogden incorporated a personal experience into his fictional writings. I was surprised to discover in the interview that he was, in fact, the older brother. The recurrence of this scene in both books leads me to believe that this is in fact a biographical detail and telling it from his younger brother's perspective reads as an attempt at atonement: the elder Ogden gives his brother the gift of empathy. He shows him how much he understands his disappointment, how sorry he is over it. This is the power of literature – words create worlds but also have the power to heal.

No happy ending

The end of Novel B, like the end of Novel A, is tragic.

As time passes, Damien becomes more and more haunted. When someone from their past discovers their incestuous home and threatens to expose them and rattle their daughter's world to its core, Damien is pushed over the edge. After their mother dies and Erin comes back into their life, he fails to assuage Damien's fears. He descends into deep paranoia, and the outside threat only echoes the threat from within. He feels that he and Catherine have grown apart over the years, that they both focused on their daughter and the only thing that can save their daughter from their disgrace is if he disappears from her life.

Ogden could have chosen to end his novels a few paragraphs before he did, but his choice to bring disaster upon his characters actually activates the reader. We are made to think in a way that is not only psychological, but moral as well: it seems a person cannot kill and commit incest without retribution. These taboos cannot be violated without severe internal punishment [guilt] and external punishment [by society and the law].

In both novels the family is a type of hell, and in both the protagonists battle for the right to hold onto the fantasy that the family was supposed to be a safe haven. It seems to me that the law of the mother only applies if the mother is "good enough"; if she isn't, and has no love to give, her children will develop ways to evade this truth to safeguard their sanity.

Often, as in the books discussed here, children replace their abusive mothers or absent fathers with brothers or sisters. This substitution is often found to be temporary and ultimately disappointing, or even dangerous in that it pushes them to break the most basic taboos and pay a high price for doing so. In both of Ogden's novels, the attempt to stabilize horizontal relationships as equally important to vertical relationship ends negatively. Ogden seems to conclude with the pessimistic message that damage caused by parents' sins cannot be healed, and the attempt to create a 'substitute home' with siblings might end in tragedy.

As for my own story, after my brother was born, my fantasy of being the lead actress in my world shattered, but my image of my mother as perfectly suiting my needs cracked as well. I accused her of preferring my brother, an accusation which held a grain of truth because he was an infant whose care took precedence and because my mother was part of a generation that viewed boys as more important than girls. And maybe, though it is difficult for me to admit, they suited each other better than we did. Despite our painful beginning, my brother and I developed a deep bond over the years. For many years I lived with my husband and [only] son in Amsterdam and I used to amuse myself with the question, if I had one plane ticket to fly someone to Amsterdam from Israel, who would I choose? And the answer was always, my brother.

Before her death, when she no longer had many words, my mother repeated, like a mantra, the sentence: "Take care of each other." It was like she understood that her death might leave an opening for the old resentment to arise. Despite her warning, after her death, my brother and I fell into conflict. It is possible that our age-old battle, buried beneath a blanket of appeasement, once again stood naked between us. Contrary to Ogden's heroes, my brother and I were raised with good enough parents, and though we let discipline slip for a moment, my mother's will echoed inside us, that we were eventually able to bridge the gaps between us.

Perhaps there is yet something to be said for sibling love. Like the good fit found between some infants and mothers, so may there at times exist such a fit between siblings. Human ties emanating partly of genetic affiliation and partly of a sympathy to the other, which precisely provides one's needs. My brother and I, ultimately, represent such a case. Our shared likenesses and shared predicaments accumulated over the years into a love for each other that we did not want to let go of.

Bibliography

Ashuach, S. (2012). Am I my brother's keeper? The analytic group as a space for re-enacting and treating sibling trauma. *Group Analysis*, **45(2)**: 155–167.

Freud, S. (1921 [1958]). *Group Psychology and the Analysis of the Ego*. London: Hogarth Press.

Mitchell, J. (2006). Sibling trauma: A theoretical consideration. In *Sibling Relationships*, ed. P. Cole. London: Karnac: 155–174.

Mitchell, S. A. (2002). *Can Love Last?: The Fate of Romance Over Time*. New York: Norton & Company.

Ogden, T. H. (2018). *The Parts Left Out*. Sphinx London: Fort Da.

Ogden, T. H. (2018). *The Hands of Gravity and Chance*. Sphinx London: Sphinx.

Ogden, T. H. and B. H. Ogden (2013). *The Analyst's Ear and the Critic's Eye: Rethinking Psychoanalysis and Literature*. London: Routledge/Taylor & Francis Group.

Winnicott, D. W. (1968 [1974]). The use of an object and relating through identification. In *Playing and Reality*. London: Pelican.

Winnicott, D. W. (2018). Ego distortion in terms of true and false self. In *The Person Who Is Me*. London: Taylor & Francis.

1.4 A new take on Joseph and his brothers

Siblings as a potential rescue from parental destructiveness

Robi Friedman

Group analysis' lesson from a horizontal secure space as a defense against the vertical axis

Joseph, the Bible's dreamer, almost lost his life by sharing his dreams in the family. Fortunately, his siblings' repetition of Cain and Abel's envy-based tragedy did not end in his homicide. On the other hand, the plot of a murderous enactment in their sibling relations could have also ended in a constructive development, if Joseph's dream's hidden messages would have been understood. Such a more constructive opportunity actually happened later in Egypt, where the sibling/horizontal axis created a new safe space for the cure of the relations among the siblings. The earlier conflict between the horizontal and the vertical/intergenerational family dynamics reopened and was negotiated better. Their father Jacob's absence helped; he had been emotionally manipulating his family, infecting them with his firstborn Relation Disorder. In Canaan, the young Joseph, who was unfortunately chosen by his father to compensate with his own inferiority, had dreamt these "deposited" (Volkan, 2010) megalomaniac motivations and told them to his family. His dreams unconsciously communicated a beginning elaboration of a familiar shared "preoccupation" with Jacob's "complex". By telling these dreams, rather than making his already known father's open preference public, Joseph asks to be rescued from his father's grip and the split in the relations with his siblings.

By having provided Joseph with the "striped coat", Jacob inevitable recreated his past vertical, intergenerational inherited, relational rejection disorder in the present through the horizontal children's relations. Not only was Joseph existentially threatened by this re-enactment in his sibling's relations, but also by the hidden threat of the birth of his brother Benjamin. Joseph, and all around him, knew that Jacob could never resist his urge to coronate his loved second-born and feared he would be himself sacrificed[1] by his father. Is the fear of the firstborn to be sacrificed by his parents in the favor of the second-born a "foundation matrix dread"?

Unfortunately, his sharing dreams as a request for containment, as a cry to be freed from an impossible and destructive intergenerational mission could not be heard. He also couldn't find in his siblings the kind of partners to work

DOI: 10.4324/9781003220060-6

on the scapegoat process, even if he seemed to be deeply dependent on them. The transgenerational contagious poisonous virus took Dreamtelling into more sickness. Jacob's vertical "Relation Disorder", re-enacted and repeated in the horizontal sibling axis, proved destructive rather than curing.

Only in Egypt, more than two decades later, did the siblings succeeded to become partners. Joseph's final rejection and almost murder in Dothan, his slavery, his brothers' emigration to land of the Nile and the elaboration of retaliation were steps toward healthier siblings relations. The "game changer" seemed to be the achievement of a distance from their father's vertical influence, which facilitated a horizontal/sibling relational development. The scapegoating/rejection patterns were cured. Can we see here a group-analytic paradigm?

Dreams and Dreamtelling

There is nothing like dreams to connect the past and the present, the vertical and the horizontal. Dreams cast the "long shadow of the past", the vertical, "on the present", (Sandler, 1987) on the horizontal. And for me, there is nothing like a good Bible story in order to dream and re-dream the human condition. Like Dreamtelling, reading biblical stories in a curious state of mind can show fascinating ways of coping with "preoccupations" emerging in relations.

Such is Joseph's story (Genesis 37): the horizontal perspective, the here and now, is that a very gifted young man shares his provocative and omnipotent dreams with his older and bigger brothers and parents in what seems to be a suicidal state of mind. Genesis 37:7: He said to them, "Listen to this dream I had: We were binding sheaves of grain in the field, and suddenly my sheaf rose and stood upright, while your sheaves gathered around and bowed down to mine." (8) "Do you intend to reign over us?" his brothers asked.

The Bible often takes vertical, historical equivalent perspectives as an "unthought known" (Bollas, 1987), information that stays in the subconscious until it is made explicit. While from a religious orthodox point of view, Joseph's dreams communicate to his brothers his future godly sovereignty, to those of us who connect dreaming more with a personal process than with a divine influence, this Dreamtelling process points to worrying secrets in the family relation's unconscious. What "preoccupation" is Joseph dreaming (digesting)? Are these "preoccupations" only personal or are they shared and delegated unto him to elaborate? To what end does he "need" his audience for? This is a preferred child in a difficult familiar situation, who seems to invite his antagonistic brothers to "dream the dream" he shares.

The possibility that Joseph was stupid, or a suicidal autistic person, must be discarded in order to understand that there is a family history of generations of sibling disorders, which is carried by this young man's shoulders. His father Jacob was poisoned already as a child by his inability to accept his older brother Esau's firstborn right. But cheating him and his own father Isaac in order to achieve firstborn rights didn't cure Jacob. Thus, he re-enacted this drama often in his life,[2] and now repeated it by preferring the youngest sibling Joseph and providing him with the "colored coat". Joseph was delegated (Stierlin, 1981) to cure his father's vertical complex by rising over all his brothers, no matter the emotional/relational price he and his family payed on the present, horizontal as a scapegoated and rejected member of the family.

Dreams told have a powerful communicative value, because of their import/export of containment value. They are often created as a result of relationships that have digestion difficulties and import this "preoccupation" onto the dreamer. He, in his turn, later exports his digestion efforts back into relationships. Partners who help to elaborate a dream co-create a space in which to "request containment" promotes psychic development. Can we also consider Joseph as requesting help in both the elaboration of his "preoccupation" about his family role as a result of his father's manipulation, as well as his inability to elaborate his father's problems? Preferring one child over the siblings-group almost automatically puts him in danger of becoming the envied, hated and rejected scapegoat. After having considered these dynamics, would the reader who is prepared to step into Joseph's shoes be proud of his dreamt future glory or rather terrified of his destiny in the family and his personal well-being?

The horizontal and the vertical

In a personal interview I conducted with Yalom (2005), he asserted that "the" most significant moment in his professional life was when he joined his first experiential group, while still in psychoanalysis. When he tried to share his thoughts about the reasons and history of why he reacted with anxiety to another participant, the group leader stopped him. She demanded only a "here-and-now" comment on his present and actual relations with participants in his group. Yalom seemed to say that much of his later theorizing was an attempt to explain and support this "event" and his group leader's avoidance of the "vertical" aspects of contents and processes.

Foulkes (1973) addressed his experiences as psychoanalyst and group analyst:

> In comparing the psychoanalytic and the group-analytic points of view of the individual and of the individual processes, the analogy of a differentially magnifying microscope is useful. The psychoanalytical view takes the individual mind as the unit of observation and tries to understand all mental processes in terms of this individual mind. This makes it particularly useful for its special purposes, namely the vertical analysis of the individual in a chronological, historical sense. Seen from the psychoanalytical approach, new relationships are brought about essentially by transference, and counter-reactions by the transference of the other people concerned act as modifiers on these now different relationships. Ultimately this means that they can be understood as results of the original family relationships of each individual.
>
> By contrast, a group analytic view would claim that vertical and horizontal interactional processes play in a *unified mental field* (italics RF) of which the individuals composing it are a part. Group analysis is the method of

> choice for the observation and for gaining effective influence in both the horizontal sense – this means in view of the present participants' different characters and reactions, and in the here and now of present life. The point I wish to stress is that this network is a psychic system as a whole, and not a superimposed social interaction system in which individual minds interact with each other. This is the value of thinking in terms of a concept which does not confine mind, by definition, to an individual.
>
> (p. 226)

What is this "unified mental field"? It seems to be a transitional space where past influences meet and converge with the present co-created relational dynamics. The vertical, with which a member enters a group, includes the individual history and experiences together with transgenerational transmission. The vertical influences the horizontal axis, which is the changing interactive space between group members. The group's conductor is also fully part of this "unified mental field", where the vertical and horizontal converge. I understand Foulkes' "unified" as being together, not united but rather meeting in one space, which is the co-created Dynamic Matrix.

The group-analytic concept of a matrix means a net of communication and relations where individuals and groups find meaning and are reciprocally influenced. Nitzgen and Hopper (2017) describe a tri-partite matrix model of the social unconscious. The Dynamic Matrix represents a group's communication and culture, "co-created" by interacting Individual Matrices and in addition influenced by a traditional, basic Foundation Matrix. Examples for the Foundation Matrix would be their shared history and culture or other aspects that seem to be "given" (as opposed to "co-created) like the "firstborn rights". Thus the "unified mental field" is the meeting area between the vertical and the horizontal. Here, past familiar/relational experiences, as the story of Cain and Abel, and Jacob's stealing Esau's traditional birthrights, emerge and wash in the present family waters, creating a shared mental space, which may cause fixation or change.

In our biblical passage, there are two meetings between Joseph, the troubled dream-teller, and his family in "unified mental fields", where the vertical and the horizontal converge. In the first one his proud, vulnerable and manipulative father Jacob and his rejecting brothers listen to Joseph's Dreamtelling. I suggested that we understand this meeting as a request for containment, as an effort to enroll his brothers to help digest and change his scapegoat role in the sibling's clan by exposing his father's delegation. Unfortunately, his father's favorizing had already generated their hate for him, his exclusion and later rejection, all typical of the scapegoating process.

In the second meeting, in "Dothan", when Joseph met with his siblings after having been sent to them by his father (Genesis 37:15), they already had lost almost all shame, guilt and empathy. The scapegoating process, can be considered a co-created dysfunctional pattern, which I called Rejection Relation Disorder (Friedman, 2007), which is when a subgroup ready to annihilate

(Hopper, 2003) a scapegoat in fantasy of the efficiency function and under the powerful influence of hate.

Unconscious aspects of the meeting between vertical and horizontal processes make it difficult to differentiate between them. For example the lethal conflict between Cain and Abel may be seen as a basic model of sibling' interaction. Every individual matrix and every group dynamic is influenced by this foundation matrix – it becomes a "given" which is co-forged in the collective mind of familiar interactions.

"Vertical" heritages, which are usually disordered relations transmitted for generations (Volkan, 2010), have "horizontal" bearings in the here-and-now. The sentence: "The fathers have eaten sour grapes, and this has set the children's teeth on edge" (Jeremiah, 31, 29) is a classic example. Pathology is located not in the individual alone but between connected humans, in the emotional co-created "horizontal" space of the Relation Disorders (Foulkes and Anthony, 1957; Nietzgen, 2010; Friedman, 2007). In a transgenerational transmitted disorder such as in Joseph's family case, we seem to be with one foot on the horizontal axis, and with the other foot standing on the relations with living or dead figures, ancestors, chosen heroes or past devils who are not past at all. Pathology is located in the relations and between the generations (the vertical axis).

A "condenser event" as the crossroad between the past and the present, the vertical and the horizontal: what is condensed?

Foulkes (1957):

> The term "condenser" phenomena is used to describe the sudden discharge of deep and primitive material following the pooling of associated ideas in the group. The members' unconscious conflictual interactions seem to activate emotions with a tendency to discharge in a special moment. This accumulation of pent-up emotions evoked in the group relations is condensed in a "collective unconscious".
>
> (p. 199)

This collective unconscious is deposited in a dreamer, with whom a shared group event called a dream is co-created. Later, because of only partial ability to contain the "preoccupation" alone, the dream returns the collective unconscious by being told with the group. Thus, Joseph's dreams very ably create the act of condensation between the horizontal and the vertical processes and because of the creativity, like any other piece of art, it takes the audience by surprise.

While Foulkes (1957) thought that the concept of condensation bore "some relation to Bion's 'emergence of the basic assumption' and to Ezriel's 'common group tension'" (p. 200), for me it shows the result of the reciprocal influence in the powerful chemistry between the collective past and the shared present.

Joseph was infected by his father Jacob's inferiority virus, which resulted in his cheating his brother and father for the seniority. His father's contagious illness continued until the end of his life. Jacob inflated Joseph's (his then youngest son) narcissism and provoked social madness by providing him with the colored coat, maybe shortly creating a "father-and-son" Relation Disorder. Was it a "folie a deux" (Bleuler, 1972) in the presence of a group? Family favoritism immerges a whole family in an Exclusion Relation Disorder. The unconscious "transpersonal" boundary less inter-communications of emotions (Foulkes, 1948; Volkan, 2010) reciprocally influences everyone. By unconsciously delegating Jacob to elaborate his father's inferiority feelings, fears of rejection and scapegoating fantasies, he manipulates also his son's siblings, restaging a 40-year-old play. While the vertical was expected in the horizontal, here the unconscious "non-rejection promise" (Friedman, 2018), a familiar security pillar, was not functioning any more. The moment the siblings reacted with hate and rejection toward Joseph, the effort to cure Jacob's unconscious effort to cure himself failed. The horizontal prevailed over the vertical; the paranoia, deprivation of rights and rejection pathology were already firmly located in the space between Joseph and his brothers and in the vertical space between Joseph and his father.

The development of mental digestion in Dreamtelling: the vertical in with the horizontal?

Dreamtelling includes a four-step process from the moment a need for digesting excessively threatening or exciting emotions emerges, until an interpersonal and transpersonal elaboration process is ignited by telling and listening to a dream. Dreaming is first ignited as a *shared* "preoccupation". In a second step the preoccupation is dreamt and in a third step it may become the object of reflection and some further elaboration if remembered. Finally, in the fourth step, provided there is a partner ready to participate in a shared digestion, the elaboration is continued, the dream is shared.

At the first step there is the meeting between the vertical and the horizontal. In our example, Joseph, the child, gets "preoccupied" by the already described intergenerational influence: his father's difficulty to contain inferiority and his acting-out. But Joseph's preoccupation was not his individual worry, and was surely shared by his brothers, who were themselves victims of their mother Leah's marginalization by their father's Jacob preference of Rachel, her younger sister. We guess that it was the (horizontal) siblings' group itself which provided the brothers some consolation.

An enlightening example of the horizontal and vertical is found in the experiments of Palombo (1992) with "dreaming". He described that our mind tries to cope with "preoccupation", with comparing excessive present threats and glories with endless past similar personal experiences and relations. It seems thus meaningless to try to understand dreaming only in the horizontal or the vertical axis, because the dream itself is a creation of the "unified space of mind".

Dreaming seems thus as an effort to digest the vertical in the horizontal, partly by later communicating the dreams unconscious emotions to the horizontal axis for further elaboration. Dreams told carry for the listeners both a request for containment of yet undigested emotions and a demand for (future) influence. We deduce that the transmission of Joseph's father's relational primogeniture disorder, on the one hand, and his being rejected and scapegoated by his brothers, on the other, were too difficult for Joseph to contain alone and resulted in requests for containment to them.

"A dream told is a letter to be opened"[3] (Talmud, Brachot 55), thus suggesting an interaction, an influence and needed help to contain. But bible interpreters had difficulties to understand the unconscious relational message carried in dreams. Joseph's dreams could only be a cry for help to his siblings. He needed help to separate from his father's "birthright complex" and his scapegoating position.

This Jacob's relation disorder was never to be healed. When Joseph visited him at the end of his life, in order to have his two sons blessed, Jacob could not bring up anything different than his usual favorizing the second-born son. Just before dying, Jacob repeated his own envious "firstborn right" drama with his brother Esau. Genesis 48:12: "Then Joseph removed them from Israel's knees and bowed down with his face to the ground". 13: "And Joseph took both of them, Ephraim on his right toward Israel's left hand and Manasseh on his left toward Israel's right hand, and brought them close to him". 14: "But Israel reached out his right hand and put it on Ephraim's head, though he was the younger, and crossing his arms, he put his left hand on Manasseh's head, even though Manasseh was the firstborn".

But this time, a now separated and dis-identified Joseph was aghast by his father's act: 17: "When Joseph saw his father placing his right hand on Ephraim's head he was displeased; so he took hold of his father's hand to move it from Ephraim's head to Manasseh's head". 18: Joseph said to him, "No, my father, this one is the firstborn; put your right hand on his head." 19: "But his father refused. . . . So, he put Ephraim ahead of Manassah".[4] While Joseph's own transformation did not influence his unchangeable father, his favorizing the younger over the older one had no deeper consequences. Joseph was aware of this.

Two aspects of a scapegoating process: cure by re-inclusion and coping with (semi-unconscious) fears of retaliation

Joseph's development is most interesting and complicated enough to fill some chapters of this book. He grew further than only to accept the "firstborn rights" of the rest of his original group. Joseph and his siblings' rich journey may open second thoughts of what the results of a Rejection Relation Disorder (scapegoating) could be.

Scapegoating, or the rejecting of a small or median group member, and a subgroup of a large group, is one of the conscious and unconscious dreads in the life of any community. It may be a real sickness, in the end hurting and scarring all participants. Joseph was first marginalized and then hated by his siblings' group. Group workers are familiar with this dreadful process, which includes an unconscious communication between one side that feels disdain and hate and finally death wishes (the "Dothan event") and the other side (Joseph) that deeply connects and communicates his being ever-more dependent on being included. More: the brothers' open hate not only doesn't distance Joseph, but he seems more eager than ever to belong to them. This need for inclusion is typical for a scapegoat and is described succinctly by the Bible: Joseph is provided an excuse to avoid his hating brothers, but he insists on finding them. Although this could surely have informed his brothers of his needs to belong, as in every scapegoating process, rejecters seem to progressively loose shame and guilt and they become less empathic. They could only feel contempt when they spotted him from a distance:[19] "Here comes that dreamer!" they said to each other. [20] "Come now, let's kill him and throw him into one of these cisterns and say that a ferocious animal devoured him". This unconscious relation between hating and dependent participants of a disordered relation is almost too much to bear.

Scapegoating contradicts the "promise of non-rejection" (Friedman, 2018), a basic assumption in the foundation matrix of families. This vertical basic assumption will influence the horizontal process by making the scapegoater as well as the rejected group participant feel sick.

Curing rejection processes?

Can a rejection from the family, or the small group, be cured? Is there treatment for an emigrant expelled from his country, forced to leave behind "the familiar" and having to meet the "uncanny".[5] Becoming an "Egyptian" seemed not to have cured Joseph's rejection, because when he meets again his brothers it's clear that he "longs to belong" (Schlapobersky, 2015). In my experience, no social success, no powerful position, no superiority feelings could cure Joseph from his traumatic ejection from the family. For him, the vertical trauma and its influence on the horizontal were far more significant than the glory in the new community. As a result when we go deeper in the individual dynamics we find that in spite of the effort that the horizontal cures the vertical, re-inclusion fantasies of immigrants, especially those rejected, testify to the possibility that ejection is never really cured.

This is an enormous challenge for group analysis, a therapy that claims personal and social maturation is achieved by participating in a group where three processes can unfold: "outsight" – understanding and accepting the horizontal processes; "insights" – understanding vertical, historical (personal and intergenerational) transmitted past difficulties, like his father's intergenerational heritage and his father's manipulation. For example, the "Dothan event", Joseph's final rejection by his brothers, taught him a lesson about his brothers' suffering and hate, under his father's discrimination, as well as an understanding of his own needs and acting.

The third element of this development that may cure scapegoating is training, practicing different behavioral patterns. Foulkes (1948) thought insight and outsight provide for guidelines to change relations, by "ego-training in action". This training happens in the horizontal here-and-now, where present relational patterns, which have been influenced by the past vertical processes are influenced toward new patterns. Pages started to be turned by being the victim of rejection and slavery. Interestingly, Joseph's development seemed to have started in jail, as if he were practicing more egalitarian relations in a therapeutic group, where he got a chance to participate in his "siblings'" relations. He became the prisoners' address of their dreams (Friedman, 2002), responding to his inmates' requests for containment. Foulkes (1975) describing[6] what it takes to be a conductor: a person who doesn't silence his resonance to those in need is in a leadership position.

If we really look for change, we have to consider change of the rejecters, too. His siblings, the perpetrators, had to repent the rejection of their scapegoated brother. We read that guilt, shame and empathy seemed to be reintroduced. In addition to having learned to live with these feelings, fear of retaliation also seems present. Fear of retaliation is found in many bullies and especially bystanders after the scapegoating process has "terminated".

For almost a decade, from 2012, we[7] have organized a conference where German descendants of perpetrators meet Jewish/Israeli descendants of Holocaust victims. One of the interesting aspects of this is the fear of more than a few German participants to be the victim of retaliation violence. My German friend shared his father's repeated saying: "they will do to us what we have done to them". They have to overcome fears to come to Israel and are reminded all the time by their parents' fears to have earned the treatment they perpetrated on the Jews in the concentration camps. Most often it is voiced by their extreme surprise in how nice Israelis are toward them. This unconscious relation is not psychotic – the victims of rejection/annihilation are really in the grip of these two tendencies – to wish the rejecter will actually wish them back, reincluded, and, at the same time, their wish to retaliate. The vertical should be sorted out in the present. Normally, the rejected cannot forget nor forgive past traumas in the horizontal, the here-and-now. On the other side, the bully and perpetrator would like absolution because they made a change: they reintroduced the repentance feelings, the mental suffering when guilt, shame and painful feelings enter again into the relations. The horizontal should protect them from the past, from the vertical, and only open meetings can achieve this.[8]

When Joseph, incognito, met his brothers in Egypt, who had escaped a draught in Canaan, the vertical, the past, suddenly forced itself on the horizontal, threatening the present encounter. To stay only in the horizontal was impossible, and the vertical, the horrendous past between Joseph and his brothers, had to be handled. It seems to me that no reconciliation between rejecters and rejected can be achieved without dealing with the vertical. This is especially true when the rejected, the scapegoat, has felt to be part of, or even dependent on, the community from which he was ejected. This new independence is a very significant element in the renewed relation between rejecters and rejected. One-sided forgiveness, without elaborating the relations, does almost never seem to be enough. It needs a real meeting, where in a first step semi-conscious wishes and fears for retaliation are encountered, in whatever setting. In a second step, re-inclusion wishes must be felt and communicated by the siblings, who are all caught in the crossroad between the vertical and the horizontal.

Finally, scapegoating relations are seldom over, because the bullied and scapegoated child or adult who suffers from this Rejection Relation Disorder will forever chew on this vertical bone in their throat. The unspoken aggression that was impossible to express directly toward Jacob resulted in the destruction of Joseph, together with his hated colored coat. Sending the coat stained with goat's blood back to their father seems to me an enormous expression of hate toward their father, the vertical. Overly strong or charismatic (Lieberman, Yalom and Miles, 1973) authority, which is untouchable by angry group participants, results in the transportation of aggression toward the scapegoat. Accordingly, one of the ways to cure scapegoating is opening a possibility to criticize and redirect aggression toward the authority. In the "Dothan event" aggression toward the father, the authority, is communicated through symbols as well as by killing the favorite of the oppressor.

Joseph's decision not to harm his brothers, from an initial omnipotent position that potentially enabled his vengeance, came only after the meeting with his siblings' leader Yehuda. This brother "went up" (שגיו) to him, and found the main way to re-include Joseph in the group. By meeting with him, he addressed Joseph's humanity and moved him from the retaliation position. After weeping, Joseph became again part of the group. Without the presence of their father, the horizontal aspects of the here-and-now relations enabled an egalitarian, inclusive solution. Joseph also became the ejecting group's savior, which often is the scapegoat's hope and fantasy.

After the horizontal relations cured the vertical, the main familiar relational pathology, the need to rule over brothers, or to steel the "firstborn right" was not needed. Instead of restaging conflict and war, Joseph and his brothers had overcome the vertical trauma in the interest of co-creating a horizontal healthy relation.

Notes

1 Going to Shechem to meet his hating brothers, Joseph seems to be re-enacting Isaac's agreement to be sacrificed by his father Abraham. Similarly to Isaac, who must have known on his way to Moriah that his father sacrificed his brother Ishmael, he "knew" he would be himself sacrificed in order to obtain God's love. Joseph must have "known" it too.

2 For example, I regard his wish to marry Rachel, the second born, before her older sister Leah was married, as of the same pattern.

3 The full citation is "Rabi Chisda said, "An uninterpreted dream is like an unread letter."

4 Not that it did really matter, because history showed that both Ephraim and Menassah became part of the ten lost tribes. But a now critical and independent Joseph could handle this.

5 Freud (1919): Das Unheimliche.
6 (p. 1).
7 Every 18 months, two Israelis and two Germans have organized four conferences in Israel and one in Germany.
8 Scapegoating only seemingly makes a monolithic subgroup of rejecters. In reality most of the bystanders stand somewhere between the bullies and the victim. This subgroup includes some participants who are less comfortable with this rejection and extermination. On the other pole of the continuum, usually there are bystanders who collaborate with the scapegoat's liquidation. This heterogeneity is often the reason why such an ejection from the group may not only become traumatic for the victim but also for the rejecting group as well.

References

Bleuler, E. (1972) *Lehrbuch der Psychiatrie*. Heidelberg and New York: Springer.

Bollas, C. (1987) *The Shadow of the Object: The Psychoanalysis of the Unthought Known*. London: Free Association.

Foulkes, S.H. (1948) *Introduction to Group Analytic Psychotherapy*. London: Heinemann. (Maresfield Reprint, Karnac Books, London 1991.).

Foulkes, S.H. (1973) The group as matrix of the individual's mental life. In: Foulkes, E. (Ed.), *Selected Papers*, pp. 223–234. London: Karnac.

Foulkes, S.H. (1975) *Group Analytic Psychotherapy: Method and Principles*. London: Gordon and Breach, reissued Karnac 1986 and 1991.

Foulkes, S.H., & Anthony, E.J. (1957) *Group Psychotherapy: The Psychonalytic Approach*. London: Penguin.

Freud, S. (1919) The 'uncanny'. In: *The Standard Edition of the Complete Psychological Works of Sigmund Freud, Volume XVII (1917–1919): An Infantile Neurosis and Other Works*, pp. 217–256. NY: Vintage.

Friedman, R. (2002) Dream-telling as a request for containment in group therapy – The royal road through the other. In: Pines, M., Neri, C., & Friedman, R. (Eds.), *Dreams in Group Psychotherapy*, pp. 46–67. London and New York: JKP.

Friedman, R. (2007) Where to look? Supervising group analysis – A relations disorder perspective. *Group Analysis*, 40(2): 251–268, Sage.

Hopper, E. (2003) Incohesion: Aggregation/massification; the fourth basic assumption in the unconscious life of groups and group-like social systems. In: Lipgar, R.M., & Pines, M. (Eds.), *Building on Bion: Roots*. London: International Library of Group Analysis 20, Jessica Kingsley Publishers.

Lieberman, M.A., Yalom, I.D., & Miles, M. (1973) *Encounter Groups: First Facts*. New York: Basic Books.

Nitzgen, D. (2010) Hidden legacies. S.H. Foulkes, Kurt Goldstein and Ernst Cassirer. *Group Analysis*, 43: 354–371.

Nitzgen, D., & Hopper, E. (2017) The concepts of the social unconscious and of the matrix in the work of S.H. Foulkes. In: Hopper, E., & Weinberg, H. (Eds.), *The Social Unconscious in Persons, Groups and Societies: Volume 3: The Foundation Matrix Extended and Re-Configured*. London: Karnac.

Palombo, S. (1992) The eros of dreaming. *International Journal of Psychoanalysis*, 73: 637–646.

Sandler, J. (1987) Interpretation: The past in the present. *The International Review of Psychoanalysis*, 14: 126.

Schlapobersky, J.R. (2015) *From the Couch to the Circle: The Routledge Handbook of Group-Analytic Psychotherapy*. London: Routledge.

Stierlin, H. (1981) *Delegation und Familie*, Beitrage zum Heidelberger familien-dynamischen Konzept. Frankfurt: Suhrkamp.

Volkan, V. (2010) *Psychoanalytic Technique Expanded*. Istanbul: Oa Publishing.

Yalom, E. (2005) *Video Interview by Robi Friedman*. Haifa University.

1.5 Transferences in Groups and Organizations

Definitions and Clinical Value

Einar Gudmundsson

Introduction

Transference in therapy is probably one of Freud's most important discoveries. Transference, in short, means that the patient unconsciously transfers roles and feelings belonging to a significant person in his past to his therapist in the present. The patient may even start to treat the therapist as if the therapist is that person from his past. Because transference is unconscious, the patient himself is unaware of it's occurrence. On the other hand, the therapist's awareness of transference in the therapeutic relationship is often crucial for a successful outcome.

The original type of transference, described by Freud as early as 1912, is lately referred to as a parental/authority type of transference, or a vertical transference (1). Freud's therapeutic focus was mainly on individual psychotherapy, or rather psychoanalysis. As far as the author knows, he did not study other types of transferences. Other transferences, often referred to as horizontal transferences, are much easier to recognize in a group environment.

For theoretical and practical reasons, especially when working with groups and organizations, it is important to be aware of the four main types of transference:

1. **Transference** in the classical sense, which is used to describe a parental/authority type of transference. Also referred to as a "vertical transference" (Freud's original transference).
2. **Sibling transference** mainly describes transferences that can occur between group members in therapy and/or colleagues in organizations. Also referred to as "horizontal transference".
3. **Family transference** mainly describes a "whole family transference" occurring in groups and/or organizations. It is best described as a "horizontal-vertical transference".
4. **Peer transference** describes mainly a non-sibling peer transference. It is often referred to as a type of "horizontal transference".

The first transference type, the parental/authority type of transference, or the vertical transference, originally described by Freud, has gotten much acceptance and

DOI: 10.4324/9781003220060-7

covering since it was first published. It is the authors belief that further clarification in this chapter is therefore unnecessary and will add little to the body of knowledge already existing. The focus of this chapter will therefore be on transference types 2 through 4, as before mentioned, frequently described as horizontal transferences.

Sibling Transference

Sibling transference is similar in nature to the parental/authority transference, except the object/person from the past is not a parent, or authority, but a sibling (2, 3, 4, 5). Usually the transference receiving person, the person the transference is directed at in the present, is similar in age to the patient. Age difference is therefore important in the definitions of the horizontal transference versus vertical transferences. For those similar in age, the transference is likely to be horizontal. An older person is more likely to receive a vertical transference. A much younger person might be receiving a horizontal transference, like a younger sibling transference.

Sibling transference can theoretically occur anywhere in life, but for practical purposes this chapter focuses on vignettes from (a) group therapy and (b) organizations.

(a) Sibling Transference in Group Therapy

Vignette 1

In spring Mrs. A announced that she was leaving her therapy group during the summer break after about a year in the group. In the following group sessions after her announcement, Mr. B, a young male in the group became increasingly anxious and depressed. He could not explain or understand why he suddenly was so emotionally unstable, but he was quite sure it had nothing to do with Mrs. A leaving the group. Rather he found the idea absurd. The therapist inquired for similar experiences from his past, but Mr. B was sure there were none. Sessions passed and his condition worsened. He got antidepressants from his general practitioner, but it did not seem to help much. The therapist insisted that there must have been a similar experience in his past that was keeping him from working through his present situation, but Mr. B could not see any similarities, and continued to deny the possibility. He pointed out that all his family was alive and well. When the therapist was analyzing the relationship between the two of them, it was clear that Mrs. A was the group member who had most frequently shown interest in Mr. B, usually in a caring way. It then came to the therapist that Mr. B had, in one of his group-preparation interviews, mentioned that he had an older sister, of which he had never spoken in the group. The therapist asked about his sister and it turned out that she was approximately the same age as Mrs. A, around 15 years older than Mr. B. They grew up in a rather isolated area, and his sister had been the only one in their family to show any interest in him and care for him as a child. When he was about ten years she went to live in the

Far East. No one understood what she had really meant to him and what he had lost. He was told that he should be happy that his sister was starting a life of her own. After she left, the home they grew up in felt empty and he was lonely and depressed. He had nowhere to go with these thoughts and feelings. Understanding that Mrs. A had evoked feeling in him that belonged to his older sister became a major breakthrough for Mr. B in the group. Mrs. A clearly became an object of his sibling transference, an "older sister transference". The fact that Mrs. A herself had a younger brother, her only sibling, may have contributed to her interest in Mr. B. She could have been experiencing a "younger brother transference". Alas, there was no opportunity to explore this, since she had already left the group.

Vignette 2

Mr. D was an active member of a slow open and stable group. In the beginning of the groups fourth year a new female member, Mrs. C, entered the group. Although Mr. D liked the new member and welcomed her warmly in the beginning, he later on began to have mixed feelings towards her. As time passed, he began to overlook her and showed little interest in what she was bringing to the group. When he finally became aware of this, he did not like it, and shared his feelings with the group. Exploring this he became aware of similarities from his past. He was one of many siblings, all rather close to each other in age. When he was a teenager, his widowed father brought a woman to the home and she became his stepmother. His mother had died years ago. The stepmother brought with her a young girl. This was Mr. D's much younger sister on his father side. He had only seen her sporadically. He was at first happy to have her in the home, but the stepmother was overprotective and jealous, which made contact with the little sister difficult. This eventually led Mr. D to lose interest in his sister and keep a distance for the years to come. Mrs. C had re-evoked his ambivalent feelings towards his youngest sister, a "youngest sister transference". This discovery led to intensive work on his relationship with his youngest sister and stepmother, with good results.

(b) Sibling Transference in Organizations

Vertical transference is well-known in organizations were authorities often become the transference receiving objects. Sibling transference is also common in organizations. "People that cannot work together" or "how things change when a new colleague starts at work" are two examples of possible sibling transference. Age difference, which commonly affects transference, can often be diminished in organizations by the colleague status. Colleges, young or old, can be experienced as siblings, but the boss is most often experienced as the parent, even independent of age. The following vignettes highlight how sibling transference can appear in organizations:

Vignette 5

Mrs. X and Mrs. Y were highly qualified nurses, liked by all, except each other. Mrs. X was the head nurse, but Mrs. Y was older and more experienced. Everybody knew that they had problems working together, but they could never really explain why, and both could sometimes on a good day admit that they respected each other's qualities as professionals. Mrs. X was the younger of two sisters and spent her youth competing with her older sister without much success, while Mrs. Y was the older of two sisters. Her younger sister was the favourite. Working together seemed to create an "older sister transference" in Mrs. X and a "younger sister transference" in Mrs. Y, with all the difficult feelings that belonged to their past sibling rivalry.

Vignette 6

Mrs. G was the third in the row of four sisters. She was a teacher and had moved quickly to a leadership position where she flourished. When she joined as a singer in a female quartet, she noticed that she was withdrawn and was not so active in decision making in the quartet. She did not like it but felt that she could not change it. In the quartet two "prima donnas" did the decision making and the fourth girl was considerably younger. In her family of origin, her two older sisters were fighting all the time for leadership and it was wise not to take part in their wars, or else they would turn on her. Her youngest sister did the same. When she realized that she had unconsciously been repeating her sibling role, she was able to break the spell and become more active in the quartet, which was much welcomed by the others.

Family Transference

The concept of family transference is that of a "whole family transference". It means that the patient unconsciously finds himself back in his family of origin, assigning the roles of a parent to the therapist, and some of the group members are assigned the role of his siblings, and he himself returns to his own old role in the family, good or bad. Although a group member can experience different types of transference at different times in group therapy, the concept of family transference should be confined to a simultaneous horizontal and vertical transference, a kind of whole family experience (6, 7). For the therapist to be aware of, and to observe this, can be extremely helpful in understanding the dynamics of the group. Since family transference is in reality both horizontal and vertical, the term horizontal-vertical transference is probably the most descriptive of its nature. Family transference can occur both in (a) group therapy and (b) organizations.

(a) Family Transference in Group Therapy

Vignette 3

An elderly man was the therapist of a slow open group where Mr. K was an active member. Mr. K spent a lot of time and energy arguing and fighting with

Mr. H who was the oldest male group member and a few years older than Mr. K. Still, Mr. K was not happy when Mr. H announced that he was going to leave the group during the summer break. Mr. K tried to convince him to stay on in the group without success. When Mrs. J became a member of the group after the summer break, Mr. K suddenly became increasingly anxious and depressed. This led to extensive work on the loss of his mother who died young when he was only about eight years old. He was the second oldest boy in a large sibling group and had a bullying older brother who constantly made him miserable, and whom he had tried to stand up to, without success. Finally, his older brother (at the age of 20) was thrown out of their home by their father. The brother refused to contact the family ever again. After some strong emotional sessions it became clear that the group had become like Mr. K's original family, where the father was distant (as Mr. K experienced the therapist), mother was absent (died) and the troubled older brother was behaving as the head of the family (as Mr. H had tried to do in the group). Mr. K's older brother left the family (as Mr. H had left the group), but since he deep down loved his older brother, he was sad to have him leave the family (so he did try to get Mr. H to stay on in the group, as a way of repairing the loss of his brother). Then the arrival of Mrs. J was like having his deceased mother coming back to the family after all those years of absence. Mrs. J was closest to the therapist in age, being the oldest woman in the group, and had some physical resemblances to his mother. Also, she almost immediately showed Mr. K caring interest in a motherly way. The rest of the group became to him as his many younger siblings, who were too young to understand what was going on and therefore not that helpful. Understanding his family transference helped Mr. K to see and understand the role he had taken on in the group and was also a breakthrough in the mourning process concerning the losses of his mother and his older brother.

Vignette 4

Mrs. U joined a slow open group of young people with a male therapist. Mrs. U was the oldest daughter with many younger siblings and grew up in a foreign country. It was often her job to babysit her younger siblings. Her father had sexually abused her from early age. When she at older age spoke of the abuse, she got little support from her family and left home in anger, and later left her country. After almost two years in the therapy group she left, also in anger. Afterwards the therapist saw more clearly what had happened in the group. Mrs. U had focused on the therapist watching his every move, demanding much of his attention, but quick to point out his shortcomings when his interventions were not to her liking. Thus, recreating her love-hate relationship with her father. This is not uncommon in parental transference. What was also important here is that she had treated the other group members with almost total lack of interest. Every session she waited until they had finished (as if the younger siblings need attention first) and then she took the scene and usually was not interested in the other group members' comments, and was quick to point out their shortcomings in helping her, and gave the message that they really couldn't understand her. The group slowly started withdrawing and making it the therapist's job to deal with this angry woman, who no one really dared to take up a fight with. Focusing on how she treated the other group members as "ignorant younger siblings" (as part of the family transference) could have opened up for her, and for the group, a way out of the stuck father (parental) transference focus.

(b) Family Transference in Organizations

Vignette 7

Mr. N worked at a clinic were Mr. P was his boss. Mr. P had a younger brother the same age as Mr. N, and Mr. P was the same age as Mr. N's older brother. Mr. P was his parents' favourite, and Mr. N was more popular in his family than his older brother. Mr. P got a promotion and Mr. N took over his old position and his old team, in which Mr. P had been a popular leader. Mr. N soon became quite popular with the team. This Mr. P didn't like at all. In a staff meeting where Mr. N was present he took his anger out on his old team. He conveyed feelings of betrayal, blamed them for incompetence, and made unfair demands on the staff. The staff was hurt and had problems defending themselves. Mr. N was unusually helpless in the situation, although he made some vague attempts to defend his staff. In a later supervision session, Mr. N broke down when he realized that he had experienced the same helplessness in defending his younger siblings from his aggressive older brother. Also, his old fear for his older brother was evoked in the situation and paralyzed him. Thus, the Family and Sibling Transference Mr. P and Mr. N were unconsciously experiencing was greatly interfering with the function of the organization. The knowledge of this made working through possible.

Peer Transference

One of the most frequently asked questions, when introducing the topic of sibling transference is "What about the only child, where there are no siblings"? The importance of this question will probably become greater in the future, since childbirth on the whole is decreasing in Western societies and growing up with siblings is less likely in the future.

Peer transference is a type of horizontal transference and is valuable to explain transferences that occur towards non-sibling peers. It is observable when a group member, who is an only child, develops transference towards one, or more, of the other group members, as is highlighted in the following vignette.

Vignette 9

Mr. O was well liked by his therapy group, which was a part of a training program. He was a good listener and gave space for the others and seemed to like the group. The group members where all actively using the group for personal matters, except Mr. O, who seldom sought help for himself from the group. Although friendly, he never allowed any member to get very close to him. Many really did make an effort to get closer to him with meagre results. On the other hand, he would more easily open up to what the therapist had to say and seemed to value the therapist's interventions much more than those from the other group members. This difference was sometimes pointed out to him, but he usually dismissed the idea quickly. When there was a natural break in the group's life, he decided to leave the group, and thus only partially completed the training. Since Mr. O was an only child, his behaviour in the group may be seen in the light of that fact. He never really seemed to get the feeling of belonging to the group, although he obviously liked it. It is likely that for him, unconsciously, the group became a group of peers to be with, learn with and have fun with, but not for opening himself up to, or using to help with personal problems. His rather early departure from the group may also be explained from the unconscious feeling that other group members were coming to a level of intimacy and openness he was not familiar, or comfortable, with. The unconscious desire for such intimacy, and desire for the "sense of belonging" one has the possibility to find in groups, may have led to his participation in the group in the first place. On the other hand, there clearly was a positive parental/authority transference towards the therapist.

Discussion

As far as the author knows, Freud was unaware of sibling transference and family transference. The most likely reason is that observing sibling transference and family transference is much easier in group therapy, and in groups at large, than in individual therapy.

Concluding from the preceding it is understandable that therapists doing individual psychotherapy have shown relatively little interest in the issue of siblings. Foulkes spoke of diluted transference by the horizontal dimension. Lately this seems to be changing because there is a dramatic increase in publications dealing with the subject of sibling transference. Sibling rivalry is probably the subject that has had the most attention amongst professionals through the years, as it is mentioned in numerous publications (4, 8, 9). Sibling rivalry (Vignettes 5–7) may often be seen re-enacted in groups and organizations, but it is important to keep in mind that sibling love and affection (Vignette 1), or indifference (Vignette 2, 4), is also common.

Taking the preceding into account it is also understandable how easy it is to overlook family transference. The concept is still seldom mentioned in group literature. Although the concept of family transference is not used as described earlier, some authors are aware of the importance of the family of origin in group therapy. In his renowned book, *The Theory and Practice of Group Psychotherapy*, Yalom speaks of "the Corrective Recapitulation of the Primary Family Group" and its importance in group therapy. He draws an important conclusion when he argues that using both male and female group therapists is likely to enhance the corrective recapitulation, or rather family transference (10).

Conclusion

As is explained earlier, it is important to divide transference into four main categories:

1. Parental/authority transference, which is Freud's classical transference concept (also referred to as vertical transference).
2. Sibling transference (also referred to as horizontal transference).
3. Family transference (also referred to as horizontal-vertical transference).
4. Peer transference (This concept should be confined to non-sibling peers). It is also a type of horizontal transference.

This distinction has proved to be of great clinical value in group therapy. Its understanding can also be helpful in individual therapy when patients report problems at work, or in groups outside the therapy room. In organizational consultation those concepts have proved to be valuable tools in understanding relationships and conflicts in organizations.

Finally, reduced birth rate in Western countries with consequent lack of sibling experiences may affect groups and organizations in the future. Further research is advocated.

References

1) Freud, S. (1912) The Dynamics of Transference. In *Standard Edition*. Vol. 12, pp. 97–108. London: Hogarth Press.
2) Gudmundsson, E. (1993) *Elaborating on Different Phenomena Observed in the Group Analytic Setting*. Diploma Paper (unpublished). London: Institute of Group Analysis.
3) Gudmundsson, E. (2013) Sibling Transference and Family Transference in Groups and Organizations. *FORUM, 6*: 143–152. https://doi.org/10.3280/FORU2013-006014
4) Karterud, S. (1999) *Gruppe Analyse og Psykodynamisk Gruppepsykoterapi*. Oslo: Pax Forlag.
5) Shechter, R.A. (1999) The Meaning and Interpretation of Sibling-transference in the Clinical Situation. *Issues in Psychoanalytic Psychology, 21*(1–2): 1–10.
6) Walrond-Skinner, S. (1976) *Family Therapy: The Treatment of Natural Systems*. London and Boston: Routledge and K. Paul.
7) Hamori, E. and Hódi, Ágnes (1996) Reflection of Family Transference in Group Psychotherapy for Preadolescents. *Group Analysis, 29*(1): 43–54.
8) Kaplan, H.I. and Sadock, B. (1993) *Comprehensive Group Psychotherapy*. Third Edition. Baltimore: Williams & Wilkins.
9) Kahn, B.S. (1980–81) Freudian Siblings. *Psychoanalytic Review, 67*: 493–504.
10) Yalom, I.D. (1985) *The Theory and Practice of Group Psychotherapy*. Third Edition. New York: Basic Books.

1.6 Otherness in groups

The nursing couple and Oedipal relations

R.D. Hinshelwood

The topic of horizontal relations with siblings as having formative influence as well as the vertical relations of the Oedipus complex has begun to be address recently (Mitchell 2003; Coles 2003, 2006). But there has always been a psychoanalytic awareness of the dynamics between individuals within the setting of a group, going back to Burrow (1927). The various ideas compiled in these works have on the whole tended to be drawn from individual work in psychoanalysis.

It is true that the two major conceptual traditions of group dynamics have also been predicated largely on the intra-group relations and tensions between members (Bion and Rickman 1943 [1961]; Foulkes 1948). These traditions have however been adapted from the psychoanalytic session, albeit with debts to gestalt psychology and to social field theory (Lewin 1936). They are group-as-a-whole traditions which take a somewhat aerial view of the group as an entity in itself, generalising group phenomena at a higher level of abstraction. So, the notions of a matrix (Foulkes) or of the proto-mental basic assumptions (Bion) are models these astute observers used in their position as facilitator, conductor, therapist or consultant.

It is important to recognise however that it is not just the mind of the person running a group who seeks or applies conceptual models of group behaviour. In fact, all the members of a group make their own assessments, with whatever models they themselves have in mind. In a psychoanalysis, too, the individual analysand has a metapsychology of his own, as well as the analyst. Of course, we tend to call the analysand's metapsychology his 'transference', but there is a much better understanding today than in Freud's time of a meeting of the intra-psychic systems of the two parties in the activities of a psychoanalytic setting. A group therefore is not just an anonymous entity that is somehow alien to the individuals who come into it. All participants in groups of two or more have their own anticipatory expectations, conscious and unconscious. There may well be *anonymised aspects* of the group, but they are so because the existing membership have themselves, through unconscious processes, collaborated to anonymise them (see Bion's 'Experiences in Groups II', in Bion 1961).

In this chapter I propose to investigate one fairly general factor in the way members of the group perceive and cooperate with each other in their group interaction. These common aspects will be the experiences that come simply

DOI: 10.4324/9781003220060-8

from having a human mind. Such endowments are brought out by being in the context of other minds. I start however by drawing on a particular set of observations derived originally from the individual psychoanalytic setting. These observations are about the very first group we all encounter in our development – the infant in the family.

Freud described a transition in the earliest days of life from 'his majesty the baby' (Freud 1914, p. 90), where the dominant pattern was a hierarchy ruled by an infant's demanding crying (and blissful satisfaction), to the complicated threesome modelled on Sophocles' play *Oedipus Rex*. The latter is a difficult turmoil as the dynamics of an intruder supervene on the original two-person innocence.

The third position

Britton (1989) in developing the dynamic understanding of the Oedipal conflicts emphasised these two different positions for the infant vis-á-vis the parents. His paper is a chapter in a book called *The Oedipus Complex Today* (Britton et al. 1989). Britton took up Klein's writing on the Oedipus complex, and described how the capacity for developing the reality principle develops hand-in-hand with the depressive position, If that principle is not established, the infant lives with delusions and illusions (and later the adult may too). Apart from recognising the rivalrous love and murderous jealousy of the Oedipus complex there is the prior step to relinquish a preceding state:

> The initial recognition of the parental sexual relationship involves relinquishing the idea of sole and permanent possession of mother and leads to a profound sense of loss which, if not tolerated, may become a sense of persecution.
>
> (Britton 1989, p. 84)

The experience is that he is excluded from the nursing couple of which he had previously been an exclusive member. Relinquishing the exclusive possession of mother is a traumatic step, difficult for the immature ego to take. So that fully reconciling oneself often takes much of a lifetime. Some of us never fully make it. The rather comforting saying, 'Two's company, three's a crowd', conceals the full pain of recognising the exclusion.

Britton writes of that painful threesome:

> The primal family triangle provides the child with two links connecting him separately with each parent and confronts him with the link between them which excludes him.
>
> (Britton 1989, p. 87)

The first experience is the mother and infant exclusively together. Then, this has to be succeeded by the excluded position in which mother and father have their own link together. Further major steps in development are then possible; as he says:

> If the link between the parents perceived in love and hate can be tolerated in the child's mind, it provides him with a prototype for an object relationship of a third kind in which he is a witness and not a participant. A third position then comes into existence from which object relationships can be observed. Given this, we can also envisage being observed. This provides us with a capacity for seeing ourselves in interaction with others and for entertaining another point of view whilst retaining our own, for reflecting on ourselves whilst being ourselves.
>
> (Britton 1989, p. 87)

Britton's paper does two things; first, it is an update of Melanie Klein's early writing about the Oedipus complex, and, second, it focuses on the important transition of the object-relations out of the paranoid-schizoid position.

The development of the ego

His picture of the 'nursing couple' is an absolute and uninterrupted exclusiveness, a complete possession of mother and her breast and the satisfactions she brings. This cannot last as the awareness of the reality of a third presence with mother intrudes as a challenging new scene. Someone else is there who turns mother away from the infant, and towards a new couple from which the infant is now excluded. The infant has then the work of recognising two others, typically mother and father, as the couple (but equally frequently it is the birth of a younger sibling). And this couple the infant now sees as excluding him/her. It is a painful move from exclusiveness to excluded; from inclusion to occupying a third position.

When Klein herself qualified as a psychoanalyst in 1919, Freud and psychoanalysis were committed to the Oedipus complex as the central dynamic of the human unconscious mind. In the course of her career, Klein developed her ideas about the unconscious and described what she called the 'deeper layers'. In many respects this moved her ideas away from the Oedipus complex, although she initially described her modifications as only minor changes. In fact there were important new elements. And eventually she found herself discussing the dynamics involved in the very formation and coherence of the ego – rather than the conflicts which could occur within the ego once it has satisfactorily developed.

There has been much debate about the validity of the strategies used by the early ego, and the relics of them in later life. While it will not be relevant to describe the debate here, it is worth noting that both classical and Kleinian analysts have focussed on the strength and weakness of the ego. Britton used as evidence, adult psychoanalytic material from patients who have not been successful in their progress and are still struggling with the issues of a basic self-observing ego.

Accommodating the parental couple as different from the nursing couple is the beginning of a more realistic view and it is not just painful, it is developmental. So, to respect the real world of the others in his family group involves a good deal of emotional work and pain. The infant's work is to begin to see itself in a new way, moving from *being a part of* the nursing couple to *witnessing* the parental couple – that is the crux of the reality sense. It is the beginnings of the ego's capacity to observe and recognise itself.

It is a position from which thought can begin. The triangular space created by this observing is known as the space for reflection, the reflective space. By reconciling himself to the position of observing, the capacity for self-observation can also begin.

This is clearly of interest with the constant pressure from certain patients to restrict themselves exclusively to the analytic couple, to shut down on observation and reflection, and to spare the pain of jealousy and intrusion into their exclusiveness. If the analyst makes attempts towards observing what happens in this move, the patient may violently resist. One of Britton's patients screamed 'stop that fucking thinking' (Britton 1989, p. 87). Thought itself means the exclusion from the nursing couple. The capacity to think and observe necessarily requires adopting the third excluded position. This step is felt by the patient as a violent assault.

Now this has relevance way beyond individual therapy, out into everyday life and experience. The intruding other (in terms of gender, ethnicity, etc.) has become a powerful eruption in the politics of the 21st century, for instance. But it also contributes to understanding what happens in group therapy.

Group positions

I suggest that this is an interesting and important model for thinking about a patient's clinical material, not only in a psychoanalytic sessions but in therapeutic groups as well. In fact, we might expect more opportunity in a group than in a psychoanalytic session to examine this crucial step in development and how far a group member has proceeded. In a group, members do intrude into each other's conversations and connections with each other all of the time. Whatever the wish for exclusive relations, the pain of being excluded is potentially a much more open, accessible and immediate problem in a therapy group than in a psychoanalytic couple.

These descriptions of two kinds of couples are key alternative horizontal relations between group members. The seeking of exclusiveness in a group is a forlorn hope and the experience of intrusion is a constant experience, or at least a constant threat.

Each individual member in a group appears to have the option of experiencing one or other of these positions. However, in small groups there is a tendency for the members to create a group culture in which they have, and give each other, similar experiences – good, bad, therapeutic, anti-therapeutic.

For instance, here is a group in which each has the experience of feeling out-of-it, or excluded:

> In this group a woman, 'X', described an event in which her husband had had a row with her mother. Another woman, 'Y', waited just until this story had finished, and immediately asked for the dates of a forthcoming holiday break. They had been announced recently. The therapist pointed out how 'Y' had cut across the first woman's story. She had also cut out her own memory of the dates. 'Y' immediately turned to enquire of someone else. A man started to talk about his mother-in-law, seemingly following the first woman, though clearly absorbed only in his own tale – more to do with seeking out a mother for himself because in childhood he had spent long periods separated from his own mother.

This is a culture in which the group can be said to fail to contain the individuals in a satisfactory way (Hinshelwood 2003). The relations between the members does not connect them; it disconnects. The members seem isolated in their own stories. What connections there are seem tangential, on a more cognitive level, without reading each other's feelings. And there is a considerable cutting across each other's communications, or using another's communication in order to divert to one's own thoughts without linking into the other person's state of mind. The link to the mother-in-law problem for X's wife, and for the last speaker, is not accurate; they are different stories with quite different affective tone. There is here talk that aims at others, but falls flat. The constant repeated disruption of an intimate connection provides a repeated experience of exclusion and then a quiet resentment about it. One person's disrupted connection with the group or with another member is followed by a disruption of the next story.

There is no real observation of others, and no capacity for self-observation. In discussing a group somewhat like this Bion said:

> I reflect that from the way in which the group is going on its motto might be: 'Vendors of quack nostrums unite.' No sooner have I said this to myself than I realize that I am expressing my feeling, not of the group's disharmony, but of its unity. Furthermore, I very soon become aware that it is not accidentally that I have attributed this slogan to the group, for every attempt I make to get a hearing shows that I have a united group against me. The idea that neurotics cannot co-operate has to be modified.
>
> (Bion 1961, p. 52)

The group together formed a culture in which each is excluded from close interest or acknowledgement. There is no regard for the opportunity of a reflective space together.

The relevance for this discussion is that there is a circulating experience of exclusion as someone butts in. Resentments occur and get expressed as further interruptions and intrusions. The culture becomes self-sustaining. These resentments at feeling excluded provoke a comparable response, a revenge almost. They feel an immediate need to pass on the feeling to others. It can be seen that the response to feeling that one's contribution does not succeed in gaining an entry into someone's full interest leads to a denial of someone else's need for exclusive attention. Each member appears to make his contribution as if from outside, from an excluded position, whilst others are involved in thoughts and interests elsewhere. The sense of being in the unwelcome excluded position seems enforced. And the result is not a culture of reflection, but the opposite; it is a reciting of a story that gets nowhere. The relations of each member to each other, that is, the horizontal dimension, is a forced exclusion which is resisted, and no moves succeed in getting proper observation and reflection going.

Such a culture suggests a need to deal with and contain the experience of feeling unaccompanied and excluded, the loss of a nurturing mother-infant couple to be part of. Despite the seeming hopelessness of the situation, one could say that in a therapy group there is adequate opportunity to examine and work with this sense of loss, and the yearning for something exclusive. By adopting the model of the exclusive versus excluded relationship, we gain a focus for helping the members understand and learn about their need for exclusiveness, even though it is not really on offer, or it can only be realistically found in some modified form in groups.

Moving then to what a more realistic group might be like here is a moment from another group. This time it is possible for members to engage in a way where they are not struggling for exclusiveness but can accept a position in which they do witness others' experiences, without being too disruptive, and they can contribute self-observation in a more relevant way. It is not without friction, but the members are connected and those connections feel different from the previous group:

> Two men in a group were discussing a trivial detail about some maintenance work on a car that belonged to one of them. 'A' described his difficulty with a rusty bolt. 'B' talked about how he had once had the same problem and had solved it by hitting the bolt with a hammer; he seemed pleased with himself. Another, third man, 'C', gave a slight laugh and remarked on 'B's hint of pride. 'A' looked startled and then a little angry, as he realised that he had given 'B' the opportunity to be pleased with himself. He told 'B' that it was no solution to hit the bolt with the hammer and explained why. Clearly he now wanted to put 'B' down. Two women in the group were looking on with some fascination at this male sparring. One said 'Men!' with mock exasperation. The other said her husband had returned from a football match recently with a bruise on his cheek which he had refused to talk about.

In this group, the participants seemed much more able to grasp the importance of what was being described and *felt* emotionally in ways which connected them to each other. They exchange experiences of rivalry and prowess which was responded to by the men and the women each in their own way.

The five people involved seemed willing to tune in, in their own characteristic ways, to the male rivalry and psychological bruising which was going on. The talk was not necessarily harmonious, respectful or friendly. But they were reading each other accurately and it is this quality of being 'in tune' which I am emphasising, each feeling the tune of the one who is speaking. They are excluded – but *can* observe. They function in a third position but can nevertheless *accompany* each other. The resentments at feeling the loss of exclusiveness can be tolerated, expressed and observed, although not necessarily comfortably. Here is a capacity in the group to tolerate the exclusion, not without resentments of course, but with a preservation of observation and self-observation.

The exclusive position

Though it seems rare, it is possible to find reference to a group culture in which an exclusive relationship occurs typical of a nursing couple. The most striking description is the following:

> I thought that some patterns of behaviour were recurring and, in particular, one that went like this: two members of the group would become involved in a discussion; sometimes the exchange between the two could hardly be described but it would be evident that they were involved with each other, and that the group as a whole thought so too. On these occasions the group would sit in attentive silence – rather surprising behaviour in view of the neurotic's impatience of any activity that does not centre on his own problem. Whenever two people begin to have this kind of relationship in the group – whether these two are man and woman, man and man, or woman and woman – it seems to be a basic assumption, held both by the group and the pair concerned, that the relationship is a sexual one. It is as if there could be no possible reason for two people's coming together except sex. The group tolerates this situation, and, although knowing smiles are interchanged, the group seems prepared to allow the pair to continue their exchange indefinitely.
>
> (Bion 1961, pp. 60–61)

This description was Bion's introduction of the pairing group basic assumption. The quality of exclusiveness of the conversation, whatever it is about, was the culture that Bion was trying to convey. He likened it to the intimacy of sex, and even attributed it to sexual expectations. It could equally be the intense intimacy of the nursing couple, possibly more intimate and exclusive even than sex. Bion introduced this description by saying: "I wish I could give concrete examples, but I cannot record what was actually said" (p. 60); it is as if the incident was almost too private to keep in memory. The point I make is there may be a group position in which the culture expresses and enacts this longed for exclusive intimacy. It would be basic assumption pairing.

Concluding reflections

The development of the idea of the triangular space for reflection presents us, therefore, with an array of three possible states that a group member may establish for himself:

- The *excluded third*, with a resentful reaction at having to witness others seeking the 'parental couple' and its exclusiveness, and then finding themselves disrupted when they attempt it themselves
- A culture we might call the *accompanying third* when there can be a genuine interested witnessing, observing and reflecting on other's relations
- And a visible connection demonstrating the pairing of an *exclusive couple*, maybe a merged couple, comparable to the mother-infant 'nursing couple' that excludes the world around

The slipping between these different states may be quite frequent, but there appears to be a collaborative quality in which the members of a group move collectively between these group cultures. Each state may persist due to self-sustaining feedback processes.

These three positions are arrived at from considerations of clinical psychoanalytic observation. However, they do have a resonance with descriptions arrived at from observations made specifically within groups. I have drawn on Bion's (1961) pairing group as a group which is dominated by the exclusiveness of a nurturing couple. It may be that the basic assumption flight/fight group corresponds to the group where members are struggling resentfully with the state of being excluded. And indeed the group I have called the accompanying third (as opposed to the excluded third) seems to correspond to Bion's work group.

I am also reminded of the descriptions that Pierre Turquet (1975) made of the possible states an individual can occupy in a large group event at experiential group relations conferences. He also described three states of the members but defined them by their sense of identity in the group. The three kinds of identity he noted in the large group were:

- The 'singleton' who exists in the group as if not a part of it – coping, by avoidance we might say, with this expression of feeling threateningly excluded.
- The 'IM', is short for the 'individual member', who can come to find a way of expressing himself in the context of others – making a link, as an accompanying third.
- The 'MI', is short for the 'membership individual' in which he plays a role defined by the group, rather than by himself; so that his identity has merged with the group dynamics and he is no longer separate – someone who perhaps does find an exclusiveness through merging with the given role.

The fact that something similar comes from both the 'individual' work of psychoanalytic therapy as well as from therapeutic groups and also from the experiential study of large group dynamics does suggest some degree of consistency to the generalisations being described here.

One can reflect here on the importance for psychoanalytic work, where there is no actual intrusion from a third. In fact, ends of sessions, weekends and holiday breaks all represent the intrusion though it is often missed in therapeutic work. Then there can be a collusion between both analyst and analysand to exclude those beyond the room. It is not difficult then to indulge in the exclusive couple as if replicating the nursing mother with baby, for most of an individual treatment. That is not a mistake so easy to be drawn into in a group setting. Perhaps too, in individual work it is possible to recognise the equivalent of a stilted group that fails to make real contact. Often one gets the impression of a patient playing the part of a patient and giving an apparently intimate account, but it fails to move and engage. We might wonder about that pseudo-connection as a reaction to, and holding back from, the risk of real pain from feeling excluded.

The group therapist in turn has to accomplish his own capacity for thinking whilst under the extreme pressures of these cultures. His work is to invite the patients to join him in this observation. Instead his mind is required to accommodate – that is, contain – the experience of a violent assault which the patient feels is made on his/her own position within the *nursing* couple. The very capacity to perform the role of thinking about this is itself an assault on that position of exclusiveness which is aimed for. The group facilitator embedded in one of these group cultures, is not in a vertical relation of dominance, but is as much affected by the culture as the other members. His one resource is that he knows about the powerful pressures on himself, on his sense of relatedness and difficulty to reflect and on the distortions of his own identity in the group context of the moment.

This chapter has been an attempt to consider that being in a group provides an experience that is close to one of the first hurdles in life. That is, it offers an opportunity to examine the first major assault that an infant has to cope with, as well as each person's means of coping. It is after all an experience we repeat over and over again as we enter and leave groups all our lives.

References

Bion, W. R. (1948) Experiences in Groups: II. *Human Relations* 1: 487–496. Republished in W. R. Bion (1961) *Experiences in Groups and Other Papers*, pp. 41–58. London: Tavistock.

Bion, W. R. (1961) *Experiences in Groups and Other Papers*. London: Tavistock.

Bion, W. R. and Rickman, J. (1943 [1961]) Intra-Group Tensions in Therapy. In W. R. Bion (Ed.) *Experiences in Groups and Other Papers*, pp. 11–26. London: Routledge.

Britton, R. (1989) The Missing Link. In R. Britton, M. Feldman and E. O'Shaughnessy (Eds.) *The Oedipus Complex Today*. London: Karnac.

Burrow, T. (1927) *The Social Basis of Consciousness: A Study in Organic Psychology*. New York: Harcourt, Brace.

Coles, P. (2003) *The Importance of Sibling Relationships in Psychoanalysis*. London: Karnac.

Coles, P. (2006) *Sibling Relations*. London: Karnac.

Foulkes, S. H. (1948) *Introduction to Group Analytic Psychotherapy; Studies in the Social Integration of Individuals and Groups*. London: Heinemann.

Freud, S. (1914) On Narcissism: An Introduction. In *The Standard Edition of the Complete Psychological Works of Sigmund Freud, Volume 14*. London: Hogarth.

Hinshelwood, R. D. (2003) Group Mentality and 'Having a Mind'. In Malcolm Pines and Bob Lipgar (Eds.) *Building on Bion: Volume 1, Roots*. London: Jessica Kingsley.

Lewin, K. (1936) *Principles of Topological Psychology*. New York: Mcgraw-Hill.

Mitchell, J. (2003) *Siblings*. London: Polity.

Turquet, P. (1975) Threats to Identity in the Large Group. In Lionel Kreeger (Ed.) *The Large Group*, pp. 87–144. London: Constable.

1.7 What happens when you cut a worm? Group members as peers

Joanna Skowronska

This somewhat puzzling title of my chapter is a quote from one of my group sessions, one of those that tends to bring to mind an intriguing yet undeveloped idea by S.H. Foulkes (quoted by Luis Ormont in the movie *Personal Encounter with S.H. Foulkes*, Brunori, Knauss, 1998) about a particular kind of regression that can be observed in small analytic groups: a regression caused by finding oneself among equals, like in peer groups. From this perspective, he described the group as "an instrument constantly moving forward," freeing participants of the past burden by ongoing experiences with equals. This notion is of particular interest to me because, in the course of my group practice, I occasionally experience moments that remind me of the atmosphere of a playground – a rich space full of potential where exchange, experimenting, mirroring, being mirrored, and experiencing a sense of interrelatedness are all ever-present.

Henry Grunebaum and Leonard Solomon (1980) postulated the need to form a peer group psychotherapy theory. They pointed to a surprising inconsistency: although in their espoused theory (the theory one says one does follow), group therapists are concentrated on members' or the group-as-a-whole's relations with the therapists, their theory of action (what is done) is usually peer-oriented, focused on member-to-member relationships (Grunebaum, Solomon, 1980). Hubert M. Rabin (2011) blamed for this the tradition of thinking rooted in classical individual psychoanalysis, claiming that all goings-on in a group are a derivative of Oedipal and pre-Oedipal situations; hence, the only transformative interventions are the ones referring to member-conductor transference (e.g., Ezriel, 1973). Rabin insists that we should treat "relatedness to peers not as a derivate of parent–child relationship but as having separate developmental lines" (Rabin, 2011, p. 286). In his view, neglecting peer relationships has essential consequences: (1) patients' peer relations are not sufficiently explored; (2) peer transference is rarely examined in the group; and (3) lack of peer relationship theories within the group therapy paradigm.

E. James Anthony described the "group analytical phase" (1967, p. 61) as "based on family and peer group" (1967, p. 65). Foulkes describes group analysis, in contrast to vertical psychoanalysis, as horizontal analysis that goes on here and now, within the circle of peers (Foulkes, Anthony, 2014, p. 62). Do we then have a group-analytic peer theory or not?

DOI: 10.4324/9781003220060-9

Sibling relations have recently enjoyed a degree of interest in psychoanalysis and group analysis. Such authors as, for example, Profecy Coles (2003), suggest that they should be treated as a separate developmental path with all its consequences, including being sensitive to the specific kind of transference in psychoanalytical psychotherapy.

While relationships with siblings are played out in the shadow of relationships with parents, peer relationships are initiated and maintained with selected playmates and are based on voluntary interactions that often are equal and mutual. They vary in duration and frequency compared to the relatively stable relations with adult family members and siblings. They are sources of new meaningful experiences with others, of new vital self-experiences, and they allow the child to see themselves in a new way. Later, we tend to make and keep relationships with non-familial age-mates during our lifespan.

If looking at our patients, we mostly think about their experiences with their parents and other family members, and we naturally focus on their current relations with authority figures, their dependence, autonomy, competitiveness, separation, and individuation. The horizontal transference among group members is often seen as the outgrowth of the relationship with parents or siblings. Would it not be interesting to see what sort of space opens when we view the horizontal dimension as powered by peer experiences, a multi-person space, and apply it to the multi-person psychology of group analysis.

> Once, working with a mature group, I realized that I had enjoyed myself very much working with this group. I appreciated their cooperativeness and was reluctant to the change that would occur due to my much-needed intervention. I realized that the group had become my refuge from disappointing relationships with my colleagues. A friendly atmosphere in the group, once an achievement, now became a hurdle preventing the continued growth and further development, and my personal needs played a role in this dynamic. I had to relinquish the status of the group member. My intervention undertaken from the conductor's position ruined the group's cohesion but enabled the process of individuation of the group participants.

I was only able to overcome this impasse by reflecting on the importance and meaning of peer relationships for me in the conductor's role and on the interrelationships between horizontal and vertical relations in my group.

A lot of what brings patients to group therapy has to do with their current peer relations: lack of friends, inability to realize their professional ambitions due to poor social skills, or difficulties in building satisfactory romantic ties. If we view peer relationships as a separate developmental line, we need to consider how what happened among their peers bears on the lives of group members and their relations in the group.

> X., who was considering his therapy's termination, brought the subject of an electronic device used to alleviate phantom pains. In his thirties, he was

an only child, brought up in a multigenerational family consisting mostly of women: mother, grandma, and sisters. His father, having a life-threatening disease, was treated as a hero representing all male members of that family that spilled their blood in numerous wars over the generations. Someone said: "Listen, I wonder: is it true that when you cut a worm in half, the pieces will go on living." Someone else added: "That would depend on whether you cut it length – or cross-wise." This opened many evocative associations, metaphors containing unformulated thoughts, unarticulated feelings concerning the fleeting nature of life, death, and the sense of life, all eliciting from childhood memories. Towards the end of the session, X. spoke about the lack of support from the peer group in his lonely childhood. Now he felt contained by the group, and he experienced vividly the void this lack of the peer group created in his life and was able to grieve this loss.

Peers matter

> Peer relations are a basic part of our shared human nature. We are social beings. Nearly all of us live, work, and function in social groups. Experiences in friendship and groups can begin as early as the first year of life . . . experiences with peers are an enduring and meaningful part of human experience across the lifespan.
>
> (Bukowski et al., 2018, p. XIII)

For developmental and social psychologists, peer relations are simply an aspect of an inborn human ability "to form the larger social units of which they are part, whether the dyad, family, or the group," as Schermer postulates, referring to studies on mirror neurons (2013, p. 31).

Peer space is the source of essential skills that cannot be acquired elsewhere. That space is characterized by equality and is governed by the rules of play. Winnicott was the one who appreciated the developmental value of children's play. While at play, they can experiment with alliances, emotional relationships, and expressing aggressive urges without fear of retaliation since they are expressed in play form and not as an outburst of rage (Winnicott, 1969).

Engaging with other people of equal status and power, children develop their operational thinking about being in the social space (Piaget, 1932). By participating in co-construction, they learn to rely on the resources of others, and they realize that together they can achieve more (Vygotsky, 1978). Grunebaum and Solomon write: "The quality of peer relationship and self-esteem . . . better be regarded as different perspectives of a single phenomenon, the person-in-the social-world" (1987, p. 476). Behavior oriented model of development states that "via processes of rewards, punishments, and imitations, peers 'shape' each other's behavior along multiple dimensions of actions ranging from aggression to altruism" (Bukowski et al., 2018, p. 11). Peter Fonagy writes: "Peer group interaction should increase the opportunities the child has for simulation, imagining what he would see, think, feel, etc. if he were in another person's situation," and as such, together with pretense and talking, mediate the growth of the reflexive function and mentalization (Fonagy et al., 2004, p. 50). So, quoting Bukowski again:

> Without peer relations, healthy human development would be very unlikely, if not impossible. Peer relations are not an ephemeral luxury: they are a necessity. To understand development, one needs to understand peer relations.
>
> (Bukowski et al., 2018, p. XIV)

Peer relations follow a predictable trajectory. Already in the first months of life, one can observe the mutual exchange of attention between babies and one-year-olds gaze at other children for a longer time than at adults. Toddlers enjoy playing with peers, and they imitate them more often than adults. In mid-childhood (6–11 lat), there appears a new form of social relations: groups of peers transform into peer groups.

Peer groups provide children with self-creating and emergent social context. "Self-creating" means that cooperating children co-create rules and norms of being together. They hold and limit each other. "Emergent," because as a group, they can do and achieve more and differently than each of them could on their own. Peer groups are a space that intermediates between the family and the broader social context, and they offer a potential space. Social games with peers that require pretense and cooperative problem solving add up to an ability to share symbolic meanings: intersubjectivity and contribution to the emergence of the theory of mind, which can lead to improving social skills and more positive peer experiences. Children's social and emotional connections while playing are a vital source of support, emotional regulation, and adjustment. In short, the ability to engage in age-appropriate play has a crucial role in development.

> A group member in his late thirties grew up in a chaotic home full of tensions. In his mid-childhood, he spends a lot of time "outside" with his peers, engaged in age-appropriate games and plays, especially the physical ones – exercise play and rough and tumble as well as pretend play. These kinds of plays have affiliative nature, and they let children experience a lot of positive emotions, so they act as a means for emotional regulation. The peer group became his safe haven against his family life's insecurity and unpredictability. Further upheaval in his family caused him to lose his group of pals. He idealized these relationships and missed them even in adulthood. His avoidant personality style found expression in acting and pretending, psychological functioning specific to mid-childhood, and his fantasies allowed him to lead a life that kept him cut off from his emotional experiences. The same set of tools served him later to deal with the shame of not having appropriately mature social skills. As an adult, he complained about unsatisfactory relationships with others he experienced as superficial and had a constant feeling of missing out on things.

Peer theory of group-analytic psychotherapy

With few exceptions, peers have not sat well with psychoanalysis. Peers' developmental significance has been somewhat neglected. But they feature prominently in the attachment theory. To Bowlby, the need to find safety and trust in close and stable emotional bonds with others "continues from the cradle to the grave" (Bowlby, 1979, p. 129).

Do peers sit well with group analysis? Foulkes was ahead of his time with his many observations and hypotheses, which nowadays are fully incorporated in relational and intersubjective approaches in psychoanalysis, such as "the field of mental processes" or "mind between people" (Foulkes, 1984, p. 86). I feel he left us also a "peer theory of group-analytic psychotherapy" written in invisible ink.

Here are some of the traces of this hidden theory:

In his "Introduction to Group Analytic Psychotherapy," Foulkes explains to a hypothetical doubter how putting in a group setting several people with mental health issues would work:

> suppose you have to wash a number of dirty shirts together, and the water is not clean, and perhaps you have not even soap? . . . even then, you can get the shirts reasonably clean, albeit you add dirt to dirt, by using them for mutual friction upon each other.
>
> (1949, p. 29)

He goes on to form the law of group dynamics: "collectively they constitute the very Norm, from which, individually, they deviate" (1949, p. 29). Our practice shows us that this "norm" boils down to the sense that tells you how to be in a group. I understand this law as follows: just as in the parent–child dyad, there is an implicit relational knowing how to be in this relation (Stern, 2002; BCPSG, 2014); "the very Norm" refers to such implicit knowing how to be in the group, the prototype of which is formed based on experiences with peers. Through interactions, games, and plays, peers get into each other's bodies and minds, and the group members somehow know how to "make" a group.

Another element of this theory consists of therapists stepping out "into the open" and finding themselves on the same level with group members as a "participant observer" (Foulkes, Anthony, 2014, p. 29).

> He treats the group as adults on an equal level to his own and exerts an important influence by his own example. . . . The conductor represents and promotes reality, reason, tolerance, understanding, insight, catharsis, independence, frankness, and an open mind for new experiences.
>
> (Foulkes, 1984, p. 57)

By introducing a unique form of being together: "free-floating discussion" – which is a nonhierarchical, non-goal-oriented way of communicating – the conductor "helps to create a special situation": a "dynamic field of experiences" and an "aggregate of interactive and interdependent factors of personality and circumstances" (Foulkes, Anthony, 2014, p. 29). This space is characterized by spontaneity, flexibility, and the spirit of permissiveness. From it, everything follows "as if they were self-generated by the nature of the situation, which, to a great extent, they are" (Foulkes, Anthony, 2014, p. 100).

In a similar vein, Schlapobersky has recently written:

> In the group analytic model, play is a key to work, for it is done through free-floating discussion. Through its play with words and the play of experience that may have no words, a group can provide both an arena for containment and a platform for exploration.
>
> (Schlapobersky, 2016, p. 393)

Does it not sound as if we were assuming that placing strangers in a group, inviting them to engage in a free-floating discussion, having the conductor take up a participant's position, results in a self-creating and emergent environment, one for which a peer group would be the prototype? In it, just as during development, the participants will be acquiring age-specific social and psychological skills (tolerance and appreciation of individual differences . . . reality, reason, tolerance, understanding, insight, catharsis, independence, frankness, and an open mind for new experiences; see Foulkes quote earlier), and both improvement and further development are possible.

Limitation of peer theory of group-analytic psychotherapy

If we were to make full use of the peer space we co-create with group members, shouldn't we be aware of what goes on in genuine developmental peer relationships and what happened to our group members in their peer relationships? There is no reason to assume that a person who entered such a relationship under-equipped will be able to make the best possible use of the peer group space that they are offered. Sigmund Karterud writes:

> They might comply on a more superficial level to basic group rules, acting, so to speak, on deeply ingrained reflexes for group behavior, while mentally being preoccupied with how to survive in the here and now. In the conjoint individual therapy, patients can tell how they can go totally blank in the group, or experience extreme bodily discomfort, becoming dizzy and unable to think, or starting to dissociate in order to survive.
>
> (Karterud, 2011, p. 361)

A peer group's rich developmental environment is not equally available to everybody. The fact that a peer group has no hierarchy does not automatically mean everybody can use its resources equally. The better the children are endowed to relate, the better they are to benefit from the peer group.

Developmental and social psychology and neurobiology unanimously show that humans as a species are "hardwired" to prefer prosocial partners for their interactions. Others better like children with prosocial skills, more often chosen as playmates, so they have more opportunities to polish their social skills. The less-skilled children fall even further behind. Failures in relations with peers, in the space of crucial importance for building one's self-esteem, have a lasting impact on self-representations.

One's status – being liked, accepted, popular – in the peer world is particularly important for psychological well-being. Studies show that a child's position among peers impacts their social behaviors, self-image, development, acquiring new skills, and even neurogenesis (Prinstein et al., 2018). Authors cite empirical evidence to claim also that "children who peers like enjoy lifelong adjustment advantages, and those who are rejected have problems with physical and psychological adjustment even decades later" (Prinstein et al., 2018, p. 630).

Social rejection is "akin to the brain's reactions to the experience of physical pain" (Prinstein et al., 2018, p. 620). The experience of social pain constitutes a risk not only on the biological level within the central and peripheral nervous systems but also shapes the cognitive attitude toward social rejection and increases the social stress for years to come.

Bullying, systematic abuse of power against someone to harm them, is a form of rejection. Bullying is a co-product of certain personality traits, group, and social environment. The most prone to bullying are children with poor social skills and ineffective emotion regulation mechanisms (mainly through externalizations) and low status in the group. It's enough that a child has just one friend and their risk of being bullied diminishes.

Numerous studies cited by Christina Salmivali and Katlin Peets (2018) confirm the reciprocal relation between bullying and internalizing problems such as depression, anxieties, low self-esteem, and interpersonal difficulties such as rejection and lack of few friends. In the book *Bullying Scars* (de Lara, 2016), people who experienced bullying in childhood or adolescence report its consequences in their later life. Ellen Walser de Lara describes the universal indifference with which the social system meets bullying, making its victims internalize the feeling of being inferior or even evil. Health issues, mental problems, and difficulties in relations experienced even after many years show that being subject to bullying is a traumatic experience.

> Two group members, a man, and a woman, got into an interaction that made the woman uncomfortable. Another woman admitted to being scared she might become his next victim. The exchange she observed made her painfully recall the period when in early primary school, she had been bullied. Helplessness, fear, anger, and above all, shame came flooding back when she spoke about these experiences. Group peers expressed their support and anger towards her past abusers. In this atmosphere, she understood past events and the bullies' motivations, which stemmed from the external circumstances and not from, as she used to think, from her being broken.

> She realized that her current peer relations: at work, with friends, and in the group were all underpinned with anxiety, preventing her from being authentic.

Fonagy admitted that "peer abuse is far more prevalent and more painful than abuse by adults" (2020) and the traumatic character of these events makes them psychologically unavailable.

Why keep peers in mind?

Without diminishing the importance of other issues present in the group mental space, I would like to postulate at least three reasons that make keeping peers in mind quite worth our while. Keeping peers in mind helps us assess the new group members' ability to use and benefit from the group's peer space. L. Alan Sroufe posits that the secure attachment in the early relations equips children with a specific set of expectations toward others, gives them interactional skills and the ability to regulate their emotions that are the prerequisite for successful peer relationships: (1) expectation of connectedness, (2) expectations of responsiveness, (3) exploratory and play capacities, (4) capacities for arousal and emotional regulation, and (5) empathy and expectation of mutuality (Boot-LaForce, Groth, 2018).

> This group member who "got stuck" among his buddies tried to recreate in the group the action-oriented atmosphere of the group of pals with an "as if" state of mind. He loved to engage the group in his fantasies about brave actions, wild acting outs that they would all participate in. The group appreciated him, and some fearful members admitted that going along with his fantasies helped manage their anxieties. While they were discussing what these "wild stories" meant for them, he was unable to engage in the conversation and succumbed to depressive ruminations. He had no idea about connectedness, responsiveness, and mutuality, and his emotional spectrum ranged from excitation to withdrawal and isolation. If viewed from that perspective, we can see that he could only take over the stage but felt threatened and unable to participate in a free group discussion leading to emotional liveliness and connectedness. Before he could benefit from the "mutual friction upon each other," he needed some help fixing his primary interpersonal resources through sensitive attunement and metallization of his states and more mature relations as friendship.

Friendships in childhood serve several vital functions. They are a security source outside the family environment, which allows for exploring the self in the world. Friends teach us about ourselves safely; they give us opportunities for self-esteem enhancement and positive self-evaluation. And finally, it is friendship that promotes the growth of interpersonal sensitivity; and offers prototypes for later romantic and parental relationships.

If the therapist allows that peers cross her/his mind, the group's co-creation of meaning opens to peer experiences. Nuclear idea (Billow, 2014) is one of the conceptualizations describing the work done by a conductor striving for understanding and giving meanings to goings-on in the group. The nuclear idea emerges from the:

> intersubjective forces and locations that cannot be fully specified yet may be possible to observe, name, and utilize clinically. They arise from the indeterminacy of the network of communications and interactions, that is from within the dynamic matrix (Foulkes, 1964) or "culture" (Whitaker and Lieberman, 1964) of the group, co-created by therapist's participation and influence and expressed in the group's idiom (Bollas, 1989) and discourse (Schlapobersky, 1994), its particular language, symbolization, and enactments.
>
> (Billow, 2014, p. 92)

In the "worm cutting group," the story about a tool used to alleviate phantom pains told by the member preparing to leave became the "call for containment" (Friedman, 2004), and it evoked the response of the group containing his unformulated and unexpressed experience. His final comment, an "unconscious interpretation on the part of the patient" (Foulkes, 1986, p. 119) illustrates how a therapist's *nuclear idea* embodied in the feeling of being on the playground allowed for a sort of group enactment. The patient linked the current peer relations with the other group members with the lack of such ties in the past, which left him in the world still "peopled with giants" (Coles, 2003, p. 88), in shadow of the tragic history of his family. In the final stages of his therapy, this helped him place and view his fate in the context of his family and time.

The permission for peers to cross your mind is even more critical as some of the instances of peer experiences can be traumatic and hence "unspeakable" (Herman, 1992, p. 1). As such, they can only be acknowledged, when expressed, and discussed by somebody else.

Conclusion

Relationships with peers are an expression of the human need for companionship and community. It seems likely that the mirror neuron systems, which have been detected in multiple locations all over our brains, are a neuronal mechanism creating the unity of self and others:

> the precognitive "instant recognition" inherent in mirror neuron activity may explain why some group formation can occur in short order, pointing to "grouping" as being, like primary attachment, a "wired-in" tendency of our species.
>
> (Schermer, 2013, p. 32)

Paying closer attention to the peer space in the group goes hand in hand with a more profound interest in the procedural, implicit relational domain. The concepts such as "schemas-of-being-with" (Stern, 2002), implicit relational knowing (BCPSG, 2014; Stern, 2002), built on the observation of dyadic relations between a caregiver and a small child, may very well have an equivalent in a group of peers. We are biologically determined to form close emotional attachments to others to keep our nervous system in equilibrium.

Just "belonging to a group" can create central nervous system homeostasis and stabilization, which reduces cortisol to more manageable levels, thus combating the debilitating effects of chronic stress, which interferes with learning and memory (Grossmark, Wright, 2015, p. 171).

"Implicit memory is the eternal present past" (Badenoch, Cox, 2013, p. 5). Still, present mutual regulation in the group can change its participants' implicit memory, as findings of interpersonal neurobiology (IPNB) suggest (Badenoch, Cox, 2013). Concepts such as "moments of meeting" (BCPSG, 2014) that describe the transformative power of spontaneous, authentic, and personal therapist reactions within the co-created emergent space of therapeutic relations deserve more attention from group analysts. They may just be the thing that makes a group "an instrument constantly moving forward, freeing participants from the past burden by present experiences between equals."

References

Anthony, E.J. (1967). The generic elements in dyadic and group psychotherapy, *International Journal of Group Psychotherapy*, vol. 17, pp. 57–70.

Badenoch, B., Cox, P. (2013). Integrating interpersonal neurobiology with group psychotherapy, in S.P. Gantt, B. Badenoch (eds.), *The Interpersonal Neurobiology of Group Psychotherapy and Group Process*, London: Karnac Books.

BCPSG (2014). *Change in Psychotherapy: A Unifying Paradigm*, New York, London: W. W. Norton & Company.

Billow, R. (2014). Developing nuclear ideas, in R. Grossmark, F. Wright (eds.), *The One and the Many, Relational Approaches to Group Psychotherapy,* New York and London: Routledge.

Bollas, C. (1989). *Forces of Destiny: Psychoanalysis and the Human Idiom*, Northvale, New York: Janson Aronson.

Boot-LaForce, C., Groth, A.M. (2018). Peer-child attachment and peer relations, in W.M. Bukowski, et al. (eds.), *Handbook of Peer Interactions, Relationships, and Groups*, New York, London: The Guilford Press: 349–370.

Bowlby, J. (1979). *The Making and Breaking of Affectional Bonds*, London, New York: Routledge.

Brunori, L., Knauss, W. (1998). Personal encounter with S.H. Foulkes. A Movie by Group Analytic Society.

Bukowski, W.M., et al. (2018). *Handbook of Peer Interactions, Relationships, and Groups*, New York, London: The Guilford Press.

Coles, P. (2003). *The Importance of Sibling Relationships in Psychoanalysis*, London, New York: Karnac.

De Lara, E.W. (2016). *Bullying Scars: The Impact on Adult Life and Relationships*, New York: Oxford University Press.

Ezriel, H. (1973). Psychoanalytic group therapy, in L.R. Wolberg, E.K. Schwartz (eds.), *Group Therapy, An Overview*, New York: Intercontinental Medical Book Corporation.

Fonagy, P. (2020). www.bbc.co.uk/sounds/play/m000dpj2?fbclid=IwAR3X_5NsIiB3I8O Ho48CSeq2Kiedf4YcvBpTAKeMbJCgqL97XHslZKrS7ig

Fonagy, P., Gergely, G., Jurist, E.L., Target, M. (2004). *Affect Regulation, Metalization, and the Development of the Self*, New York: Other Press.

Foulkes, S.H. (1949). *Introduction to Group Analytic Psychotherapy, Studies in Social Integration of Individuals and Groups.* New York: Grune & Stratton.

Foulkes, S.H. (1971). The group as matrix of the individual's mental life, in E. Foulkes (ed.), *Selected Papers of S.H. Foulkes, Psychoanalysis and Group Analysis*, London: Karna Books, 1990.

Foulkes, S.H. (1984). *Therapeutic Group Analysis*, London: Karnac Books.

Foulkes, S.H. (1986). *Group Analytic Psychotherapy: Methods and Principle*, London: Karnac Books.

Foulkes, S.H., Anthony, E.J. (2014). *Group Psychotherapy, the Psychoanalytic Approach*, London: Karnac Books.

Friedman, R. (2004). Dream-telling as a request for containment – Reconsidering the group-analytic approach to the work with dreams, *Group Analysis*, vol. 37, no. 4, pp. 508–524.

Grossmark, R., Wright, F., ed. (2015). *The One and the Many: Relational Approaches to Group Psychotherapy*, New York, London: Routledge.

Grunebaum, H., Solomon, L. (1980). Toward a peer theory of group psychotherapy, I: On the developmental significance of peers and play, *International Journal of Group Psychotherapy*, vol. 30, no. 1, pp. 23–49.

Grunebaum, H., Solomon, L. (1987). Peer relationships, self-esteem, and the self, *International Journal of Group Psychotherapy*, vol. 37, no. 4, pp. 475–513.

Herman, J. (1992). *Trauma and Recovery: The Aftermath of Violence – From Domestic Abuse to Political Terror*, New York: Basic Books.

Karterud, S (2011). Constructing and mentalizing the matrix, *Group Analysis*, vol. 44, no. 4, pp. 357–373.

Piaget, J. (1932). *The Moral Development of the Child*, London: Kegan Paul.

Prinstein, M.J., et al. (2018). Peer status and psychopatology, in W.M. Bukowski, et al. (eds.), *Handbook of Peer Interactions, Relationships, and Groups*, New York, London: The Guilford Press: 617–637

Rabin, H.M. (2011). Peers and siblings: Their neglect in analytic group psychotherapy, *Group*, vol. 35, no. 4, pp. 279–288.

Salmivali, Ch., Peets, K. (2018). Bullying and victimization, in W.M. Bukowski et al. (eds.), *Handbook of Peer Interactions, Relationships, and Groups*, New York, London: The Guilford Press.

Schermer, V.L. (2013). Mirror neurons: Their implications for group psychotherapy, in S.P. Gantt, B. Badenoch (eds.), *The Interpersonal Neurobiology of Group Psychotherapy and Group Process*, London: Karnac Books.

Schlapobersky, J. (2016). *From the Couch to the Circle: Group-Analytic Psychotherapy in Practice*, London, New York: Routledge.

Stern, D.N. (2002). *The First Relationship: Infant and Mother*, Cambridge, MA: Harvard University Press.

Vygotsky, L.S. (1978). *Mind in Society: The Development of a Higher Mental Process*, Cambridge, MA: Harvard University Press.

Whitaker, D., Lieberman, M. (1964). *Psychotherapy Through the Group Process*, Chicago: Aldine.

Winnicott, D. (1969). *The Child, the Family, and the Outside World*, Baltimore: Penguin Books.

1.8 Mature Adult Siblinghood

Suzi Shoshani and Pnina Rappoport

Behold, how good and how pleasant it is for brethren *to dwell together in unity*!

(Psalms 133: 1)

Introduction

The members of the Journal Club have a long-shared history: together we learned, specialized, and gained a lot of group analysis experience over the years. We have established the Israeli Institute of Group Analysis where most of us served in key positions and were members of the teaching staff. We have developed enriching initiatives for the curriculum and organized conferences and seminars. After ten years of the institute's activity, we gradually passed the baton of leadership to the next generation, graduates of our training program.

After a while, we felt that we needed something for ourselves – a framework that would satisfy our needs in the current time of our lives.

The initial purpose of the Journal Club was to expand our professional knowledge in the study of group analysis by looking at related fields of life. Soon we realized that the Journal Club was much more than a meeting place for the expansion of knowledge. The group relationship has become stronger and more important for each of us, especially during the spread of the COVID-19 pandemic. We have created a network of security within this group of "brothers and sisters" based on social and ideological solidarity.

There is a magical atmosphere in the group that is often difficult to explain. The fact that we are all mature adults, educated and experienced, with an established professional standing connects us and creates a group that gives confidence and allows freedom of expression to all its members.

There are currently 24 members in the Journal Club. We meet seven times a year for lectures and discussions. In between we connect through a WhatsApp group. This project has great importance in all of our lives.

We rely on our experience as group conveners to describe the special close relationships developed between its members during its five years of existence.

DOI: 10.4324/9781003220060-10

The Journal Club as a Median Group

You could say that the Journal Club is a median group without a conductor, accompanied only by two conveners. The group's goal was to develop a dialogue and discuss broad cultural and civil issues, or as De Mare (1994) called it "external insights". The conveners encouraged the members of the group to share their opinions and beliefs with the others based on their personal and professional life experiences. The emphasis was placed mainly on forming a dialogue. These experiences, when described within a median group of mature adult members, received emotional significance, gained recognition, and clarified our social opinions. They mainly strengthened the connection between us, or in the words of De Mare ([1994] 2010): "provides an opportunity for each member to have his say within a reasonable time; it is a good setting for learning to talk and think, and for direct access between psyche and society (p. 203).

As one of the group members noted, this group resides at the seam between the personal and the communal. It allows enough room for the development of a unique identity without losing the common ground. In fact, this group expands the common ground and enriches it.

Mature, Adult Siblinghood

Professional literature almost doesn't discuss this topic and concentrates mainly on siblings at a young age. Siblinghood serves as a platform that enables and encourages the development of multiple identities and expands the world of the individual by sharing creative games, fantasies, and long-term intimate relationships. It is the basis for relationships of friendship and love. And yet, sibling relationships are also a fertile area for competition and pain, especially when the possibility of a close and friendly connection is not fulfilled or when it is destroyed, gets disconnected, or is fatally injured (Ashuach, 2012).

In our opinion, mature and adult people are motivated by two main aspirations: belonging to a group that accepts them as individuals, protects them, and allows them to have emotional and intellectual expression; and finding a platform for further learning and growth. When these aspirations are fulfilled, they help the individuals in their self-realization.

Foulkes and Anthony ([1957] 2003) emphasized belonging as the first and most important aspect that group therapists deal with, and according to which they build their concepts. It is impossible to think about mental health without group affiliation, and belonging to a group of mature and adult siblings is doubly important.

When we established the Israeli Institute of Group Analysis we were all relatively young. Today, most of us are in our late sixties or seventies and are approaching older age. In the past, most of us had small children. Today, the children have left the house. In the professional field as well, "our children", our young students, began to feel more and more central and influential roles in the institute. As a result, some of us felt pushed to the margins. Although we emboldened the students and encouraged them to take charge, the fear of exclusion and loss of our central status existed in most of us consciously and unconsciously.

These concerns, which are common in our age, prompted us to search for a membership group, a containing group where we could share joys and sorrows with others; a group in which we would be understood through the personal experiences of each of us and which would give us support and encouragement; a group in which mirroring, reciprocity, and exchange among its members would strengthen us; a sharing group, raising its members' self-worth; a group that creates trust and an experience of faith in both the personal and the group's ability; a group that would serve as a shield against the threat of disappearing.

As shown by Friedman (2015), the fear of annihilation, rejection, and exclusion is one of the contributing factors for cohesion in the group. Belonging to our group of siblings is an act against loneliness and against the anxiety that stems from lack of control and physical and mental death (Friedman, 2015).

In our view, the "horizontal (sibling) axis" of Mitchel (2017) is of great importance. The horizontal axis makes it possible to manage multiple parallel communications that include the conscious and the unconscious, emotions and thoughts, and influences from different directions. The horizontal axis is enabled in our group since the conscious and unconscious common authority (the vertical axis) is the common theoretical knowledge, values, attitudes, and norms that are at the basis of group analysis and characterize us all.

Therefore the communication is characterized by reciprocity and a lack of hierarchy and can be positive, helping, and supportive, but can also be negative and dangerous (Berman, 2019). In the Journal Club group of adult people, the positive aspects of the horizontal axis predominated and overcame the negative effects. At our age, appreciation and admiration for the other replaced jealousy and competition. Encouragement to reciprocity and exchange grew and contributed to a sense of well-being and security in the entire group.

Reaching an advanced age means coping with the void, with physical losses as well as losses of identity such as centrality or meaning. The ambition to build something out of nothing, the desire to be happy, to live and enjoy, the will to keep moving and not to give up connects us all, associates us with our group, enhances the strength and importance of each individual in the group, and makes the whole membership group meaningful in mature adult age, which was especially true during the COVID-19 pandemic.

In addition, in advanced age, when we can somewhat step away from the vast investment of raising children, establishing a career, and forming our own identities and unique places in society, there comes a need to share our mature inner emotional and intellectual worlds with a wider world, and in particular with professionals who we perceive as equal to us. According to Mitchel (2003), if these conditions are met, the individual manages to resolve their initial sibling conflict and get to be different from their brothers, but equal to them. That is exactly what happened in our group, in spite of the fact that it was not a therapeutic group.

Furthermore, the need for enrichment and the desire to strengthen professional identity (Gerada, 2019) only grew and were used as fertile grounds for the Journal Club, so we can say that we formed a group that will strengthen our professional identity; a group one might call an identity membership group of mature and adult siblings.

Mature Adult Siblinghood in the Journal Club

The Journal Club may not be a therapy group, but we, its members, have been professional colleagues for many years. We have met in the past in various settings, including therapeutic and supervisory frameworks, and have accumulated experience together.

In the past, there were many times when our opinions were divided. We competed with each other for our place, sometimes hurting each other. Today, later in life, when each of us has a solid status, we turn our libido to construction, love, partnership, and connection, not destruction. Competition and jealousy have not completely disappeared, but they are minor now. Instead, encouragement, admiration, and equality have become dominant and contribute to the pleasant atmosphere between us.

These aspects characterize the mature siblinghood in this group of adults. As Foulkes and Anthony (1957) explained, we have created a large hall of mirrors used as a platform for sharing pain and expressing enjoyment from our accomplishments, a platform that can be relied upon and rejoiced in both large and small touches/experiences/elements/things that it offers.

Indeed, this group contains a rich variety of formative experiences: one member is a Holocaust survivor and other members are second generation to Holocaust survivors. Some members grew up in communist Eastern European countries or in South American states under a dictatorial regime where they had firsthand experience of exclusion, rejection, discrimination, and fear, and later immigrated to Israel to find a home and openly redefine their identities and affiliations. Some members were born in Israel right after the establishment of the state and have witnessed their parents' efforts to build the country. There are also members who fought in Israel's wars and have lost their loved ones. On top of that, unfortunately, over the years we also experienced the loss of three group members who died unexpected. The meetings dedicated to the processing of the grief and emptiness that remained helped us all.

It is possible that the pleasant atmosphere in this group is also linked to the friendship siblinghood which is, as emphasized by Friedman (2015) in "Soldier matrix", a part of the Israeli experience in particular and the Jewish experience in general. All of us served in the army; we all have brothers, sisters, or friends who served; and we have all experienced this special togetherness in times of peace and in times of war. Most of us immigrated to Israel from the Diaspora, where we suffered persecution as a Jewish minority. The Jewish tradition in the Diaspora maintained the cohesion of the people to protect it from enemies and help it survive disasters. For this reason, apparently, the value of fellowship and the value of mutual help described in Alexandre Dumas' (1844) well-known phrase "all for one and one for all", is deeply imprinted in the Israeli personal and social unconsciousness (Hopper, 2002). We all know what group cohesion and coherence means.

The siblings in our group serve as "witnesses" (Berger, 2012) to the suffering or traumatic experiences of the other within us, that arises during an in-depth emotional discussion revolving around a particular topic. Thus, for example, the story of one member about the traumatic experiences of his mother, a Holocaust survivor, or the despair another member expressed about not being able to see her mother in her nursing home during the COVID-19 pandemic, or the heavy fear expressed by one of the members regarding the restrictions imposed on the whole population due to the pandemic, resulting from her traumatic experiences under a communist government, or the fear of losing the freedom of speech in our country and the fear that the government would become dictatorial expressed by another member – were all listened to, gained recognition, empathy, and resonance, and evoked sharing of similar experiences. The "witnesses" in the Journal Club served as firm support and allowed sharing of difficult experiences. The members felt heard. In other words, we felt that witnessing is the existence of one in the mind of the other, as described by Stern (2012).

In Berger's (2012) terms, it can be said that the willingness of our members to be there with attentive empathy for the other without judgment but to merely be present allows mutual recognition and provides a kind of public approval (Roiphe, 2000) for the injury and injustice they experienced, which gives them and our entire group validity and healing value.

Thus, witnessing in our group has a meaning by its very existence. It releases the narrator to some extent from the burden of feelings they carry, consciously or unconsciously, and serves as the basis for change, for hope and for faith in the other. This "favorable witnessing" (Stoller, 2018) considerably reduces the sense of exclusion, rejection, and loneliness in a person and helps them feel present and meaningful in their life and in the life of their community (Berger, 2018).

This healing value was felt more strongly in our group at the untimely deaths of three members. The sudden death shocked us all. Each member who passed away had a few close friends in the group who experienced the death in a more traumatic way than the rest, but we all felt that a void had opened up within the group. We met together to process the grief and each of us spoke about their relationship with the deceased, their personal memories, and pain. Free associations came up and with every new story told, the pain increased, growing the healing power of the group at the same time. The group's embrace helped us digest the trauma we experienced and our fears of illness and our death to come.

The Journal Club WhatsApp Group

At the first year of the Journal Club we started a WhatsApp group whose goal was to deliver organizational information to members. However, over the years, and especially during the COVID-19 pandemic, group chat on WhatsApp has become much more than a communication channel for transmitting information. Initially, group members began sharing their feelings and thoughts on WhatsApp in conventional ways: sharing family experiences, sending wishes to their friends and congratulating them for publishing, providing information about lectures and conferences, and asking for recommended professional therapists. Later they were consulting each other on the procedure of receiving patients during the pandemic, shared anxieties and dilemmas regarding the change of therapeutic setting during this period and expressing personal fear, concerns for relatives and for the members of the group. All of these found a sympathetic ear and an empathetic heart in the WhatsApp group and gave us the feeling that we are not alone.

The Journal Club WhatsApp group became a place for immediate listening, support, understanding, and containment of the many anxieties that arose during the COVID-19 period. At a time when we felt uncertainty and instability, when we needed to change our behavior both personally as well as professionally, with social distancing and isolation from our family, friends, and "siblings" at the Journal Club, and with economical, health, and political insecurity – the WhatsApp group provided an immediate answer. Every message from any one of us received many responses, reducing the feelings of loneliness and chaos we felt. The feelings and experiences we exchanged calmed our anxieties, increased our sense of belonging, and gave meaning to this group of mature adult siblings. As conveners we took care for everyone who wrote something to get a response.

In addition, the WhatsApp communication became a platform to express our dissatisfaction with the way our government was functioning, especially during a time of pandemic and war. It angered us and made us disappointed in our "parents" who led us in devious ways and failed to maintain our physical, mental, and financial health. Interpretation of political and social events that took place at this time found a place in the group of mature and adult siblings.

The Journal Club Conveners

The Journal Club was initiated and established by us, the two group conveners. Both of us are group analysts and among the founders of the Israeli Institute of Group Analysis. We are also experienced individual therapists. It can be said that our role has expanded and become clearer during its five years of activity in which a kind of group self was formed, and we simultaneously served as the representatives and as the conveners of the group. As a saying attributed to Alexandre Auguste Ledru-Rollin: "I must follow them, for I am their leader". And indeed, we saw ourselves, in the spirit of our teacher Foulkes first and foremost as the instrument and the servants of the group (Foulkes, [1948] 1991, p. 139).

It was clear to us that this is not just a learning group or a friends group, and not a family with blood ties. However, as the group conveners, we have invested many hours over the years in planning group meetings, searching for suitable lecturers from all aspects of culture, and routing their lecture towards group analytical content, providing answers and clarification to any group member, arranging zoom meetings, sometimes with lecturers from abroad, and running the meeting itself.

All this holding of the matrix helped to develop the cohesion in the group and as Yalom (1975) mentioned, the cohesion of the group is represented by its attractiveness to its members; it is the invisible force that holds group members together in the face of emotional conflicts, which can lead to a deep acceptance of each other and to meaningful relationships.

The first meetings in the first year helped us to increasingly define the nature of the role we took upon ourselves. These meetings opened with an attempt to define the roles of the group conductor, as Foulkes and his successors defined it. In fact, the entire first year was devoted to learning, thinking, and discussing the characteristics of the analytical group conductor and the nature of their relationships with the group and with society as a whole. In retrospect it is clear to us that this was not a coincidence.

We suggested to expand the scope and look together at models of guidance as they appear in various life cycles. We examined the diverse role of the group and social conductor/coordinator/manager/leader through an encounter with different worldviews: sociology, philosophy, history, and economics. Many subjects came from the fields of literature, theater, and music. These fields were inspiring and promoted the group process and the connection between the mature and adult siblings. In the words of Pisani (2012) as cited in David, 2016:

> the group analyst [or the convener] is "a creative acting person" like a conductor of the orchestra, in a democratic style whereby in each session "the theme is always new and un-repeatable. Each session is a piece of "music" without a score", and his art is expressed through his personality . . . in a word his creativity within a scientific framework.
>
> (p. 254)

Although our group was not defined as a therapeutic group, we tried to read the group unconscious and find innovative and interesting topics that would consolidate the group, meet the different needs of its members, and make it a healing and growing force. And thus we have formed coherence in the group, in the terms of Pines (1998).

Over the years we have always tried to listen to all the voices of the group members, to identify the different tunes they played and to follow their requests and suggestions. We offered many of them an opportunity to lecture us on ideas in the field that concerns them and led emotional and experiential discussions. We tried to see each member of the group and to make room for them, to turn to each of them and take an interest in them, and to treat everyone as equal and belonging even when one of the members was not easy for us to accept. We listened to criticism and served as a voice for the group unconscious. Thus, according to Klain (2009 as cited in David, 2016, p. 254). we served as "'a kind of amplifier' – who receives meanings and emotive contents from the communications and works on them through his emotional participation".

Together with the members of the group we created a culture of acceptance, of tolerance, and of unity. We can say that we created a kind of "relational bubble" (Ullman, 2014), a bubble of connection between professionals who knew each other in the past and knew how to protect and preserve each other. We strived to support and encourage each other out of a belief in our shared ability to get through the pandemic and the difficult period both health-wise as well as mentally.

Conclusion

In this chapter we discussed the characteristics of the phenomenon of a mature and adult sibling group.

We believe that the Journal Club formed a social matrix that encouraged and invited exchange. Many personal topics were discussed thoroughly through the diverse lectures we organized. The resonance in the group, including its WhatsApp group broadened each of the group members' world view as well as the view of the entire group.

In retrospect we can say that what made this relationship so unique and strong is the ability to communicate in two levels: The first level is common between professionals as they share their understanding and experience, learning and enriching professional abilities, and especially as they create a culture of multidisciplinary discourse that encompasses wider areas of knowledge, experience and treatment, in the spirit of group analysis.

The second level was very personal and touched on emotions. It manifested specifically in the WhatsApp group during the COVID-19 pandemic, at a time of political crises and war in our country. The messages expressed our longing for belonging, for touch and for empathy, and especially for sharing our deep inner feelings at this stage of our lives.

Man is a creature who seeks meaning. Likewise, especially at our age, we want to live in a world that we have created and that has meaning and values, a world of inner harmony. This world can contain conflicts, which form laws and order. As the group matrix of the Journal Club became more cohesive, communication within it and the ways of finding meaning for all of us became more developed and more coherent. The group members were able to see the world through the eyes of others, as suggested by Oscar Wilde in 1889 regarding seeing the London fog through the paintings of Monet and Pissarro.

> To look at a thing is very different from seeing a thing. One does not see anything until one sees its beauty. Then, and then only, does it comes into existence.

And so has our view of ourselves and of the group formed.

The WhatsApp group allowed each "brother or sister" in the group to express themselves, recount memories to their siblings, memories that until now were kept only for themselves, share their thoughts, feelings, and experiences, and mainly their anxieties, fears, and dilemmas.

No doubt that the group formed with our mature siblings, who are able to understand us, has become over the years a safe place to wonder, think, share feelings, and understand important events in our lives together. It continues, if you will, our therapeutic journey and growth from deeper insights on to new events and new learning. We may say that this is a group that we were glad to belong to. And perhaps, as one of our group members described it:

> The partnership in the group, which grew stronger, testified most of all, and in retrospect, that the need to establish it was one of survival, a vital need, spiritual and mental survival for all of us.

In different parts of the world there are programs and activities designed for citizens of the third age, but these revolve around specific topics. In contrast, the way we built the Journal Club group offers a model of belonging to a group of mature academics in the field of mental health who, apart from the professional interest and aspiration to learn and develop they have in common, are driven by a desire for belonging and a common emotional interest.

We hope that similar groups will be established among similar professional organizations around the world.

Yoram Teharlev's words are able to convey what we believe took place in our group very well:

> Be my friend, be my brother
> Lend me a hand when I'll call out
> Be my friend, be my brother
> Lend me a hand at times of trouble
> I am your brother, don't forget it
> Be my friend, be my brother
> (Yoram Taharlev, "Be My Friend,
> Be My Brother")

We thank the members of the Journal Club without whom this enterprise would not have existed: Shlomit Alon, Mira Bar, Meir Berger, Miriam Berger, Shosh Briner, Avi Berman, Nurit Goren, Anka Detroi, Bracha Hadar, Rivka Harel, Diana Topilsky, Anat Yogev, Orenia Yaffe-Yanai, Elena Laor, Yehoshua Lavie, Ruth Lavie, Oded Navé, Galia Nativ, Gila Ofer, Enav Karniel, Aliza Rosen, Batya Rosenthal, Elisabeth Rothschild, Shlomit Schindler. And our departed friends: Herzel Yogev R.I.P., Esti Sofair R.I.P., and Sarah Kalai R.I.P.

References

Ashuach, S (2012). Am I my brother keeper? The analytic group as a space for reenacting and treating sibling trauma. *Group Analysis, 45*(2), 155–167.

Berger, M. (2012). 'The brother's keeper': Witnessing as a moral presence in group analysis and beyond. A response to 'Foulkes lecture'. *Group Analysis, 45*(4), 459–471.

Berger, M. (2018). *What happened – Happened: Witnessing as a crucial stance in the process of healing wounds of war* [conference presentation]. Civilians at War, Prague.

Berman, A. (2019). Therapeutic semi-safe space in group analysis. *Group Analysis, 52*(2), 190–203.

David, M. (2016). The group analyst's role when facing the group. *Group Analysis, 49*(3), pp. 249–264.

De Mare, P. (1994). The Median group and the psyche. In D. Brown and L. Zinkin (eds.), *The psyche and the social world: Developments in group- analytic theory* (pp. 202–210). London: Jessica Kingsley.

Dumas, A. ([1844] 2010). *The three musketeers.* The French of August Zolder. Frankfurt/H.: Fischer.

Friedman, R. (2015). Die Grouppe in der soldaten matrix in Gruppendynamick. Zeitschrift fuer theory and praxis der Gruppenanalyse. Heftherousgaben; Lamott, F. *Miesa, 51*(3), 191–205.

Foulkes, S. H. ([1948] 1991). *Introduction to group analytic psychotherapy: Studies in the social integration of individuals and groups.* London: Karnac Books.

Foulkes, S. H., and Anthony, E. J. ([1957] 2003). *Group psychotherapy: The psychoanalytic approach.* Karnak classics.

Gerada, C. (2019). The making of a doctor: The matrix and self. *Group Analysis, 52*(3), 350–361.

Hopper, E. (2002). *The social unconscious: Selected papers.* International Library of Group Analysis. London and New York: Jessica Kingsley Publishers.

Mitchel, J. (2003). *Siblings: Sex and violence.* Oxford: Polity Press.

Mitchel, J. (2017). *Cambridge, core concepts: From sibling trauma to the law of the mother* [Conference presentation]. Siblings in Individual and Group Psychoanalytic Psychotherapy. Tel Aviv University, Israel.

Piners, M. (1998). *Circular reflections: Selected papers on group analysis and psychoanalysis.* International Library of group Analysis. London and Philadelphia: Jessica Kingsley.

Roiphe, A. (2000). Brief communication other views: A discussion on a memoir of early childhood loss. *International Journal of Psycho-Analysis, 81*, 1011–1014.

Stern, D. B. (2012). Partners in thought. In L. Aron and A. Harris (eds.), *Relational psychoanalysis. vol. 5: Evolution of process* (pp. 381–406). Relational Perspectives Book Series. New York and London: Routledge.

Stoller, E. (2018). "Sibling witnessing" as a therapeutic factor in Group Analysis. *Final presentation of the diploma course of the Israel Group Analysis Institute.*

Ullman, C. (2014). The personal is political: On the subjective of an Israeli psychoanalyst. In S. Kuchuck (ed.), *Clinical implication of the psychoanalyst's life experiences* (pp. 98–111). New York and London: Routledge.

Wilde, O. (1905 [1889]). *The decay of lying.* New York: Brentano.

Yalom, I. D. (1975). *The theory and practice of group psychotherapy.* New York: Basic Books.

1.9 Kinship and Sibling Dynamics in Organisational Consultancy

Gerhard Wilke

Introduction

The intention is to reflect on how we can conceptualise consultancy work with lateral and vertical social differentiations in mind. It is our internal relationship matrix that gets transferred from the family of origin into the work context. This internalised relationship matrix is on the vertical level dominated by the quality of the interaction with mother and father and the siblings, as well as grandparents and the wider network of kin. On the lateral level our internal working model of being an actor in a social network is deeply shaped by our siblings as well as cousins and other kin. From my point of view, we have internalised a triangular parent–child relationship matrix and we tend to unconsciously fall back on the experience with uncles and aunts and the two tribes of blood relatives and in-laws. In other words, in relating to other at work, we reference internally a nuclear family and a generational and kinship relationship matrix. Last but not least, some have an internal sense of being an only child with imagined siblings and possess the best internal knowledge of how to manage the parents. Children can be alone, one among equals or a location point in a sibling status hierarchy, from eldest to youngest and first- to last-born.

Psychoanalytic consultants have worked preferably with the parent–child and leader and group transference within an organisations that it conceptualises as an abstract social system. Many colleagues have therefore argued that family metaphors are inappropriate in an institutional context. The denial of the influence of family and kinship dynamics on teams and organisations needs to be challenged culturally, sociologically and psychologically.

Rethinking Siblings and Generations in Organisational Consulting

The psychoanalytic model of the transference relationship between parent and child, as well as a primary task and unconscious defences against it, is shared by many consultants. In this picture the leader and the group form a parental couple. The group, from the leader's perspective, is an 'as if' single object of 're-socialisation'. What is missing in this picture is the exploration of the dynamic

DOI: 10.4324/9781003220060-11

between group members as rivals, competitors and as brothers and sisters in arms. Equally absent, is the perspective of our department, as a kinship tribe of insiders and outsiders. My thesis is that the link of 'as if' relatives and in-laws between functional divisions in the workplace are left out of our 'imagined' organisation – yet unconsciously everyone at work carries inside themselves a vertical three generational and lateral family and kinship relationship model to deal emotionally with a team, several departments and an organisation as a community.

Juliet Mitchell (2008) has rightly argued that psychoanalysis needs to complement its focus on the vertical transference between parents and children with a lateral sibling transference concept. Equally, she asserted that siblings amongst themselves and in relation to the parents learn about family dynamics as well as the social world, in which people are different and the same, separate and linked. What Mitchell plays down in her work is that siblings are divided by a vertical social structure, based on the birth hierarchy. In group analysis the implicit way of seeing a team or organisation is primarily in lateral terms, focusing on small or large group dynamics, with reference to the group as one unified object. The vertical birth order, the hierarchy of the organisation and the lateral intergroup dynamic between subgroups, with different amounts of political influence, is psychologised and defined as undesirable. In such a preconceived picture the group is idealised, and the social structure and the division of labour as well as the hierarchy of power and expertise is denigrated.

It becomes apparent that the true complexity of the inner world, which people transfer into a work context, is hard to name, describe and analyse. For this reason, 'reductionist' and 'simplistic' ways of conceptualising what is going on in a work group or organisation are prevalent. The exclusively psychological view of social interactions in a work group has made it possible that analytic consultants can maintain the tradition of making group interpretations, identifying shared group themes and describing developmental and malignant mirroring processes, as if they were shared by all group members at the same time.

This established view of a work group suffers from 'psychological as well as sociological blindness' because analytic consultants pay attention to the relationship between group members in an 'equivalence modus' – where all group members are assumed to be the same, perhaps to maintain the ideal of the analyst, who like Freud believes that social groups can be explained in terms of individual psychology. More convincing to me is to see this stance as a defence against the realisation that the relationship network in a group, working with and for each other is 'literally' indescribable. Max Weber (2020) struggled all his life to find the missing link between lived experience and abstract descriptions of what goes on in an institution and society. In the end he came to believe that sociologists can construct an *Ideal Type* of what characteristics an institution has, but we can never assume that this amounts to a description of the lived reality inside an organisation. Instead, an *Ideal Type*, can help consultants make sense of what it means for people themselves to work together in an institution. Weber's sociology of *Verstehen* (sense making) is indispensable to my consulting work, which I would describe as a combination of 'joint and pragmatic sense making', ethnographic participant observation and analytic free association in 'live' work situations. Client and consultant focusing on what helps and hinders the process of working together (Wilke, 2014).

In the vertical perspective, siblings are excluded from the minds of many consultants. In the lateral perspective, the sibling differences, the birth and status order are ignored. Both perspectives serve the 'ruling paradigm' in analytic consultancy that we can talk about the group as if it were a fused imaginary community of equals and a single, easily describable psychological object of identification, idealisation and transformation. We need a sibling transference model in analytic consultancy that is not a model for total inclusion and equality, but a sociologically inspired conceptualisation, which allows us to understand the hierarchical differences within an organisational relationship network and its capacity to cooperate across divisional boundaries. Equally, what makes it possible for rebellious small groups to challenge authority, habitualised work practices and trigger helpful change.

Work group members in a 'sibling-like' experience move in and out of connected and differentiated role positions and into familiar and unfamiliar patterns of social interaction within a status hierarchy. Team-siblings can, due to their unconscious knowledge, become the location point for the re-enactment of a sense of helplessness and failed dependency. This kind of role suction is associated with the endless reorganisations and leader changes typical in current organisations. Unconsciously, the second generation is liable, just like in history, to get sucked into post-traumatic reparation processes, unconsciously 'designed' to restore respect and pride to a humiliated organisation and the parental and grandparental generation within them.

Vertical and Lateral Consulting Work

A central idea in my group analytic consultancy work is that our internal relationship matrix serves everyone as an inner template for how each of us engages in a group and takes up a role in an organisation. The way we related upwards, downwards and sideways inside the family of origin and outwards to the extended kinship system is transferred into the group context in interactions with colleagues, managers and members of other groups. Our internalised relationship matrix serves to assess what is familiar and unfamiliar in the interaction rituals of daily life. We compare and contrast unconsciously new experiences with what we already know from our internalised world view of vertical and lateral interactions with parents and siblings and kith and kin.

This 'repetition compulsion' of comparing the emotionally familiar and unfamiliar is heightened in intensity during periods of transition, moral panic and uncertainty in organisations. In a context of rapid change, outbreaks of sibling rivalry and solidarity in organisations act as a defence against perceived existential threats to survival. Sibling phenomena are a symptom for a betwixt and between state in teams and organisations. As organisational changes are imposed from the top, sibling preoccupations surface to prevent the working through of the breakdown of relations between the 'institutional parents' and their dependants, but also between teammates, who unconsciously embody 'collaborators' or 'competitors'. In situations perceived as existential, 'team-siblings' also form sisterhoods and brotherhoods to protect themselves from unfair, overpowering and threatening bosses, competitors or market forces.

In the present historical context of "dis-embedded social structures" (Giddens, 1991) "permanent transitions and change" (Wilke et al., 2017) and a sense of living in "Liquid times" (Baumann, 2008) in organisations, authority figures are often experienced like borderline or absent parents, who evoke sibling solidarity, denying the vertical status differences between siblings. Instead, the work group gets gripped by the idea that they are an imagined equal band of brothers and sisters. This dynamic has functioned to deny the guilt and the fear of retaliation associated with fratricide and matricide committed during 're-engineering' processes and generational change. In such contexts the whole spectrum of internalised interaction models from the family of origin is unconsciously triggered and shapes the response to 'disruption' of familiar social interactions at work. For instance, a very strong unconscious urge to seek out organisational parents and to find shelter in sibling solidarity.

If analytic consultants could see the organisation as a multilateral and trans-generational kinship structure, they could do interpretive work with the internal family matrix of each group member, the maternal group 'Matrix' of the work group, the group 'Patrix' of the organisational hierarchy (Wilke, 2017). In addition, the complex restructuring and merger processes in and between organisations could be compared to shifting alliances within the kinship system with its trans-generational and repeated insider-outsider dynamic. This is not too difficult as such multilayered relationship networks make up the internal social map of leaders, managers and employees. A multiple transference perspective in respect of status and role holders would protect analytic consultants from simplistic and fetishised thinking and from natural science explanations like systems or complexity theory. They have their place but not in a context of making sense of emotions and unconscious defences and the desire for connection and a containing authority (Volkan, 2004).

We live in an age where business schools preach self-management of teams, flat hierarchies and an 'un-holy trinity' of strategy, change management and charismatic leadership. In reality this 'orthodoxy' gives birth to permanent disruption of teams, departments and the whole organisation. With 'permanent transitions' existential anxiety is born, and a predictable career and a sense of an organisational home gets lost. This state of insecurity is meant to invoke more productivity and creativity. Emotionally, it triggers a sense of disorientation and detachment from the formal organisation as well as inner rage, resentment and helplessness.

In this social context, compliance to the endless stream of new strategies and forms of self-organising in open space offices has generated a deep longing for 'organisational parenting', 'sibling solidarity' and 'protective tribalism'. If solidarity does not work, people fragment and become singletons and rivalrous siblings, or they become a mob and follow a 'saviour' leader. In this context of flux and transition without end, the functional subgroups of an organisation become us and them tribes and can threaten the integrity of the organisation. Internally, many people have experienced death, illness, divorce, remarriage, inheritance rows and the like and use this lived experience to make sense of the 'designed disruption' of their sense of place and position at work. It helps them cope but reinforces a collective sense of existential insecurity.

Social and Psychological Roles in Work Groups

The participants in a team meeting have many different agendas when they come together, as each member's internal needs do not necessarily comply with the overall task. They will also bring personal issues to the table. For instance, to sit it out, to make peace, to seek attention, to pick a quarrel, to fulfil a socially unconscious role, delegated to them by another member, or to seek shelter in the shadow of the leader. Unconscious roles such as fool, victim, warrior, persecutor, rescuer or provocateur emerge regularly. These informal roles help the individual cope but can easily hinder the work that needs to be done. What is certain is that the role takers separately and together 'shape' the positive and negative energy flow in every work group. What an analytic consultant can do is to change the energy flow in work groups from negative to positive and help the group and leader work with and for each other, practically and emotionally.

In the organisational world meetings are the context into which the internalised vertical and lateral relationship patterns from the kinship system are unconsciously transferred by its members. At one level the group is an environmental mother, the team leader is a father figure and the members embody a set of differentiated roles akin to the birth order. At another level, a three-generational structure exists in each team as a hierarchy of experience. Last but not least, the team members really are 'as if' siblings in that they are the same and yet different.

My work has taught me to differentiate between three types of team members in the work group: those who adopt defensive and resistant group roles, those who contribute to the maintenance of the group and those who play a 'helpful' task-oriented role. The character types who help the team adapt and function well are: the *Initiator*, who suggests new ideas and ways of organising; the *Co-Ordinator*, who clarifies relationships and attempts to link subgroups; the *Information Seeker*, who ask for clarification and who knows what is missing; the *Orienter*, who locates the group in a wider relationship context and points out external dangers; the *Opinion Seeker*, who questions well-versed patterns of thinking and involves silent members; the *Evaluator, who* scrutinises the work of the group and compares it to accepted standards; the *Information Giver*, who gives straight and honest answers and embodies the reality principle; the *Opinion Giver*, who quotes previous experience and what learning is relevant for the task in hand; the *Proceduralist*, who gives advice on how to avoid legal and political pitfalls; and the *Historian*, who acts as the group memory and records what has been decided and who is responsible for what.

The following characters contribute to the psychological and social maintenance of the group as a cohesive and coherent whole: the *Encourager*, who praises, agrees and makes empathic suggestions; the *Harmoniser*, who can mediate, relieve tension and reconcile different interests; the *Compromiser*, who yields to status, admits mistakes and puts the interest of the group first; the *Gatekeeper*, who involves the silent members and opens up more exchange; the *Standard Setter*, who reminds the group of its task and professional practices; the *Group Observer and Analyst*, who encourages issues in the here and now to be compared with what has gone before and how things are done; and last but not least the *Follower*, who complies and is a witness.

The third set of roles are the most unconscious and embody patterns of resistance against the leader, the task and the team's social integration. These roles include the *Aggressor*, who attacks the group, envies the leader and is nihilistic about the meaning of the task; the *Blocker*, who disagrees and opposes without reason in order to feel important; the *Attention Seeker*, who exaggerates personal achievements or incompetence in the hope to be picked up and seen by the leader; the *Self-Confessor*, who wants to be wanted and safe but seeks attention with non-relevant issues; the *Dominator*, who seeks everyone's attention through flattery, interruption and self-righteousness; the *Playboy*, who displays rebelliousness, cynical detachment and denigration of the work; the *Help Seeker*, who is self-deprecating, seeks sympathy and spreads confusion; and the *Special Interest Pleader*, who hides insecurity by defending the rights of the disenfranchised and builds up a kind of anti-authoritarian counterculture.

In the analytic literature these 'sibling-like social roles' are excluded because the focus is on the triangle between task, leader and group as a whole. This established vertical view turns a blind eye to the wealth of experience in the group as well as the impossible demands made on the ordinary leader. In the lived experience of a work group, the different roles can best be understood with an intertwined vertical and lateral perspective: where people move in and out of different positions and contribute to an atmosphere of 'us as a cooperating team' or 'us at each other's throats'.

Despite the existence of a formal structure of power differentials and a hierarchy of experience, all members of a work group will still yearn emotionally for safety, support, protection, understanding, recognition and care. More importantly, in a real crisis the group will only feel held in the hands of a leader and the eyes of each other, after they have learnt that everyone is a person with insecurities, fears and in need of help. Only with this awareness can they acknowledge that the team needs a good enough authority, a group that functions as an environmental mother (Winnicott, 1986) and sibling solidarity, differentiation and competition. Contrary to psychoanalytic organisational theory, the employees of the 'wounded organisation' are looking for a holding parental couple as well as brothers and sisters in arms.

The way I work with adopted social roles is that I ask a work group to take part in an exercise. Group members meet in subgroups of eldest, youngest, only and middle, second born and so on, and reflect together what behaviour patterns, emotional responses in relation to their siblings and parents they repeat in their task roles and how these internalised family experiences shape their dealings with authority and predispose them to the role they adopt 'unbeknown to themselves' in a work group.

Working with the Basic Assumption Group Defences

The preceding way of looking at roles in the enactment of the social drama of a work group is challenging Bion's brilliant basic assumption theory (1961). As Bion did not really sketch out the characteristics of a work group, he fell into the Freudian trap that leader and group can be understand in terms of one-to-one interactions. In my view, we can stop pretending that a work group always defends against the task and the leader, in one fused basic assumption group. Most of the time at work, not everyone gets sucked into the same defensive psychological stance because the accomplishment of the task involves complex social mechanisms such as cooperation, exchange, divided roles, territorial segregation and mutual dependence.

Nevertheless, Bion's basic assumption defences do occur in a situation of 'existential insecurity'. In such a context it is helpful to frame what is going on in a work group in this 'classical' way and deal with the question of how to come out of it. Nevertheless, I would always link the relationship matrix in the group with the social structure of the whole organisation.

In *dependency mode* the members of the group want the leader to do all the work. Such groups make the leader feel needed in the parent role. This behaviour surfaces in a situation where group and leader are exposed to an overwhelming number of tasks.

In a context of a very busy national specialist hospital, the leader did all the work in order not to lose track of everything in every meeting. The management group went along and made helpful suggestions on the way. Unconsciously they treated this leader as an overburdened mother and behaved as if they needed to parent him to make the organisation work. The leader was aware that he could not carry on as usual, especially as he had taken on a major national and international role. I suggested that I spend a day with him and, like an anthropologist, observe what he had to put up with, and what others had to put up with him. My bluntness was designed to signal that I meant business and had understood that he was desperate. In addition, we agreed that I can come out of the observer role in the meeting with his key managers, who made things work on a daily basis. In the actual meeting he did all the work, the others answered yes and no or gave short updates of the work. As agreed, the leader stopped the meeting early in order to reflect on how the group had worked. Instead of waiting for me to open the reflective session, he asked: So, what do you think? How did I do? The group giggled, like children do when they are embarrassed for their parents. I answered: You did all the work, the room is full of world-class researchers, but you did not ask them for advice once! Whereupon the Deputy Director said: "I feel ashamed that a stranger has to come to say the obvious. You always do the work, and we feel like compliant schoolchildren. You are so busy that you no longer notice that we are loyal and that we could take lots off your plate. I would like you to see that we are here, also for you." In time this leader chaired every fourth meeting, privileging his themes on the agenda and in the other three weekly meetings people took turns to take the lead and consult on what needed to be on the agenda. The leader mainly listened and observed the different characters on the team, giving him a much better sense of what he could delegate to whom, who he could trust blindly and who needed help.

In *fight-flight mode* the group splits the world into friends and enemies, perpetrators and victims. In such a situation the group splits the world into goodies, baddies, victims and perpetrators. From the aforementioned characters, it is the aggressor or the playboy who can tip a group into this mode of dominating the others by attacking the task, the leader and the rest of the group.

In a learning set on a leadership development programme for junior and senior medical researchers one group member was a pathologist, who was world renowned but a social isolate in his laboratory. In the group he was confronted with his incompetent self, unable to express what he felt, thought and wanted. Being ashamed in this role, he prevented being exposed to the situation repeatedly, until I reminded him that he had chosen to be in the leadership programme and that he was free to leave. He then revealed that he was only in the group to please his superior. She was of the opinion that his social skills were not good enough for a step up the ladder. The group sunk into a kind of 'ironic' silence, meaning at last he says what we all know. A group member then broke the spell of him against the rest of us by asking directly: "You could use this group and our collective wisdom to find out what you really want to do with the rest of your life." In the next session I reminded him of the invitation and mirrored back to him that he had fought the group repeatedly in order to flee into his idealised lab. In my profession, I added, idealisation hides resentment and hatred of an "idolised idea, person or occupation." He began to cry and then revealed that he was tired of being a famous pathologist. A group member then asked him, what he would like to do instead? He said to everyone's surprise that he wanted to get into university politics and management. Another group member revealed that he had got into organisational politics because he was tired of inefficient management in his area and decided that doing something about it would be better than moaning and blaming. The fight-flight pathologist took up this challenge and after a relatively short time ended up being the Lead Officer on IT in his university. Happy to move from an inverse, vertical position of critical parent in the group to being comfortable with being a 'brother' scientist in the lab on a lateral level and the 'parental' IT boss of many people in a vertical role.

The third basic assumption position is pairing. Such a group is in love with its leader. The group sinks into compliance mode and is unified by its hatred of an external enemy. In that sense it is similar to the fight and flight and dependency modus. Except, the interactions all feel much more intense and manic. Anyone in the team not toeing the line is scapegoated, and certainty replaces curiosity and learning from experience. I have seen such groups most often in the upper layers of management, but they enact this position especially when representatives of the whole organisation are present. The attempt is made to level all the differences. The symptoms that appear then are that everyone uses similar buzzwords, group members are frightened to speak their mind, while the leader is hungry for more and more adulation. Psychologically, the danger is a loss of reality. Evoking unconsciously that which is feared most: the loss of thinking and the death of the organisation. The hope is that the fusion between leader and group expels uncertainty and ensures survival.

The analytic answer to pairing is triangulation and a reality test. The way I bring this about during a consultancy process is to let people stand on a long vertical line and ask them to differentiate themselves into three subgroups: the top, the middle and the bottom of the organisation. Each group is asked how their positional place in the organisation influences their perception of themselves and the others. The result is usually, after a few minutes, that the people in the middle group turn their backs to those at the bottom and get fixated on the top. The top and bottom develop a lot of energy and can be witnessed to talk and laugh a lot amongst themselves. The middle group appears overburdened, overly serious and unhappy about their situation.

In the debrief the top reveals that they give out a clear strategy for the middle to implement and impose on the bottom; the middle finds it impossible to overcome the resistance from below and turns in vain to the top for help with how to accomplish their task in detail; the bottom laughs at both the other groups and at themselves, waiting for the others to finally start listening to them in order to find a way forward, or for the boss to get replaced during the next restructuring.

This exercise has been an effective way to explore the communication flow, or lack of it, in the organisation and ends in a shared understanding that change is brought about more easily when the three layers of the hierarchy connect and explore their experience of change in each other's presence.

Working with Intergroup Dynamics in the Organisation

As the team is only one of many subgroups within a department, each employee makes use of their internalised experience of a wider kinship system. This helps them deal with boundaries, with hierarchy and the need to get connected with other 'silos', the informal relationship network and the organisation as a community. The established analytic way to work with the organisation as a living community is to offer large group work. Over time I have conceptualised large group work, especially in the medical field with the staff in lateral as well as vertical ways: the first day I work with each subgroup, like the psychologists, the nurses, the doctors, the administration and the leader(s). The second day I facilitate three large group sessions with the whole staff present. This format is repeated over a number of years, once or twice per annum.

In the large group the vertical focus of most employees on the chief doctor and chief administrator as a parental couple from whom one could demand safety, security and a sense of hope for the future is often the dominant form of interaction. However, 'looking after' each subgroup separately enables the whole staff, in contrast to a one-day session, to work better together and cope with the endless stream of public sector reforms over the last few decades in a linked-up way. The subgroups, having had their own space to reflect on what they and the organisation need, develop the capacity to talk fearlessly about their own structural differentiation as well as their sense of interdependence. In this way large analytic groups can evolve a culture of translucent boundaries and avoid the loss of energy invested in demarcation disputes and rivalrous competition between the professional groups.

What an analytically led large group can offer is a forum that breaks free of the managerial orthodoxy of seeing organisations as a system, a set of procedures and a tsunami of targets. It pays to conceptualise organisations as living communities with a conscious and unconscious mind and direction of their own. Such a 'potential space' offers a place to everyone in the organisation to express their need to belong, to connect and work with others as well as to identify with some higher purpose. Large groups also make apparent that organisations are made up of two social worlds, which might or might not be connected: the formalised institutional status hierarchy of top, middle and bottom and its attendant bureaucratic procedures and controls. In the large group this hierarchical social structure meets the informal community, made up of multiple networks of relationships. In many ways these informal networks make an organisation work on a daily basis, by a short exchange at the coffee machine, by informal meetings before or after a formalised session. Comparisons to kinship metaphors have proved helpful in my work, as large group members can without thinking relate to the emotionally associated subgroup dynamics between parents and children, between three generations, between the sibling hierarchy and the difference between 'family and in-laws'. In other words, all professional groups are familiar and alien to each other, whilst being related and mutually obligated to one another.

My consultancy practice is based on the assumption that people need to be supported in making their expert silo their organisational home and learn that professional differentiation and interdependence hold an organisation together as a community. Connecting and communicating across specialist boundaries enables a majority to retain the capacity to think and learn from their experience with their clients, their market and from each other – just like siblings, parents and relatives do at birthdays, weddings or funerals.

Years of experience have made me concur with the thesis of the anthropologist Edman Leach that all institutions are subconsciously and culturally categorised and interpreted as an extension of the "domestic household and its extended kin" (1982). The language of kinship of father, mother, brother, sister, uncle, aunt and cousins is used to test what is familiar/unfamiliar, safe/unsafe in order to mentally make sense of the functional and positional relationships at work, in politics and civil society.

Conclusion

What is missing in a traditional analytic understanding of work groups and organisations is the appreciation of the function of leadership, management and of social roles, at the sociological as well as psychological level. Emile Durkheim's (1993) insight that the division of labour makes people separate and interdependent and holds a team, department, organisation and society together by the 'factual' experience of having to rely on each other – not through having their differences and authority level – needs to be taken seriously by analytic consultants.

The notion of laterally equal human beings has been an intellectual and political ideal since the French Revolution. No living culture studied by anthropologists has been found to be equal and without hierarchy, except in the sense of 'us' being different from 'them'. The human propensity to order the social world into insiders and outsiders within and between communities poses a real problem for those who believe that all humans can be laterally equal and free from vertical power. The tension between ideal and lived reality can trap professionals into fitting what they see, feel and experience into an abstract notion of how things should work. Lateral and vertical social relationships are not an either-or in reality, neither should these intertwined concepts of "structuration" (Giddens, 1989) be in the mind of the analytic consultant.

Bibliography

Baumann, Z.: *Flüssige Zeiten. Leben in der Ungewissheit.* Hamburg. 2008.

Bion, W.: *Experiences in Groups, and Other Papers.* London. 1961.

Durkheim, E.: *The Division of Labour in Society.* New York. 1993.

Giddens, A.: *Modernity and Self-Identity.* Cambridge. 1991.

Giddens, A.: *Sociology.* Cambridge. 1989.

Leach, E.: *Social Anthropology.* Glasgow. 1982.

Mitchell, J.: *Siblings.* Oxford. 2008.

Volkan, V.: *Blind Trust: Large Groups and Their Leaders in Times of Crisis and Terror.* Charlottsville. 2004.

Weber, M.: *Charisma and Disenchantment. The Vocation Lectures.* New York. 2020.

Wilke, G.: *The Art of Group Analysis in Organisations.* London. 2014.

Wilke, G.: *Ordnung und Chaos in Gruppen.* Zürich. 2017.

Wilke, G., et al.: *Breaking Free of Bonkers.* London. 2017.Winnicott, D.: *Home is Where We Start From.* Harmondsworth. 1986.

Sibling Trauma

2.1 Exclusion on the Horizontal Axis

Smadar Ashuach

Thoughts on Exclusion

Exclusion is an experience that affects and recreates relationships not only for the individual but also within and between societies.

From the moment we are born, we are excluded from both the vertical axis and the horizontal axis. Detached from our mother's womb, we will later have to process and accept the separation from the parental couple (Britton, 2004), on the vertical axis. We will also have to accept being excluded from the idea that we are unique and special – that is, accept that we are excluded on the horizontal axis.

I contend that the experience of exclusion is universal, stemming from the role of the Oedipal task as a central developmental task in which an individual recognizes and understands that he or she is excluded from the parental couple. Exclusion on the vertical axis is a developmental task that we can see recurring in the transference relationship between the patient and the therapist.

A developmental task on the horizontal axis – the sibling axis – also requires one to recognize and understand one's exclusion from his or her unique central place in the family, a type of exclusion that Mitchell (2006) writes about and that I expand upon later. This exclusionary experience recurs in the transference relationship in the therapeutic group (Ashuach, 2012, 2019).

Every individual aspires to have a feeling of inclusion and belonging; Foulkes and Anthony (1957) posit that a sense of belonging is a component of psychic health, an integral part of the human condition.

But belonging also implies exclusion. Dalal (2009) calls it the paradox of belonging: there can be no belonging without exclusion. In other words, it is impossible to ignore the notion of exclusion when describing belongingness. As defined by OED Online (2020), *belonging* is "the fact of appertaining or being a part; relationship, affiliation; (now *esp.*) a person's membership of, and acceptance by, a group or society." Thus, acceptance by a group implies that others are excluded from that group. Again, according to OED Online (2020), *exclusion* is the "shutting from a place, a society, etc., debarring from privilege, omitting from a category, from consideration, etc." People cannot all belong to the same category – the same gender, culture, nation, religion, or any other

DOI: 10.4324/9781003220060-13

category. However, one can make an effort to thwart the negative side effects of exclusion: the lack of respect and the undermining of rights, freedoms, and equality of the excluded individuals and populations. The most extreme and conspicuous phenomena of exclusion revolve around the creation of a society, nation, religion, or sect.

Freud coined the term "narcissism of minor differences" (1918) to explain various levels of racial exclusion, race-based hatred, gender bias, and other exclusionary phenomena. In a letter to Arnold Zweig (1927), Freud described narcissism of minor differences as a component of anti-Semitism. Several years later, Freud expounded on the concept in his article titled "Civilization and Its Discontents":

> It is always possible to bind together a considerable number of people in love, so long as there are other people left over to receive the manifestations of their aggressiveness. I once discussed the phenomenon that it is precisely communities with adjoining territories, and related to each other in other ways as well, who are engaged in constant feuds and in ridiculing each other – like the Spaniards and Portuguese, for instance. . . . I gave this phenomenon the name of "the narcissism of minor differences," a name which does not do much to explain it. We can now see that it is a convenient and relatively harmless satisfaction of the inclination to aggression, by means of which, cohesion between the members of the community is made easier.
>
> (Freud, 1930)

Similar to Freud's notion of narcissism of minor differences, the French philosopher Jankélévitch's ideas on hatred and racism, as explained by Paul Berman (1994), incorporate the role played by such "minor differences": you might feel hatred "for people who, compared with you, are neither 'other' nor 'brother.' It is hatred for 'the almost the same.'" According to Jankélévitch, as reported by Berman,

> To the person whose resemblance to you is close, yet who is not really your double, you might easily end up saying, "You are almost like me. The similarity between us is so plain that in the eyes of the world you are my brother. But, to speak honestly, you are not my brother. My identity, in relation to you, consists precisely of the ways in which I am different from you. Yet the more you resemble me the harder it is for anyone to see those crucial differences. Our resemblance threatens to obliterate everything that is special about me. So you are my false brother. I have no alternative but to hate you, because by working up a rage against you I am defending everything that is unique about me."
>
> (Berman, 1994, p. 62)

These feelings are what make the narcissism of minor differences unique. Alongside scorn, hatred, hostility, and self-idealization, one fears being polluted or infected were the other to approach one. The reverse also occurs: the idealization of the other is parallel to self-hatred or a rejection of the self along with an intensive preoccupation with, and desire to accept, the other. These are recognized aspects of the fear of the disappearance of one's uniqueness and of the roots of otherness, racism, and hatred between neighboring nations, such as Israel and Palestine.

But what is the psychological origin of the phenomenon? In his 1921 paper on group psychology and the analysis of the ego, Freud argues that the transition into culture and society begins in the nursery with the arrival of a new baby: the older sibling discovers that someone has been born who is a separate individual and whom the older child cannot kill on pain of losing the mother's love. Freud did not continue his research into this axis, but Juliet Mitchell has broadened it, describing the experience of otherness that is created when a child is faced with a new sibling (2018). At this stage, Mitchell's "law of the mother" makes the newborn's transition into society possible.

Mitchell writes about what she terms sibling trauma (2000, 2003, 2006). She treats it as a universal trauma regardless of whether we have siblings. It occurs the moment we recognize that we are replaceable. According to Mitchell, we think that the infant who is on the way will be a copy of us (2003, 2006). When we grasp that the new baby is, in fact, a separate being, we experience a crisis. This sibling trauma is the ultimate ouster, the dethronement. We feel that we have been replaced and expelled by other siblings. This exclusion experience lies along the horizontal axis; we are excluded from the place that we had believed we occupied in the family and that we no longer own. In Mitchell's view, the existence of a sibling is a necessary catastrophe. In one way or another, we must have such a relationship or a replacement of it with a friend, a partner, or a colleague. We experience the compulsory acceptance of ourselves as ordinary; it does not mean that we are not special, but, rather, it signifies that all our brothers and sisters are both ordinary and unique.

Mitchell emphasizes the powerful trauma of the narcissistic ego's annihilation, the trauma of sameness and difference. Revealed, reconstructed, and imagined, the trauma is characterized by repetitive compulsive behavior in various aspects of life and psychotherapy.

The experience of exclusion recurs in relationships with peers, partners, and friends. In therapy, it is repeated powerfully, chiefly in group therapy, by transference to other participants (Ashuach, 2012, 2019).

To Mitchell, the law of the mother organizes the relationships between siblings in the family, that is, on the horizontal axis (2006). In a 2018 lecture, Mitchell explained:

> I argue that for everyone the expectation, arrival or non-arrival of a sibling (the last or "only" child) constitutes a traumatic annihilation of the one-and-only baby whom the infant has been hitherto. The mother then forbids the older child to get rid of (murder) the baby or consider that the baby and itself are one and the same being (incest). She threatens the older

> child that if her prohibition is disobeyed, she will not love, care for, or protect it. Such a threat for the still highly dependent infant is a further trauma somewhat on the model of the later castration threat to the oedipal child.

The Bible is full of stories that portray difficult sibling relationships, such as Cain murdering Abel; Jacob stealing Esau's birthright; Joseph's brothers throwing him into a pit; and Amnon raping Tamar, whereupon Absalom murders Amnon. In each case, the infliction of harm by a brother against his brother or sister occurs when, for various reasons, the law of the mother has broken down or the perpetrator's feeling of exclusion is overwhelming.

If we ignore the horizontal axis, we in fact miss or deny the social dimension in the psychology of the individual. Observing the horizontal axis enables us to understand the difficulty of accepting the other and to identify the origin of relations with the other, such as racism, hatred, and supremacy.

The analytic group is a space that facilitates work on the horizontal axis, on the acceptance of the stranger and of difference. By working on sibling trauma and the acceptance of other siblings as equal, the group helps foster solutions for prejudice, racism, belligerence, financial discrimination, social inequality, and gender bias. As a member of the analytic group, you get to know the other by entering his or her world and by enabling the other to enter your world. This is a transformative moment. You no longer recognize yourself; your identity changes, making you something other than what you were. If you take the risk of changing, perhaps the other will change, as well. The process includes mutual recognition and transformation.

The hero of Orson Scott Card's science-fiction book *Ender's Game* explains how he is affected by getting to know the other:

> In the moment when I truly understand my enemy, understand him well enough to defeat him, then in that very moment I also love him. I think it's impossible to really understand somebody, what they want, what they believe, and not love them the way they love themselves.
>
> (Card, 1985, p. 238)

To know the enemy, the stranger, and the other in such a way can perhaps be understood as intimacy.

In this context, what is intimacy? The word has its origins in the Latin *intimus*, meaning inmost (OED Online, 2020). The most common use of the word refers to the innermost aspects of a person's body and psyche – the body's erogenous zones and thoughts and feelings concealed in the psyche. In this sense, an individual's intimate thoughts and feelings are those that the person avoids exposing to others. Thus, these feelings tend to remain internal and are not externalized.

Nowadays, the word's meaning is reversed. Instead of "innermost," with the meaning of what is not exposed to the other, the word today, in fact, implies sharing with others. Sharing occurs between friends, between partners, between therapist and patient, and between members of a group. Intimacy is based on a deep acquaintanceship, which is achieved through the exposure and self-discovery of thoughts, feelings, and the personal story. Intimacy is a kind of special closeness that also includes mutual involvement and influence in relation to thoughts, feelings, emotions, and behavior. Feelings are an essential component of intimacy; individuals who share their feelings with each other exchange roles in a dynamic, spontaneous way. They are able to place themselves in the other person's psyche.

When we talk about intimacy in a group, we go back to the paradox of belonging: by definition, belonging implies exclusion, and it follows that intimacy cannot exist without exclusion. In every group, we can see this movement between the allure of belongingness and the sense of exclusion. Intimacy is located on the border between belonging and exclusion.

As noted earlier, the relationships that are reconstructed, reenacted, and created in an analytic group are sibling relationships (Ashuach, 2012). As such, the participants build an intimacy system in which there is a constant movement between belonging and exclusion, between similarity and difference. In a group setting, processes transpire constantly, involving variation and differentiation in the development of personal identity, as well as comparison to others and the development of an intimacy that recognizes likeness and difference. Most important of all, the group space is closed to others – that is, the world outside the group is excluded. Intimacy is created by the exclusion of the other. As a patient in my group said, "The last time we met, I felt uplifted, a sense that I can lay myself bare to this group, that I can allow myself to share things that I cannot share in almost any other place."

Clinical Case

The therapeutic group that I am writing about is an analytic group that has been running for 13 years. Today the group consists of four men and four women, 40 to 60 years old, who have been working together for over a year. The participants have a strong sense of connection and intimacy.

The vignettes that I describe here occurred from February 2020 through July 2020, during the COVID-19 pandemic. In February, I moved the group from a clinic setting to online sessions (using Zoom meeting software) until the end of April. The participants were very unhappy and pressured me to reinstate the clinic meetings. Their interpretation of the change in venue was that I was afraid of catching the virus or infecting them, a concern that they thought had no basis. They did not consider the instructions from the health authorities as laws that they should comply with, and they saw no substantive reason to switch to virtual sessions. As the conductor, I felt that the group was opposed to both the law of the father and the law of the mother. For me, collaborating with the group meant endangering them and not protecting them, especially given that two participants are in a high-risk group because of their medical history and three participants are over the age of 60, including me.

The meetings that took place during this period demonstrated, to my astonishment, how much the pandemic was intensifying and exacerbating the participants' experience of exclusion; as a result, close, intimate work was made possible. At the same time, I was amazed to see that in almost every virtual session, someone reported a dream. Over the years, discussing dreams with the group has always been an unusual event.

In the first online meeting, two participants, Avi (a man) and Rina (a woman), left the group. They said they felt unable to participate in an online meeting, even though they wanted to continue treatment. I can understand that feeling but have difficulty seeing how they could disconnect themselves from the group without grasping the emotional impact on them and on the others. Only when they returned could their reenactment of childhood trauma be understood by the group. Both Avi and Rina had experienced a painful and sudden disconnection from their parents, and both were forced out of the original sibling group in their own families.

Even before moving to the virtual meeting format, the group was preoccupied with substantive questions of intimacy in their relationships with each other and in their personal lives, with their spouses and children. The participants all felt that the establishment of intimacy carries with it exclusion. Eli was concerned about intimacy with his wife and children; he was feeling rejected, isolated, and lonely. He reacted most strongly to Avi and Rina's leaving the group and was very angry with them. When they returned, he spoke of the feelings of abandonment that he had experienced by their leaving the group, as well as during his childhood – feelings that were very powerful for him. Tamar talked about the close relationship between her partner and their daughter, a relationship that excludes her and makes her feel hurt and angry.

The move to online sessions brought with it difficult experiences of alienation, loss of privacy, abandonment (incurred by the two participants who left), and exclusion, in addition to the loneliness of participating from one's own home and not in the social atmosphere of the clinic. During these sessions, the spouse and children outside the door were too close, on the one hand, and on the other, they felt excluded and angry and found all sorts of excuses to interfere. Anat forgot to attend one of our meetings because she was engrossed in a television series about social exclusion in the ultra-Orthodox world. The group thought in retrospect that the television series embodied the experience of exclusion in the group.

On one occasion, while I was explaining that the group abandonment experience was connected to the recreation of traumatic experiences in the past, I found myself facing frozen images on the screen (due to a technical glitch). I realized that the video had stopped, but I continued to hear the group talking about my interpretation and commenting that now I have abandoned them, too. Reality connects to all the emotional themes.

Yael, who was in the process of breaking up with her partner, recalled a dream: she is driving to the most beautiful place in the world to give packages to the needy and then sees that all of the packages are empty because her partner has taken everything. Eli connected to this dream in pain and told the group how his partner is taking their children away from him. Anat said that her partner is an alcoholic and shuts her out. Tal revealed his feeling that his partner is excluding him from their relationship because he lost his job. Feeling excluded by her father, Tamar shared with the group that, as in Yael's dream, her father had "emptied out her car."

In the next session, Tamar reported a dream after she felt that the group did not understand that she deserved having her father and brother break off contact with her. In the dream, she comes to a group meeting with a good friend who will help her talk to the group; Tamar is sitting next to me – the conductor – but she cannot speak, because four new participants, two of whom are good friends of Omer, have joined the group. Tamar continues relating the dream, in which she says that because of the new participants, she cannot reveal her feelings, and Omer tries to defend his friends. Yael joins Tamar in blaming me for not coordinating the entry of the new participants with the group, and as a result, I hurt Tamar. Avi (still in the dream) wears a condescending smile, and Tal, an understanding smile. Tamar cries terribly, and I say to her, "You're acting like a little girl. It's your choice whether you stay in the group or not." Then she leaves the room, and in the last part of the dream, the whole group gives up on her. The dream was very powerful. It made clear how important a role the group plays in Tamar's world and demonstrated the intense anxiety that she feels of being left behind, as her father and brother did to her.

The virtual meeting setting also enabled us to talk about previously unrevealed traumas. Eli recounts an incident in Lebanon during his military service, when he found himself in enemy territory with a trapped, frightened team. He was later wounded and taken to a hospital, but he was traumatized by the idea that the team had been forgotten, that nobody was coming to rescue them. The other participants talked about difficult experiences that their children had gone through in the military, and Omer joined in with a description of his military-related trauma. I thought how lucky we are to be hearing these stories in an online session, rather than experiencing the pain of discussing the traumas in person.

In a later meeting, Tal reported a dream in which he joins the group, which is huge, and people whom he does not know at all are participating. Some of them were in the group in the past, and others were not. He asks me, "What is this?" I reply that this is what I decided on and I don't see what his problem is. It is not up for discussion. The group in the dream conducts a dialogue that they do not really understand, a conversation at a reunion of all Smadar's patients, past and present. Talking about this dream, the participants related to the experience of being excluded from the group and from the others at home and at work.

At the next meeting, Omer told the group of a dream in which he is called up for reserve duty. He is aware that at his age, he should have already been released from reserve service, but because he was called up, he reports for duty. He reaches the barracks and goes from room to room, but nowhere is a bed available. He can't find a place to sleep. Finally he goes to the office and gets angry at the liaison officer for calling him up but not providing a bed. She replies that he is right and he can go back home. To Omer, the dream represented his feeling that he has no place in life and has difficulty finding a place in the group; and he is angry with me for that. The members of the group thought that the rooms in Omer's dream stand for the squares in the online meeting software, where it is hard for all of them to find a place.

The group was wondering what would happen when we returned to face-to-face meetings at the clinic. It is clear that a strong experience of intimacy was created precisely in the online Zoom meetings. People shared dreams, fears, feelings of loneliness, and feelings of exclusion, some of which were directed at Avi and Rina when they left. The question arose as to whether we should include them in our clinic meeting. Omer wanted us to get together without them first. He sensed that something had happened when they were not with us, and therefore it would be impossible for them to make an uncomplicated return ("they didn't have a room," as in Omer's dream). But the others felt that Avi and Rina still belonged to the group, so meeting without them would be hurtful and insulting. They worried that Avi and Rina would feel excluded and would misunderstand the situation, thinking it was a case of revenge. I struggled with myself, asking what I should do in light of the law of the mother. How could I protect all of them?

In the end, Avi and Rina returned to face-to-face meetings at the clinic along with everyone. The first session began with the members asking about the others' well-being, but very quickly anger took over. In a detached, condescending manner, Avi said that in his mind, he had already parted from the group. Rina claimed that she did not want to return at all but, after a conversation with me, she understood that it mattered whether she came or not. During this session, I became very angry at Avi and Rina and felt that they were hurting the other members of the group. The participants kept silent, and I insisted that they share their feelings. Slowly, they brought their experiences of hurt, abandonment, and exclusion out into the open.

Rina is the middle daughter in a family of seven children. From a young age, she felt different from the rest of the family, and it was easy for them to give up on her. On the one hand, she felt that she was more successful than her siblings, while on the other hand, she felt like an outsider, isolated and rejected. This experience has stayed with her in all the groups that she has belonged to. For her, the online meetings were a form of reenactment. Through the group work, she began to understand her role in the experience of exclusion by her siblings as well as by her partner and friends.

Avi's parents were killed when he was eight and his brother was 11. Sent to a kibbutz where they were brought up as foster children, Avi and his brother always felt different in the company of the other children in the kibbutz. At first, the bond between the brothers was very close. However, over the years, Avi felt that because he was more successful socially and was a good athlete, his brother severed ties with him. As Avi put it, "My brother erased me from his life." As a result, Avi has been seeking a close relationship throughout his life, but as soon as he feels somewhat abandoned, he turns around and breaks off the relationship. This is what he did twice to his wife, and in this way he ended his relationship with his business partner and also broke away from the therapy group.

Two months after we resumed meeting at the clinic, I rescheduled our session as a Zoom meeting because I had been exposed to a coronavirus patient and was in quarantine. Rina immediately announced that she would not join the meeting, and Avi just disappeared. In retrospect, it turned out that he had made an effort to join but was unsuccessful because of technical problems. What was interesting was that in the middle of this meeting, both Tamar's spouse and Yael's spouse came in and interfered with the discussion. They could not bear to see how deeply Tamar and Yael were connected to the group while they (the spouses) were excluded. Eli and Omer, who are both married, talked about their extramarital relationships, implying that in the virtual format they could reveal to the group things that they could not talk about in a face-to-face meeting at the clinic.

At the next meeting, Avi came back, but Eli berated him for not attending the previous meeting and said how much Avi's absence hurt. Slowly we understood Eli's reenactment in the group. He felt that he was trying hard to bond with the group, but Avi excluded him, just as Eli's wife and children do at home. As a child, Eli also felt excluded. He was the youngest son in his family and made a great effort to be good and be loved, but over the years, he discovered that there were deep secrets in the household that he did not know and from which he was excluded. Avi realized that for him, Eli represented Avi's older brother. Feeling that Eli was jealous of him, just as Avi's brother was, Avi severed the relationship with Eli. Following this meeting, Avi renewed contact with his brother and started working on reestablishing his relationship with Eli.

During this period, the relationships between the participants and the dreams that they reported made it possible to recreate, see, deal with, and treat the experiences of exclusion on the horizontal axis – to process the impact of early sibling relationships on all the participants.

It was interesting and exciting to see the emotional work that took place during the months under study. The departure of Avi and Rina triggered feelings of abandonment also in Tamar, who was abandoned by her brother and was now able to connect to how that rejection affects her and how it is reenacted in her relationship with her husband. Omer felt that he couldn't find a place in the group and saw how this feeling has been with him from a very young age, when he had difficulty finding his place at home and in the company of his peers. For him, it makes sense to feel abandoned.

Anat and Yael, both more successful than their siblings, have felt guilty about their success throughout their life. Through the events in the group, they understood how they recreate the experience of feeling abandoned by their partners.

Tal is the youngest in his family and grew up on a kibbutz. He was held back in kindergarten and, as a result, was excluded from the group of children whom he had been with from birth. He came to understand how he always recreates the feeling of being left back, especially during the pandemic, which caused him to lose his job. He sensed that he is the only one in the group who was left behind. He felt that nobody cares, a feeling that we could see in his dream.

Conclusions

Feelings of exclusion are universal developmental experiences. We must recognize that we are excluded from the parental room and from the experience that we are unique and special – that is, we undergo exclusion on the vertical axis and the horizontal axis. Unprocessed traumas are reenacted in social intercourse, with spouses and colleagues. The analytic group is the therapeutic space that allows for the reenactment of exclusion on the horizontal axis and consequently makes treatment possible.

Sibling trauma and the law of the mother are reflected in the group-analytic group. The group offers the possibility of many sibling transference relationships and is a place in which the interaction among members, that is, the group matrix, facilitates reenactment of the original sibling trauma. Thus, the group provides an opportunity to relive the past in the present and satisfy one's need to go back in order to remember.

The reenactment of sibling trauma in a group setting makes change and growth possible. Grossmark (2007) writes that all behavior in the group is a form of communication of the members' inner worlds and unarticulated experiences. The group can reach a level of understanding only if the conductor permits the full reenactment of these inner worlds within the group.

The COVID-19 pandemic, with the need for isolation and our group's transition to online meetings, intensified the participants' experience of exclusion and enabled powerful reenactment processes to occur between participants and within the group, including the conductor. I believe that the reenactment of such experiences is transpiring at all social levels, but without any of the necessary processing. As a result, phenomena such as extreme racism, social inequality, and discrimination can be observed all over the world.

References

Ashuach, S. (2012). Am I my brother's keeper?: The analytic group as a space for re-enacting and treating sibling trauma. *Group Analysis*, 45(2), 155–167. https://doi.org/10.1177/0533316411436141

Ashuach, S. (2019). Enactments of sibling relationships in a group. *Contexts*, 85(Autumn). https://groupanalyticsociety.co.uk/contexts/issue-85/articles/hope-and-group-analysis/enactments-of-sibling-relationships-in-a-group/

Berman, P. (1994, February 28). The other and the almost the same. *The New Yorker*, 70, 61–71.

Britton, R. (2004). Subjectivity, objectivity, and triangular space. *Psychoanalytic Quarterly*, 73(1), 47–61. https://doi.org/10.1002/j.2167-4086.2004.tb00152.x

Card, O.S. (1985). *Ender's game*. Tor Books.

Dalal, F. (2009). The paradox of belonging. *Psychoanalysis, Culture & Society*, 14, 74–81. https://doi.org/10.1057/pcs.2008.47

Foulkes, S.H., & Anthony, E.J. (1957). *Group psychotherapy: The psychoanalytic approach*. Karnac.

Freud, S. (1918). The taboo of virginity (Contributions to the psychology of love III). In J. Strachey (Ed.), *The standard edition of the complete psychological works of Sigmund Freud*, Vol. XI (1910): Five Lectures on Psycho-analysis, Leonardo da Vinci and Other Works, 191–208. Hogarth Press.

Freud, S. (1921). Group psychology and the analysis of the ego. In J. Strachey (Ed.), *The standard edition of the complete psychological works of Sigmund Freud*, Vol. XVIII (1920–1922). Hogarth Press.

Freud, S. (1927, July 2). [Letter to Arnold Zweig]. The International Psycho-Analytical Library, 84, 3

Freud, S. (1930). Civilization and its discontents. In *The standard edition of the complete psychological works of Sigmund Freud*, Vol. XXI (1927–1931): The Future of an Illusion, Civilization and its Discontents, and Other Works, 57–146. Hogarth Press.

Grossmark, R. (2007). The edge of chaos: Enactment, disruption, and emergence in group psychotherapy. *Psychoanalytic Dialogues*, 17(4), 479–499. https://doi.org/10.1080/10481880701487193

Mitchell, J. (2000). *Mad men and medusas: Reclaiming hysteria and the effects of sibling relationships on the human condition*. Penguin.

Mitchell, J. (2003). *Siblings: Sex and violence*. Polity.

Mitchell, J. (2006). Sibling trauma: A theoretical consideration. In P. Coles (Ed.), *Sibling relationships*, 155–174. Karnac.

Mitchell, J. (2018, February 16). *Core concepts: From sibling trauma to the law of the mother* [Paper presentation]. Group Psychotherapy Conference on Sibling Relationships, Tel Aviv University, Tel Aviv, Israel.

OED Online (2020, June). *belonging, n.* Oxford University Press. www.oed.com/view/Entry/17508

OED Online (2020, June). *exclusion, n.* Oxford University Press. www.oed.com/view/Entry/658208

OED Online (2020, June). *intimate, adj. and n.* Oxford University Press. www.oed.com/view/Entry/98506

2.2 The Horizontal Axis From Different Perspectives

The Social Significance of Siblings

Prophecy Coles

The Three Bronte Sisters

In 1846 a thin volume of poems written by Currer, Ellis and Acton Bell was published, but the volume 'caused little stir among the critics, it sank without a trace. . . . [and] A year after its publication only two copies had been sold' (Barker 1994, pp. 498–499). Currer, Ellis and Acton Bell, as is now well known, were the three Bronte sisters, Charlotte, Emily and Anne. By 1847 they were living at home with their brother Branwell and their father, and the four siblings were desperate to find a way of earning their living through their writing. They had all made attempts to earn their living by teaching children in the homes of the wealthy, but in the case of the three sisters, they had become disillusioned and ill and resigned. In the case of Branwell, he fell in love with his employer's wife, Lydia Robinson, and was dismissed, broken-hearted.

Branwell gradually slipped into alcoholism and drug taking to ease his disappointment, but, nevertheless, he was desperate to find a publisher for his work. In 1845 he had started to write a three-volume novel with the conviction that 'in the present state of the publishing and reading world a Novel is the most saleable article' (Barker 1994, p. 475). Branwell never completed his project, but in his belief that the novel was the way to make money he became 'the first member of his family to tread a new path, in seeing the potential of the novel as a marketable commodity' (Barker 1994, p. 475). For his three sisters he opened a door to a new way of earning their living and they each began to write a novel: Charlotte wrote *The Professor*, Emily wrote *Wuthering Heights* and Anne wrote *Agnes Grey*. *The Professor* was turned down, but encouraged by her publishers Charlotte wrote her second novel *Jane Eyre*, and all three novels were published by the end of 1847.

This is an unique period in nineteenth-century English literature in which a group of three sisters, sharing their work, produced three novels of outstanding originality. Every evening after their father had gone to bed, Charlotte, Emily and Anne 'wrote their books in close collaboration, reading passages aloud to each other and discussing the handling of their plots and their characters as they walked round and round the dining-room table' (Barker 1994, p. 500). The

DOI: 10.4324/9781003220060-14

creative influence they had on each other was astonishing and distinguishes them from any other literary sibling group from this period.

What enabled this astonishing collective creativity? One experience the siblings shared was the death of their mother when they were very young; this was followed by the deaths of their two elder sisters, Maria and Elisabeth, soon after. So grief and loss were part of the textures of their lives. Branwell expressed this collective melancholy well when he wrote in their childhood magazine 'Monthly Intelligence' in 1833,

> When a parent leaves his Children young and inexperienced, and without a cause absconds, never more troubling himself about them those Children according to received notions among men if they by good fortune should happen to survive the neglect and become of repute in society are by no means bound to believe he has done . . . [his] duty to them as a parent.
> (Barker 1994, p. 193)

One way of thinking about what he wrote here might be to say that they felt that their mother had absconded and left them because she was not interested in them. At a more unconscious level the suggestion might be that they believed they had a derelict or 'bad' parent, and if they achieved any success in life it would not be because they had been well cared for and loved. This would imply that there was an angry energy that fuelled their collective desire to show the world they could survive well. But does this interpretation offer a sufficient explanation for the flowering of their imaginations?

Something more remarkable was taking place. One cold winter's evening when they were all sitting around the fire and feeling thoroughly bored, a new dynamic spark was kindled. 'A play of the Islanders was formed in December 1827' Charlotte wrote (Barker 1994, p. 151). And from there they created the worlds of Angria and Gondal, peopled by characters that they read about in the newspapers, such as the Duke of Wellington and Byron. Later they were inspired by reading articles in Blackwood's Magazine. Their inspiration had also been fuelled by a box of soldiers that had been given to Branwell in 1826 by his father. Each child had at the time appropriated a particular soldier that became their own special one and 'tales of magic, mystery and the supernatural' that included corpses being revived were lived out in the minute manuscripts they now wrote about the lives of these characters (Barker 1994, pp. 160–161). Charlotte and Branwell formed one couple and they created the world of Angria with heroes and villains battling to the death. What is interesting is that their stories reveal an 'interweaving of often complex story lines . . . [that] demanded a close partnership between brother and sister' (Barker 1994, p. 195). In other words their tales were the fruit of their close collaboration. Emily and Anne seem not have been included into the world of Angria and instead they invented together another even more extravagant and gothic world of Gondal. The mesmeric quality of Gondal continued to entrance the two of them even when they were grown up. In 1845, Emily wrote in her diary of the pleasure she and Anne had had while on holiday as they became 'Henry Angora . . . Cordelia Fitzaphnold (sic) [and others] . . . escaping from the Palaces of Instruction to join the Royalists who are hard driven at present by the victorious Republicans' (Barker 1994, p. 451). Emily would have been 27 and Anne 25. These facts suggest that the writing of their fantastic tales and sharing them with each other had become part of their lives. A sibling bond cemented by their imaginative lives was as necessary to them as the Yorkshire air they breathed.

To understand further the significance of their relationships to each other, I am going to turn to Anne Bronte's second novel *The Tenant of Wildfell Hall*. I discovered that tucked away and almost hidden in the corners of this tale, Anne was addressing the crucial importance that a sibling relationship can have upon the later development of identity. This was portrayed by the relationship between Helen, the hero of the novel, and her brother Frederick Lawrence. It is easy to forget Lawrence and see him as a minor character in the drama of the failed marriage between Helen and her husband Arthur Huntingdon. But to imagine the tale without Lawrence helps one to see that the sibling relationship was the pivot that held the text together and drove it forward.

The Tenant of Wildfell Hall is in three parts. The first is in the form of letters that Gilbert Markham wrote in 1847 to his brother-in-law Halford in which he describes his encounter with a beautiful and mysterious woman Helen Graham who had suddenly appeared in their quiet agricultural village. He falls in love with her but when she rejects him, Markham beats up her brother, believing he was her secret lover. The second section is Helen's diary that she kept before she arrives at Wildfell Hall and meets Gilbert. The diary offers an explanation to Gilbert of why she must reject him. She is already married but has run away from her drunken husband with her son Arthur and is living under the protective wing of her brother Frederick Lawrence. In the final section a much-chastened Gilbert learns that Lawrence, the man he beat up was Helen's brother. A melodrama of continuing misperceptions between Markham, Lawrence and Helen follows when Helen returns to nurse her dying husband. However, in Gilbert's last letter he reveals that for the last twenty years he has been happily married to Helen.

In this brief synopsis of the novel the shadow of Helen's brother is cast across her life and we learn how essential his support has been for her survival. We might add that without him the resolution of her relationship with Markham might never have been achieved. Helen who is the hero of *The Tenant of Wildfell Hall* is the most arresting character in this novel, not least because we are never sure of her family name. She is Helen Lawrence by birth. Helen Maxwell perhaps when she is adopted by her aunt and uncle. Helen Huntingdon when she is married. Helen Graham when she runs away from her husband and assumes her mother's married name and Helen Markham when she marries her second husband Gilbert Markham. At the very least, just listing the shifting identities Helen has to assume throughout her life illustrates the complexities of the social and legal position of women in the middle of the nineteenth century. Helen's changing surnames also serve to highlight that as Helen's emotional life with her husband, Arthur Huntingdon, disintegrates, her social position comes under threat. If she leaves him, who will she become? The only recourse she has is to turn to her brother Frederick Lawrence to shore up her self-respect. This is where she can hope to find a safe harbour with one man who can be trusted.

Helen's brother, 'Mr Lawrence', makes his appearance in the first section of the novel and thereafter he peeps in and out of the early narrative, as though his delicate bone structure will scarcely bear the weight of the drama that he has to carry. He is introduced as not only delicate in build but also as 'reserved' and 'solitary', 'cold' and 'shy', living alone in his father's house, Woodford Hall, following his father's death. Lawrence was a man whose 'heart was like a sensitive plant, that opens for a moment in the sunshine, but curls up and shrinks into itself at the slightest touch of a finger or the lightest breath of the wind' (Bronte 1996, pp. 39–40).

This 'sensitive plant', it soon becomes clear, is the fulcrum upon which the unfolding drama rests. In the first place Lawrence has projected onto him the conflicting confusion that his sister's appearance at Wildfell Hall has upon all whom she encounters. As Markham gets to know Helen, he becomes increasingly convinced that Lawrence is her secret lover, and Lawrence's secretive behaviour encourages this belief. But Markham's fantasy is also fuelled by the collective misperception of the people who live in his village and who gossip about Lawrence's relationship with Helen, this mysterious woman who has come to live at Wildfell Hall. Further substance is given to the malicious village gossip by the observation that Mrs Graham's son, Arthur, looks like Lawrence and has the same delicate bone structure. That of course may be true as Arthur and Lawrence are nephew and uncle, but what this description serves to do is to augment Markham's conviction that Lawrence 'had some designs upon Mrs Graham' (Bronte 1848 [1996], p. 87). This belief takes hold of Markham with such force that he is driven to beat Lawrence across the head with his whip when they meet on horseback. Lawrence falls from his horse and Markham rides off leaving him semi-conscious by the roadside. Here we see Lawrence, this 'sensitive plant', has become a victim of the malicious gossip his behaviour has helped to incite. Lawrence incites gossip that leads to violence and then he becomes its victim, and all because of his hidden relationship with his sister Helen. This violent incident did much to harm Anne's reputation and the fate of the novel. Stevie Davies (1996) in her Introduction to the novel, wrote 'Reviewers reacted with fascinated shock to this 'coarse' and 'brutal' work, in which elite males degenerate into addicts and libertines' (p. vii). It was seen as glorifying the grotesque violence of uncontrolled male passion, and what made this event even more of an affront to male critics, and there were of course no female critics writing for well-known journals at this time, was that the novel was believed to have been written by a man, Acton Bell. This was an ironic fate that awaited a nineteenth-century female writer who could not get her work published unless she assumed the identity of a man.

It is possible, in the twenty-first century, to think differently about this violent incident and its meaning, in contrast to its nineteenth-century critics. We can look back on the social conditions of the mid-nineteenth century and in particular the place of women in relationship to men, and we can add the insights that psychoanalysis has brought to the understanding of the human mind. An important feature of the novel rests upon the misperception of Helen and Lawrence's relationship. So the question is, what was Anne pursuing when she put this sibling relationship at such a central place in the book? One answer is that Anne was challenging the assumption that a relationship between an unmarried man and a single woman was seen as necessarily sexual. This belief, or social conditioning, is what leads Markham to his violent outburst. He cannot imagine any other possibility. In the nineteenth century, young middle-class women had few opportunities to have a relationship with young men that was untrammelled by sexual innuendo except with a brother. But even such a relationship, as we see in this novel, does not provide a haven that is free from gossip. Sexual anxiety was such a powerful determining force in the way relationships between young men and women were perceived that it overrode the belief that brothers and sisters could be safe from sexual desire or enactment. William and Dorothy Wordsworth are a good example of such gossip, and even to this day they are not free from the charge that their relationship was incestuous. Byron, who was a much-admired hero of the Bronte children, was suspected of an 'unnatural' relationship with his half-sister Augusta and the gossip about them was so all encompassing that Byron left England for good. As Davidov (2006) commentated, 'The depths of emotional attachment among nineteenth century siblings – including erotic overtones – is brought out in that feature of English Victorian culture so puzzling to twentieth-century commentators' (p. 33). So we can see that these sexual anxieties in the nineteenth century did much to disturb a belief that there can be a positive side to the relationship between brothers and sisters. As though replying to that anxiety, Anne has asked us to look again at that misperception and consider that a sibling can give vital emotional support to a sibling in distress. This support does not mean the relationship is sexual even though 'The capacity to experience sibling desire may enrich our capacity for mature sexual fulfilment' (Coles 2003, p. 67). Instead, Anne is showing that siblings can step in when the outer structures of the hierarchical rules of society has made life impossible for a woman like Helen. Furthermore, Anne seems to be suggesting how diminished a woman becomes if it is assumed that the only relationship a woman could have with a man is necessarily a sexual one. This is the fundamental misperception that gives rise to the male violence in this novel.

There is another important aspect about the nature of sibling relationships that Anne explores. She shows how these relationships are constantly evolving over the course of a life, and, if the sibling relationship is creative, it has to allow in sexual partners; it cannot remain a romantic enclave. This is delicately described in the toing and froing of Lawrence and Markham's meetings following Markham's brutal attack on Lawrence. Trust has been so eroded that they do not dare to communicate their true feelings, yet they need to find a way that includes Helen. How is that possible when Markham has behaved in such a brutal manner towards his imagined rival? How can Lawrence ever imagine

Markham might become an acceptable brother-in-law? It requires a lot of emotional growth in both men for them to find a resolution. Lawrence has to finally accept Markham as a possible brother-in-law, and Markham has to accept that without Lawrence, Helen's life would have been trapped in a marriage that would have destroyed her and ruined her son. Markham does recognise this complexity in his last letter. He can hear that Lawrence did understand the potential tragedy that both he and Helen faced if Helen had succumbed to her adulterous passion. This is well summarised by Lawrence who eventually conceded that he did not want either of them to die of 'a broken heart'. Here we can sense that Lawrence is a compassionate and feeling man who both accepts their passion for each other and realised that it was doomed to disappointment while Huntingdon lived. However, he cannot resist what might be seen as a feminist barb against Markham, 'my sister's feelings are naturally full and keen as yours, and I believe *more* constant' (Barker 1994, p. 415). Was that a moment of authorial intrusion, irresistible though it might have been?

So where does all this lead? By looking at the relationship between a brother and sister in this novel, I have been led to appreciate both how original it was and how different Anne's imaginative life was to that of her two sisters, if one compares this novel with *Wuthering Heights* and *Jane Eyre*. Anne invites us to think about sibling relationships and their place in an individual life and in particular the way we may rely upon a brother or sister in a time of need. At the same time Anne is not blind to other aspects of sibling relationships; Lawrence acted like a possessive and jealous lover towards Markham, and wanted to keep him away from a relationship with his sister. In other words, Anne understood that sibling relationships are not without passions and jealousies as intense as any that are lived with partners.

Ironically, this last insight is played out in the fate of the novel after its publication in 1848. One overriding question is why is *The Tenant of Wildfell Hall* less well known than *Wuthering Heights* and *Jane* Eyre? Who remembers Helen, in comparison to Cathy and Heathcliffe, Jane Eyre and Rochester? We cannot properly answer that question without knowing what happened to the novel following Anne's death. There is substantial evidence that Anne's neglect has to do with subsequent publications of the novel that were expurgated by Charlotte. Charlotte, like several male critics, was shocked by its violence and she wanted to protect Anne's good name. Charlotte could not see Anne as her imaginative equal but only as her younger sister who was struggling to write against the difficulties of her delicate nature (Chitham 1991). Charlotte then diminished Anne's creative ability even further in a very subtle way; she believed that Anne's portrait of Huntingdon's drunken dissolution was the result of witnessing Branwell's gradual disintegration. Charlotte wrote, ' [Anne] . . . had been called upon to contemplate near at hand, the terrible effect of talents misused and faculties abused'. Unfortunately, she further assumes, Anne had a 'sensitive, reserved, and dejected nature . . . what she saw sunk very deeply into her mind; it did her harm'. Not only did it do her harm but 'she believed it to be her duty to reproduce every detail . . . as a warning to others'. This led Charlotte to emphatically assert that 'She [Anne] hated her work' and 'the choice of subject was an entire mistake' (Gaskill 1908, p. 246). In other words *The Tenant of Wildfell Hall* was not a novel of imaginative power but an autobiographical political tract, written to warn readers of the dangers of drink. The result was that Charlotte, after Anne's death, amended the novel and until the late twentieth century there was only a 'corrupt text which is highly expurgated [that] would become the basis for most subsequent British editions' (Davies 1996, p. 492). No wonder that *The Tenant of Wildfell Hall* has been seen as 'a pale version of *Wuthering Heights*'. The energy of the novel was dissipated and Anne's 'artistic and moral challenge' was transformed into a novel that was inferior in imaginative scope to that of her sisters. (Chitham 1991, p. 134). For a hundred and fifty years the public were deprived of reading the authentic novel; no wonder Helen has yet to emerge as a hero as well-known as Cathy and Jane.

This expurgation reflects something more far reaching than just a sibling dispute about whether Huntingdon was a portrait of Branwell. When Charlotte reduced the novel to autobiography and then expurgated it she was unconsciously reducing her sister's artistic power and creativity. As Tomlin (2000) pointed out, 'The power of the artist [is] to change particular personal experience into something entirely different' (p. 13). The novel stretches beyond Anne's personal biography and it opens up a door where we can appreciate Anne's insight that a sibling is not necessarily a poor relation whom we can relegate to a corner. My appreciation only came to me on a second reading of the novel. I had missed the sibling relationship on my first reading and it was not until a friend remarked on its importance that I went back and reread the novel. Then I realised that Anne had an extraordinary grasp of the social, psychological and political power of sibling relationships. My failure to see this on the first reading made me aware of how easy it is to miss siblings, whether within a text, or as we have seen, historically, within psychoanalytic theory. On first reading *The Tenant of Wildfell Hall* one is gripped by the more striking themes of drunkenness, sadomasochism, violence, pernicious gossip and marital discord. The more silent part that siblings play in the life of the family can remain unnoticed as they are less sexually dramatic. This has meant that it has been easy to imagine that sibling relationships are of limited psychological interest, not least because 'siblings have no direct effect on reproduction'. This novel has shown us that a sibling relationship can play a major part in managing a life, and our psychological theories are now recognising this to be true.

In conclusion, the Bronte sisters created an imaginative life together that led them to create some of the greatest novels in the English language. That is not to say that their relationships with each other were not without the difficulties, tensions, jealousies and rivalries we saw in Charlotte's expurgation of *The Tenant of Wildfell Hall*. But it is to remind us that the lateral sibling relationships can have as much influence and power upon our creative life as the vertical ones with parents. We must protect this knowledge and cherish it, for we diminish our understanding of human relationships if we imagine sibling relationships are less significant than the more obvious and exciting ones we may have with others.

I wish to thank Earl Hopper and Jennifer Silverstone for their contribution.

References

Barker, J. (1994) *The Brontes*. London: Wiedenfeld & Nicholson.

Bronte, A. (1848 [1996]) *The Tenant of Wildfell Hall*. Ed. S. Davies. London: Penguin Random House.

Chitham, E. (1991) *A Life of Anne Bronte*. Oxford and Cambridge: Blackwell Publishers Inc.

Coles, P. (2003) *The Importance of Sibling Relationships in Psychoanalysis*. London and New York: Karnac Books Ltd.

Davidoff, L. (2006) The sibling relationship and sibling incest in historical context. In *Sibling Relationships*. Ed. P. Coles. London: Karnac Books Ltd.

Gaskill, E. (1908) *The Life of Charlotte Bronte*. London: J.H. Dent & Sons.

Tomlin, C. (2000) *Several Strangers: Writing from Three Decades*. London: Penguin Books.

2.3 Processes of Scapegoating and Sibling Rivalry in the Context of the Basic Assumption of Incohesion

Aggregation/Massification

Earl Hopper

In this chapter I will consider some aspects of scapegoating and sibling rivalry in the context of the fourth basic assumption of Incohesion: Aggregation/Massification in the unconscious life of groups and group-like social systems, especially those which have been traumatised. Massification is supported by scapegoating processes. Sibling rivalry is an entirely neglected aspect of scapegoating. I will illustrate some of these ideas with data from one of my twice weekly clinical groups, the details of which have been changed in order to protect their confidentiality, and with data from a demonstration group at a Conference in 2017 in New York.

I. An Outline of the Theory of Incohesion: Aggregation/Massification or (ba) I:A/M

Having outlined the theory of Incohesion elsewhere (Hopper, 2003a; 2003b; Bion, 1961), I will only summarise it here in terms of the following hypotheses:

1.

Various events that cause the experience of inadequate containment and insufficient holding that can be characterised in terms of failed dependency.

2.

The fear of annihilation characterised by intra-psychic fission and fragmentation and various psychotic anxieties associated with this, in oscillation with relational fusion and confusion with what is left of and with what can be found in the other, and various psychotic anxieties associated with this, based on seeking protection against the psychotic anxieties associated with each of the two polarised conditions.

3.

The development of crustacean and amoeboid character structures, and of negative and positive encapsulations, encystment, and/or encrypment.

DOI: 10.4324/9781003220060-15

4.

The propensity towards the enactment of aggressive feelings in aggression and violence based on traumatophilia, that is, based on the sexualisation of aggressive feelings and on the use of sexuality as a defence against depressive anxieties, as seen in the development of the trauma syndrome involving addiction, somatisation, sadistic perversion, risk taking, delinquency, and criminality.

5.

Incohesion is a manifestation and an expression of the intra-psychic phenomenology of the fear of annihilation and relational forms of defensive protection against the pain of this experience. This can be seen in the primary development of the socio-cultural state of aggregation and in the secondary development of the socio-cultural state of massification, and then in the defensive oscillations between them. These socio-cultural states are manifest in those patterns of relations, normation, communication, and styles of thinking and feeling, as well as in patterns of aggression, that are typical of them.

6.

Incohesion is associated with the development of social psychic retreats such as ghettos and enclaves which are often based on subgroupings and contra-groupings associated with social identities. The subgroupings and contra-groupings within a contextual society characterised by Incohesion are likely themselves to become characterised by Incohesion and the dynamics of it.

7.

Incohesion is characterised by the development of roles that are typical of aggregation and massification.

8.

Traumatised people are especially vulnerable to the suction power of these roles, and, in turn, they are likely to personify them.

II. Massification and Scapegoating[1]

Massification is supported by the twin pillars of fundamentalism and scapegoating. When fundamentalism fails or dissipates, massification is supported by the continuous scapegoating of particular persons and subgroups. I have discussed elsewhere the dynamics of massification and fundamentalism (Hopper, in press, Ofer & Berman). I will focus here on several aspects of scapegoating:

1.

In all forms of scapegoating the members of a social system purge themselves of unacceptable and dangerous feelings, ideas, attributes, and qualities by projecting them into and onto particular people and subgroups who have been defined in terms of social category thinking and feeling. Judging them very stringently, and in absolute rather than relative terms, these people and subgroups are then perceived to be guilty of the projected violations. In turn, they are punished by being peripheralised, marginalised, shunned, and ultimately banished from the social system. They are thus deprived of the safety, support, and nurture which are available to those who remain in the social system, and who take their personal identity from their membership of it. Various other forms of aggression are also involved, including anonymisation, sacrifice, character assassination, and even actual assassination, each of which is typical of Incohesion.

2.

The motives for such projections include the need to evacuate, control the object, express sadism, turn passive into active, and even to communicate to any and all who might hear and listen to the ineffable sub-symbolic narratives that the perpetrators might wish and feel the need to voice. Scapegoating involves an unconscious attack on the father (Money-Kyrle, 1929), who is perceived to have failed the group and/or to have stopped access to the mother, and on displacements from him. However, people and subgroups who are perceived to be either obstacles to merger with a perfect group and/or as impurities within the hallucination of perfection (Chasseguet-Smirgel, 1985) are also likely to be attacked.

Ressentiment (Nietzsche, 1887; Kierkegaard, 1846; Scheler, 1933), which can be defined in terms of blaming a person or a subgroup for being responsible for one's pain, suffering, and misfortune, is a central element of such narratives. The key factor in *ressentiment* is the envy of the object who is blamed. The object of such envy can be regarded as "undeserving" and as "getting away with it", which is both a source of the *ressentiment* and a consequence of it.

3.

The victims of projections associated with unconscious shame and guilt are designated as "different", "strange", "abnormal", and "inferior". They are considered to be "dirty" and, therefore, as sources of pollution. They are also considered to be morally unacceptable and in general "unwholesome". The collective fantasy is that once such people and subgroups are excluded, the group is likely to become more "normal", "clean", "pure", and so on.

As "splinters" or "shards" of the group, scapegoats are likely to become "bizarre objects" (Bion, 1957). The collective fantasy is that once a bizarre object is extruded from the group, the group is likely to become smoother, softer, safer and more comfortable in general for those who remain in it.

The victims of such projections are often regarded as a "pseudo-species" or as a "sub-species". They not only become "enemy-others" but also inhuman (Hopper, 2003c; Erikson, 1968). The members of a pseudo-species are outside the "moral community" (Ranulf, 1964). As such, we can do to them whatever we would like.

4.

Scapegoating is an unconscious form of sacrifice. Insofar as scapegoating stems from envy (Navaro, in press; Hopper & Weinberg, Volume 4), the token of sacrifice is split into a "bad" object who is attacked and ultimately is banished, and into a "good" object who is killed and incorporated, at least symbolically, thus initiating a process of atonement (Cohen & Schermer, 2002; Maccoby, 1982). However, who and what are good or bad is rarely very clear, especially because some objects are both good and bad. For example, the objects and tokens of sacrifice might be envied for being too intelligent, for assuming that they do not need the natural protection offered by the foreskin, for believing that they are chosen people, or even for "being able to get away with it".

5.

Scapegoats are in general drawn from the ranks of singletons or isolates who lack affiliations to and protection from others. In the context of social category thinking and feeling, which is typical of Incohesion, those people and subgroups who are regarded as violating social boundaries, and even those who are regarded as "leaning" against them, are especially vulnerable to scapegoating processes. So, too, are those people and subgroups who cannot be and/or who refuse to be stereotyped in terms of particular social categories, for example, those who are characterised by status and class incongruence, those who cross social boundaries via immigration and emigration from one nation to another, via social mobility within any one nation, and via marriage between members of the main social categories of a particular society. The offspring of mixed-race partnerships are especially vulnerable, both because their offspring are not easily classified, and because they confirm that boundaries have been violated by their parents. (People who struggle with a sense of shame and guilt are likely to scapegoat themselves, which involves self-destructive collusion (Roth, 2018).) During times of socio-economic and political turmoil associated with unbridled competition for scarce resources, even one's neighbour can become a scapegoat.[2]

III. Scapegoating and Sibling Rivalry

1.

Scapegoating is often based on rivalry with siblings, which involves the wish to hurt and even to annihilate them (Hopper, 2003c; Volkan & Ast, 1997; Mitchell, 1974, 2013). The rationalisations for the denigration by older siblings of younger siblings include bad eating habits, poor personal hygiene, inability to speak clearly and properly, bad behaviour, ambiguous sexual and gender identities, and so on.

Older siblings associate their younger siblings with a variety of cute and cuddly small animals, such as squirrels and rabbits. However, they also associate them with a variety of dirty and smelly vermin, such as rats, and with stinging insects, such as wasps and hornets, who are not surprisingly yellow and brown in colour. Similarly, they love and protect some toys, but they treat others very badly. Although both sets of objects must be controlled, some can be tortured and eliminated, for example, as seen in the ways that children burn ants.

Younger siblings are sometimes associated with mice, which are a hybrid category of animal, halfway between rats, which can be dangerous, and, for example, hamsters, which can be childhood pets. Mice would seem to come in groups of three or more, and are characters in many fairy tales. Those who are paid to catch mice differ from those who are paid to catch rats. (Is this distinction relevant to understanding how psychoanalytical work differs from group analytical work?)

2.

Hurting and tormenting siblings of whom one is jealous and envious is also meant to hurt and torment those who have brought them into being in the first place, that is, their parents, which involves the desire for revenge and retaliation. This is based on a complex form of projective and introjective identification both with the parents, who are imagined to have beaten the siblings, and with the siblings themselves (Freud, 1919). Sibling are sometimes hated on behalf of parents, who comprise the Establishment of the family.

3.

It is almost impossible to distinguish siblings from particular people and their groupings within the society who are regarded as having been unjustly favoured, rewarded, and/or excused from fulfilling their obligations. This pertains to particular classes, ethnic groups, and races. Many of the words and images that are used by older siblings about younger siblings are identical to the words, images, and narratives that are used by dominant groupings about those who they wish to oppress, denigrate, and to exclude. For example, in Nazi Germany, Jews were described not only as vermin but also as viruses and parasites. They were a source of pathogens. Jews were denigrated in terms of poor hygiene and strange dietary practices, such as blood libel and the laws of kosher, as well as strange sexual practices, ranging from excessive and compulsive sexual activity to bisexual to homosexual object choices and transsexual identifications. Their malformed and distorted bodies made it impossible for them to perform military duties, to participate in athletics, and in general to become "real men" and "real women". They had kinky and curly hair, discoloured complexions, and excessively large noses (Gilman, 1991). The only way to protect the Arian race was to eliminate Jews.[3]

4.

In the context of rivalry with siblings expressed in rivalry among ethnic groups and new immigrants, the political Establishment of the contextual society is perceived to have failed to control immigration and/or to have given immigrants excessive financial support. This translates into taking revenge on the Establishment who has failed to uphold "law and order", to be indifferent towards "virtue", and to be guilty of rewarding sin. They might at least have tried birth control!

IV. Illustrations of Scapegoating in Clinical Group Analysis

In clinical work it is important to focus on the Oedipus complex and on phases of the development of it. Such processes must be understood in terms of both their vertical T and vertical CT-forms directed towards the conductor of the group, and in their horizontal t and horizontal ct-forms directed towards the members of the group (Hopper, 2006, 2007a, 2007b). These processes are almost always interrelated, and define what we regard as a "mental field". Moreover, these processes repeat the "Here and Now", the "Here and Then", the "There and Then", and the "There and Now" (Hopper, 2003a, 2018) in each sub-matrix of the tripartite matrix and in each dimension of them (Hopper, in press, Hopper & Weinberg, Volume 4).

The trauma of separation associated with the experience of the therapist taking a holiday break is virtually an archetypical source of a sense of failed dependency, betrayal, insult, and shame. The following case of "The Abusing Brother and Unprotective Parents" illustrates several aspects of this, especially with respect to scapegoating processes and sibling rivalry in the context of Incohesion.

1.

I informed this mature, twice weekly slow-open group that I would be taking a break for a couple of weeks. The group lapsed into a long silence marked by gaze avoidance. I commented on this aggregation a couple of times, referring to their "mutual isolation". They did not appreciate the irony of this observation.

The silence was broken by a woman who talked about having been a victim of sexual abuse during her childhood by her older brother, who was her mother's "favourite". She had been intending to tell us about this, but for some reason had avoided doing so. Although the abuse occurred about forty-five years ago, she now wanted to take the matter to the police, and had contacted a solicitor about doing so. The women in the group enthusiastically supported her wish to do this, and railed against the abusive power of men who could never be trusted. The men joined in this attack on unreliable men as though they were themselves excluded from this category of people.

I connected this attack on men in general to attacks on their particular fathers, brothers, and on me. I also commented that while telling us about her experience of abuse and her plans to take the matter to police, who were excluded from the category of "men", the woman seemed to have become sexually seductive and flirtatious. I wondered aloud why this was so.

The group again lapsed into silence. I suggested that the group's new silence followed my observation that the woman had become seductive and flirtatious, which had followed my comment that the group was avoiding making an attack on men and on me. I also suggested that the group seemed to be either in total agreement and solidarity with one another, or in total insolidarity and indifference to one another. Was their apparent agreement and solidarity based on being against me? Did they feel that my observation about the seductive and flirtatious behaviour of the patient who reported that she had been abused by her brother was tantamount to my abusing her? Did they feel that in the same way that her mother had not protected her from her older brother, they had failed to protect her from me?

Several people spoke up and more or less talked over one another. They asserted that first I had told them that I would be away, then I ignored what the abused and vulnerable patient had said, and then, in commenting that the woman had become sexually seductive and flirtatious, I had provoked unnecessary anxiety. In any case, they completely rejected my observations: not only had I got the sequence wrong, but they had not agreed with any of the steps of it, with the exception that I was uncaring and indifferent to them. The patient who had been abused argued that the group should "punish" me for my insensitive and intrusive comments. Another member asserted that actually I seemed to be an abusive older brother who was not really entitled to regard himself as a father, even an absent one. I asked what form she wanted this punishment to take.

Before she could answer this question, a member of the group, who was in training as a group analyst, suggested that although the process was driven by the patient with a history of abuse who also sought revenge, the issue of traumatic separation and failed dependency pertained not only to the group and to me but also to England and to Europe as a whole and their elected leaders. Another patient commented that all this could be understood in terms of people feeling badly let down by our Prime Minister and by the entire democratic political process, in the same way that I had so badly let down the group by going away for so long and without adequate preparation.

I said that whereas all this might be so, it seemed to me that it was being used as a way of getting away from the heat of anger towards me, and of avoiding going into it in a more personal way. It was an example of group analytical fundamentalism in the service of avoiding something that was very tough to chew. I said that it seemed to me that I was experienced as an unreliable father in whose absence all this could happen. It was father's fault that mother could become so enmeshed with her son, and the son could become so enmeshed with his sister.

The group was enacting several maternal functions all at the same time, and in a mashed up way. I suggested that the patient who had suffered sexual abuse when she was a child had "led" this pseudo-unanimity and pseudo-solidarity. She had become a spokesperson for this process. She had taken on a figuration of the roles of plaintiff, lawyer, jury and judge, not only on her own behalf, but also on behalf of abused children everywhere. She was becoming a kind of cheerleader for reparation and revenge, perhaps even a "leader" of those people who have been scapegoated but who now threatened to return (Hopper, 2022a). I was careful to say that my comments should not be taken to mean that I did not think that sexual abuse was a very serious matter or that her communications were "only fantasies".

The group argued that women were entitled to speak up for themselves, and that powerful men had to be held to account. I asked the group who they were arguing with or against. Who would disagree with their point of view? One woman said "Harvey Weinstein would disagree". Another said that she thought that the "casting couch" could be found in the consulting rooms of training analysts who had power over students who were applying to train as analysts. A man pointed out that there was a couch in my consulting room, and that there was some doubt whether I would support the application of a particular patient in the group who wanted to become a group analyst, and perhaps I was grooming her for some sort of quid pro quo.

I suggested that the group seemed to be devaluing the qualifications of the particular patient. I then said the group seemed to be blaming me for a multitude of sins, and for difficulties in their lives and in the group itself. Clearly, they felt that I had failed them in various ways. However, I asked what was the meaning of bringing "Harvey Weinstein" into our discussions? Was he a father, a brother, or merely a man? Did he have any particular personal and/or social characteristics that we might want to identify and discuss? I asked the group if they wanted to do to me what was being done to Weinstein?

3.

This vignette illustrates how in response to my announcement that I would be taking an untimely and a slightly longer break than usual, the group oscillated between the polar states of aggregation and massification, and how various members of the group personified the roles associated with Incohesion.

Although we did not take up various aspects of social category thinking and feeling, it is relevant that the group became preoccupied with matters of "gender", "ethnicity", and "nationality". However, the slow and steady emergence of material that was covered and disguised by various patterns of protection required careful, archaeological excavation in the sense of this classical metaphor. Ultimately, the group found a scapegoat whose sacrifice might help them maintain their illusion of massification. I was both an abusing brother and a neglectful father. The analysis of the (T)ransference was interwoven with the analysis of various (t)ransferences.

V. An Empirical Illustration of Some Aspects of Scapegoating in the Context of Incohesion in the Dynamic Matrix of a Demo Group in the Context of Both the Dynamic Matrix of the Organisation Which Sponsored the Conference and the Foundation Matrix of Its Contextual Society

The following vignette describes how as the leader of a "demo group" at an event at a group psychotherapy conference in 2017 in New York I was scapegoated in the context of the foundation matrix of the contextual society, the dynamic matrix of the organisation which sponsored the conference, and the dynamic matrix of the demo group itself. It is important to keep in mind the tripartite matrix of this group. It is also important to remember that as an American who lives in England, and as a psychoanalyst and a group analyst, which has come to be an anomaly, I was both an "outsider" and a "hybrid", and experienced as such.

The group began about fifty minutes later than scheduled. The chairman had not arranged the correct number of chairs for either the audience or the demonstration group. The two hotel technicians attached the electronic equipment to the bodies and clothes of each member of the group as in a somewhat rough and intrusive manner, at least in my opinion. This was awkward, if not actually difficult, for the women in the group, at least in my opinion. The group sat in silence and were somewhat impassive until these arrangements were completed. The two technicians were immigrants and "men of colour".

The group began by focusing on their commonalities and good feelings towards one another. They completely ignored me, both in their body language and in their refusal to take up any of my remarks. They seemed to feel hostile towards me. One after another member of the group took centre stage, seeming to want to engage with me but quickly turning to other members of the group. An Israeli woman said that she had some "leftover business" with me from another group. A gay man said that based on his experience with me in another group, he too had "a bone to pick" with me. A woman from a country in the Middle-East said that our being wired up reminded her of bombs and bombers.

I wondered aloud what was stopping the group from exploring how they differed from one another as well as their commonalities in interests, values, and motives for joining a demo group. This task would be closer to the advertised purposes of the event than to the massification of the group. This was characterised by an explicit denial of any negative feelings and thoughts towards one another and about their experience in the demo group. I suggested that they were in denial of their feelings about the social categories that were represented in the group, based on geographical regions, races, ethnicities, nationalities, genders, sexual orientations, and so on, which had been mentioned, but not taken up. Otherwise, why were they mentioned?

The group more or less ignored my remarks. I interpreted that their massification was driven by their need to deny and disavow their explosive fears that followed their experience of failed dependency on the organisation, the chairman of the event, and on me associated with the delayed and chaotic start of the group. However, the group would not take up any of this material, and I was treated as the obstacle to their sense of well-being.

In the post-mortem discussion I referred ironically to the technicians as "brothers". Consciously, I was attempting to convey several layers of meaning of the term, in the context of the foundation matrix, the dynamic matrix, and the personal matrices of the people involved: ethnic groups were "siblings"; the technicians were "brothers"; and the chairman of the event and I were often regarded as intellectual and professional "brothers". I also wanted to bring into the discussion the two panellists who were women.

In response to my "interpretation", it was loudly and almost violently asserted that not only was I an incomprehensible old-school psychoanalyst but also an old white male racist whose insensitive remarks had prevented the group from sharing a sense of their own virtue, goodness, values, and belief in racial equality, which they had felt and wanted to express. Led by a Caucasian "sister", many members of the audience walked out in protest against my use of the term "brothers", which they took to be my racially prejudiced attack on the hotel technicians.

I understood this to be an enactment of their view that I had scapegoated the two technicians, and, therefore, that if anyone should be scapegoated, it was me. I also understood this to be an enactment of a role reversal or role opposition, based on a kind of malignant mirroring, in which I was scapegoated as a defence against their taking responsibility for their own negative and aggressive wishes towards the technicians, the leaders, the panellists, and so on. I said that although I was sorry if I had inadvertently hurt anyone, the group's "virtue signalling" reflected the denial and repression of their own prejudices and hostilities towards various "minority" groups, such as Israelis, Palestinians, people of colour, Jews, immigrants, group analysts, and so on, who were represented in the demo group. These groupings were likely to be displacements from siblings, and that we were missing a chance to explore sibling rivalry. I stressed that this was also an enactment of the personal and interpersonal matrices of the people in the demo group, with some of whom I had personal histories of training experiences. It was also necessary for us to explore our relations with members of the wider audience, the dynamic matrix of the sponsoring organisation, and those of the foundation matrix of the contextual society. The enactment was a play within a play. I had in mind the Ur-themes of the great Greek tragedies in which perpetrators and victims were witnessed by a chorus. However, in the context of the United States as well as countries in the Middle-East, "brothers" also suggest the vicissitudes of continuous civil war (Berman, 2021).

During the subsequent months, in private conversations and correspondence, many colleagues suggested that although I may have been correct, I was naïve in thinking that at the present time in New York a demo group could work with these ideas in the context of the sponsoring organisation (Billow, 2018). However, the organisation continues to address these divisive issues, and to do so with conviction, in part as a result of this complex and disturbing event (Counselman, 2019). Although the leadership has become convinced that the organisation should be and should be seen to be both democratic and anti-racist, it is an open question whether the contextual and sponsoring organisation holds the professional values that are necessary in order to support and contain the process of collective self-reflection about unconscious personal and social processes, especially when they are fraught and saturated with conflicts that originate within the foundation matrix of the contextual society.

VI. A Brief Summary

In this chapter I have outlined my theory of the fourth basic assumption of Incohesion as a consequence of social trauma. As a defence against aggregation, massification is associated with and dependent on the development of fundamentalism and scapegoating. Scapegoating processes involve the projection of unwanted properties and qualities into a member of the group or subgroup who is then expelled from it, but this also involves many other specific forms of aggression. Envious scapegoating is a form of sacrifice that involves both love and hate, idealisation and denigration. Scapegoating is closely associated with unconscious sibling rivalry and rivalry among sibling-objects. These ideas were illustrated with clinical data from one of my twice weekly groups, and with empirical data from my own experience as a leader of a demo group. The data reflected the constraints and restraints of the tripartite matrix and each of its dimensions.

Notes

1 Scapegoating has been discussed extensively in several interrelated disciplines, for example field theory and systems thinking (Lewin, 1948), group dynamics (Cartwright & Zander, 1953), psychoanalytical group therapy (Scheidlinger, 1982), systems-centred group psychotherapy (Agazarian, 1997), group analysis (Hopper, 2003b, 2003c), the group analytic study of organizations (McCoy, 2012), systems centred group therapy (Finlay, Abernethy, & Garrels, 2016), cultural studies and philosophy (Girard, 1977, 1986; Cassirer, 1955), and Jungian Analytical Psychology Art Therapy (Schaverien, 1987).

2 The edict from Jesus to love one's neighbour as oneself presents a particular ethical and political problem, because if one does not really love oneself, one cannot really love one's neighbour, at least not very well. Or, to put this more precisely, if one hates oneself, one can only love one's neighbour in a perverse way, based on sadism as the eroticisation of hatred. In other words, perversion is rooted in what used to be called secondary narcissism, and secondary narcissism is rooted in traumatic experience, not only in random, idiosyncratic and personal traumatic experience but also in social trauma. In fact, social trauma might be especially disturbing, because both one's neighbour and oneself are likely to be damaged by it.

3 A bartender in New Orleans once used exactly the same language to explain to me why it was necessary to classify people in terms of the percentage of their ancestry which might be "Black": although certain men and women might look "exotic", even one drop of "Negro blood" would sooner or later have more extreme consequences. I have also been advised by a secular Jewish taxi driver during Passover in Tel Aviv not to go to a famous bakery in Jaffa: although the bread might taste good, the Arab bakers neither washed their hands after using the toilet nor ever cleaned their ovens. He did not want me to get sick.

References

Agazarian, Y. (1997). *Systems-Centered Therapy*. New York: Guilford Press.

Berman, A. (2021). Personal communication.

Billow, R. (2018). On deconstructive interventions. *International Journal of Group Psychotherapy*, 68, 3, 355–375.

Bion, W.R. (1957). Differentiation of the psychotic from the non-psychotic. *International Journal of Psychoanalysis*, 38, 206–275.

Bion, W.R. (1961). *Experiences in Groups and Other Papers*. London: Tavistock. Reprinted Hove: Brunner-Routledge, 2001.

Cartwright, D. & Zander, A. (Eds). (1953). *Groups Dynamics: Research and Theory*. Evanston, IL: Row.

Cassirer, E. (1955). *The Philosophy of Symbolic Forms*. New Haven, CT: Yale University Press.

Chasseguet-Smirgel, J. (1985). *Creativity and the Perversion*. London: Free Association Books.

Cohen, B. & Schermer, V. (2002). On scapegoating in therapy groups: A social constructivist and intersubjective outlook. *International Journal of Group Psychotherapy*, 52, 1, 89–109.

Counselman, E. (2019). Letter from the President of AGPA to its Members.

Erikson, E. (1968). *Identity, Youth and Crisis*. New York: Norton.

Finlay, L., Abernethy, A. & Garrels, S. (2016). Scapegoating in group therapy: Insights from Girard's Mimetic Theory. *International Journal of Group Psychotherapy*, 66, 2, 188–204.

Freud, S. (1919). A child is being beaten: A contribution to the study of the origin of sexual perversions. *International Journal of Psychoanalysis*, 1, 371–395.

Gilman, S. (1991). *The Jew's Body*. London: Routledge.

Girard, R. (1977). *Violence and the Sacred*. New York: Continuum (originally published in French in 1972).

Girard, R. (1986). *The Scapegoat*. Baltimore: John Hopkins University Press (original work published in 1982).

Hopper, E. (2003a). *The Social Unconscious: Selected Papers*. London: Jessica Kingsley.

Hopper, E. (2003b). *Traumatic Experience in the Unconscious Life of Groups*. London: Jessica Kingsley.

Hopper, E. (2003c). Aspects of aggression in large groups characterised by (ba) I:A/M. In Schneider, S. & Weinberg, H. (Eds) *The Large Group Re-visited: The Herd, Primal Horde, Crowds and Masses*. London: Jessica Kingsley.

Hopper, E. (2006). Theoretical and conceptual notes concerning transference and countertransference processes in groups and by groups, and the social unconscious: Part I.' *Group Analysis*, 39, 4, 549–559.

Hopper, E. (2007a). Theoretical and conceptual notes concerning transference and countertransference processes in groups and by groups, and the social unconscious: Part II.' *Group Analysis*, 40, 1, 21–34.

Hopper, E. (2007b). Theoretical and conceptual notes concerning transference and countertransference processes in groups and by groups, and the social unconscious: Part III.' *Group Analysis*, 40, 2, 285–300.

Hopper, E. (2018). "Notes" on the concept of the social unconscious in Group Analysis. *Group*, 42, 2, 99–118.

Hopper, E. (in press). "Notes" on processes of fundamentalism in the context of the basic assumption of Incohesion: Aggregation/Massification or (ba) I:A/M. In Ofer, G. & Berman, A. (Eds) *Tolerance – Coping with Painful Otherness: Psychoanalytic, Group Analytic and Organisational Perspectives*. London: Routledge.

Hopper, E. (2022b). "Notes" on the theory and concept of the fourth basic assumption in the unconscious life of groups and group-like social systems: Incohesion: Aggregation/Massification or (ba) I:A/M. In Penna, C. (Ed) *From Crowd Psychology to Large Groups: Investigations on the Social Unconscious*. London: Routledge.

Hopper, E. (2022a). From remorse to relational reparation: Mature hope. Communication, and community in our responses to social conflict and to the virus as a persecuting object. *Contexts, Issue 95, March.*

Hopper, E. (in press). The tripartite matrix in Foulkesian group analysis. In Hopper, E. & Weinberg, H. (Eds) *The Social Unconscious in Persons, Groups and Societies. Volume 4*. London: Routledge.

Kierkegaard, S. (1846). *Two Ages: A Literary Review.*

Lewin, K. (1948). *Resolving Social Conflicts*. New York: Harper & Row.

Maccoby, H. (1982). *The Sacred Executioner*. London: Thames & Hudson.

McCoy, E. (2012). A study of trauma and scapegoating in the context of incohesion: An example from the oil industry. In Hopper, E. (Ed) *Trauma and Organisations*. London: Karnac.

Michell, J. (2013). The law of the mother: Sibling trauma and the brotherhood of war. *Canadian Journal of Psychoanalysis*, 21, 1, 145–159.

Mitchell, J. (1974). *Psychoanalysis and Feminism: Freud, Reich, Laing and Women*. New York: Pantheon Books. Reprinted in 2000 in New York by Basic Books.

Money-Kyrle, R. (1929). *The Meaning of Sacrifice*. London: Hogart Press and the Institute of Psychoanalysis.

Navaro, L. (in press). Fear of envy, dispossession and scapegoating – The evil eye. In Hopper, E. & Weinberg, H. (Eds) *The Social Unconscious in Persons, Groups and Societies. Volume 4*. London: Routledge.

Nietzsche, F. (1887) *On the Genealogy of Morals*. Translated and edited in 1996 by Oxford: World's Classics.

Ranulf, S. (1964). *Moral Indignation and Middle Class Psychology: A Sociological Study*. New York: Schocken Books.

Roth, B. (2018). *A Group Analytic Approach to Understanding Mass Violence: The Holocaust, Group Hallucinosis and False Beliefs*. London: Routledge.

Schaverien, J. (1987). The scapegoat and the talisman: Transference in art therapy. In Schaverien et al. (Eds) *Images of Art Therapy*. London: Routledge.

Scheidlinger, S. (1982). On scapegoating in group psychotherapy. *International Journal of Group Psychotherapy*, 32, 131–143.

Scheler, M. (1933). *L'Homme du Ressentiment*. Paris: Les Editions Gallimard.

Volkan, V. & Ast, G. (1997). *Siblings in the Unconscious and Psychopathology*. Madison, CT: International Universities Press.

2.4 Sibling witnessing in analytic group therapy

Ella Stolper

"I had a dream about our group last night", said Rina, a woman in her forties whose youngest son died from cancer. "And in my dream", she continued in a deep voice, without looking at any of the group members directly,

> we were all sitting in this room in a circle, when suddenly a little boy, named Ben, entered. He is an unruly boy, who can't sit still like other children. Every few minutes, he gets up and wanders around the classroom and doesn't listen to instructions. In the dream, I'm very angry with you, I know that he is a complete mismatch for our group and I don't understand why you brought him here. I want to tell you this, but I can't get a word out of my mouth. Then, I notice that Natalie is angry with you, too, and it makes me feel stronger, like maybe this time I could have the courage to express my criticism directly and speak up about things I have kept inside for years. You, the conductor, spoil the group for me by bringing this new kid, jeopardizing the one place where I can really speak. For the first time, I'm seriously considering leaving the group. We can't both be here – it's either him or me.

This dream was presented in the beginning of a group session that took place four months after the arrival of two new group participants, Natalie and Avi, to a group that had been in the midst of its fifth year. During the silence that prevailed in reaction to this dream, I suddenly remembered the moment in which my firstborn son realized that his baby brother was going to stay with us for good. He walked toward me decisively and demanded that we return the baby to the hospital, "where he was born and where he belongs!", he said angrily. When he heard my explanation that his brother is our child, too, and that our home is his home, his face fell and he burst out crying.

Does the arrival of new participants cause the group members pain similar to that which was experienced by my firstborn son when his brother was born? I wondered to myself. Was I insensitive to invite two new participants at once, when one of them immediately started challenging the group order?

Natalie broke the silence in the room: "Rina, I think that I understand why you dreamt of this boy. Only two weeks ago, you said that you miss dreaming

DOI: 10.4324/9781003220060-16

of your son who died. You said how unruly he had been and how much you miss him".

"Rina, did you notice that in your dream, you were angry with the conductor?", said Hadas, "In real life, you're never angry with her".

Rina: "That's true, I really did manage to be angry with the conductor, but it was possible only thanks to Natalie, who had been angry with the conductor in the dream. I wouldn't have dared to be angry alone".

Avi (the new participant who came to this session after a three-week-long absence):

> I didn't think that my presence had been such a threat for you, Rina. I realize that I am the "Ben" in your dream. Natalie and Hadas also said that they have a difficult time with me because I travel and leave the group immediately after we have an intimate session. I'm not sure that that's always true, sometimes it's just circumstances.

Yael turned to Avi and said to him vigorously: "This behavior of yours really is annoying, you come and go as if we're a train station and not a therapeutic group".

"I've stopped paying attention to Avi," Maya said to Yael, "If he doesn't care about us, why should we care about him? As far as I'm concerned, he's an empty chair".

I saw the growing anger with Avi and the attack on his lack of commitment and devotion to the process. I thought about defending him, but this time decided to wait. In the past, my protection did not only not help but elicited more aggression toward him for receiving special treatment from me. "Trust the process", I thought to myself, remembering Foulkes's (1948) words, which helped me to stick to silence as a group intervention. Foulkes called the group a "social microcosmos" in which one can revisit and cope with issues of vulnerability, deviation from the norm, and achieve reparation. He believed that the group co-creates the matrix in which each individual establishes his own personal identity and unique subjectivity. According to Foulkes, "the basic law of group dynamics", states that "the deepest reason why group patients can reinforce each other's normal reactions is that collectively they constitute the very Norm, from which, individually, they deviate" (Foulkes, 1948, p. 29). Therefore, the group is a setting that, among other things, recreates traumatic and victimized experiences in its dynamic matrix (Foulkes, 1957) and constitutes an alternative space in which "relationship disorders" (Friedman, 2013) are expressed, but it also creates the most effective ground for their reparation.

Still, I was terrified that the group would turn on Avi and sacrifice him for all the abandonment and injustice it had experienced in the past. What about Avi made him so intolerable for the group? Would I, too, have preferred that he left the group? During my silence, I examined my own feelings.

The air in the room became thick just before Omer started talking.

Omer, who until that point used to fall asleep every time a confrontation evolved between Avi and the group, called out: "Are you serious? Why are you turning all against him? Avi, what made you think that you were the boy in Rina's dream? I'm not at all sure that that was about you!"

"Omer", Hadas called out, "How can't you see that Avi is the 'misbehaving boy' in Rina's dream?! His absences and his lack of commitment to the group hurt us all".

Natalie, who hasn't looked at Avi from the beginning of the session, joined the discussion: "I don't understand you, Omer, how can you defend him? He does whatever he wants around here, without thinking of anyone else".

Omer:

> Natalie, you're attacking Avi. Actually, not just you, all of you are. Like he is the only one here who has been abandoned. You're making me so angry! What do you mean, Hadas, when you say that "Avi *really* is the misbehaving boy??" I, too, had left the group and disappeared for three months. I didn't even come here to explain to you guys what had happened to me, and I could not have imagined how much I had hurt you all, and you turn all your anger only at Avi. It's not fair!

In that moment, in which Omer rose against the group's attack on Avi, defending him with his own body and testifying of the injustice the group did to him, at the risk of rejection, it felt to me as though the spell we have all been under has dissolved. Omer awoke himself and the group and stopped Avi's scapegoating. Through this act of "sibling witnessing" in the group "here and now", he stopped the projection of rejected parts onto Avi and led participants to share responsibility for abandonment and aggression.

Based on Bromberg's (2011) view on the patient–therapist relationship in psychoanalysis, one can conclude that participants' trauma, as pathological as it may be, would present itself on the stage of group relationships, thus providing a rare opportunity to build emotional resilience and reparation. Berger argues that the witnessing of such reparation in the group matrix builds an experience of meaning and resilience and significantly decreases feelings of exclusion, rejection, and loneliness, when the process of "talking it out" constitutes a part of the participants' struggle to become realer and more visible and present people in their lives (Berger, 2017).

We might say, then, that for Avi, Omer's behavior served as "witnessing". What is that witnessing? What is witnessing in a therapeutic group, really, and how is it different from witnessing in individual therapy? This chapter will address these issues.

Psychological trauma and its implications

Psychological trauma is damage that is caused to the psyche by a single or recurring event in the individual's life. It puts him in a state of shock, in which he is unable to cope with the situation and with his feelings. "What happened – did not happen": Berger (2017) stresses that traumatic experience is often experienced as an attack on sanity. She argues that unvalidated and unconfirmed factual reality may receive a quality of "unreality". It is as if it is erased from the recording of the events that "did happen", both in the internal world and in the external reality. This state of "non-recognition" and "unknowing" becomes a ghost-like experience, in which personal and collective events turn into a "non-presence" and even to "nonexistence". Berger argues that this state defiles the individual's psychological existence, confuses him, freezes traumatic areas in his psyche, and may eventually weaken his ability to survive.

"Unwitnessed trauma" continues to resonate in the individual's body and to sneak into reality unconsciously due to the lack of voice or expression during or after the event (Laub, 2008). "The mumbling symptom" (Foulkes and Anthony, 1957) brings to the room unconscious materials through stubborn repetitive behavior, pattern, or phrase – that don't seem to have any special meaning in the real, concrete world – but in the consulting room, they consistently mark the trauma or injury that still cannot be verbalized or mentalized.

Witnessing in psychoanalytic therapy

Witnessing in therapy, as opposed to legal witness testimony – which is a passive action performed from an observer or hearsay position – is an active, vital, and intersubjective action that involves both patient and therapist. According to Berger (2017), witnessing is a vital part of the therapeutic process, one that provides validation, confirmation, and recognition of both external reality and one's subjectivity; psychological witnessing is a vital part of mutual recognition, since it involves the responsibility to tell the truth and the willingness to face its consequences.

Berman (2017) describes the dynamics of witnessing in psychoanalytic therapy and argues that it follows a clear order of actions. He believes that in post-traumatic "self-states", it is essential that the therapist first establish his position as a "sympathetic witness", before expressing any form of "otherness", and that after such expressions, he should return to the initial position of "sympathetic witnessing". In other words, Berman suggests that the therapist should first establish concordant identification, before moving to complementary identification, and return to it after expressions of otherness in the relationship.

Witnessing in analytic group therapy

Berman (2017) believes that the group can create a temporary collective or society of sympathetic witnesses. He believes that at first, a group member who sees himself as a victim is accepted by the group members who support and protect him and show compassion to his condition. However, in later stages, that member begins to face other reactions. He eventually meets the "otherness" of the group, which is sometimes experienced as painful and frustrating.

Berman argues that there is an order to the witnessing process in a group, in the beginning of the group life. Empathy and identification with the victim's pain are the first to emerge, and only in later stages, the encounter with "otherness" becomes possible. I disagree with Berman's view of witnessing in the group space as an organized mechanism. I believe that, as opposed to individual therapy, one of the unique characteristics of group therapy is the multiple simultaneous identifications that do not necessarily emerge according to the stages of group development. I believe that the group allows one to experience concordant and complementary identifications simultaneously, whereas therapists' witnessing in individual therapy tends to oscillate from concordant to complementary identification. I posit that this situation provides conditions that are less secure for working with traumatic experiences, as opposed to individual therapy, or as Berman (2015) defined it, "the group is a semi-secure space" (Berman, 2008). Still, this process allows reviving and reliving difficult events in the group hall of mirrors, when each participant has a clear role in the re-enacted drama, while offering an opportunity to discover and experience new reparative experience. This process requires courage and changing of past patterns, and thus allows a curative process for both protagonist and participants.

In this context, it is important to emphasize another phenomenon that is unique to group therapy. Witnessing in therapeutic groups offers a unique opportunity to "witness the witnessing of the other" and thus turns witnessing into a public and shared process. This position allows the group members, according to Celan (2001), to "witness the witness", a situation that, of course, is impossible in individual psychoanalytic therapy. This opportunity allows one to emerge from stagnation and to overcome dissociative barriers that the trauma had left in the psyche, thus motivating new movement in which the witnessing of other witnesses increases the effect of the resonance of traumatic experiences and further validates the testimony.

Similarly to Foulkes's (1948) view, Hoffman argues that occurrences in therapy do not necessarily constitute transference of participants' past relationships. He argues that reality is structured by the dyad and is not only a repetition. This idea applies to both transference and countertransference. Hoffman believes that both of these processes are not one-directional repetitions but mutual influences related to a unique encounter of two subjects.

Hence, the injustices in the group result from past repetitions, as well as from a "new situation" that is created in the meeting of different subjects. Participants' witnessing of both past and present restores the individual's hope and faith in caring and "basic humanity" and increases feelings of recognition and belonging. However, we know that destructive, anti-group forces are also active in psychoanalytic groups, threatening to take the group apart; these forces can attack the individual in the midst of his sharing, as part of the repetition of traumatic experience (Nitsun, 1996). As Mitchell argued, if we want to be a part of the solution, we have to agree to be a part of the problem; thus, we enact it in the therapeutic relationship (Mitchell, 1997).

I believe that this condition, in which the group serves as means to relive and repeat past experience, a state in which constructive and destructive forces are both active, the group members' witnessing is of special importance to the curative and reparative processes of the individual. I call this form of witnessing "sibling witnessing", to note its special characteristics that distinguish it from witnessing in individual psychoanalytic therapy, as I will now describe.

Sibling witnessing

"Sibling witnessing" is witnessing that is expressed publicly by the "group siblings" regarding injustices that occur in the group "here and now", both as reparation of the patient's past experiences and as witnessing of injustices that take place in a "new situation", in the unique encounter of different subjects.

The word "sibling" refers to one of few offspring who share one or two parents. It is used in social sciences, medicine (for example, to refer to siblings who share the same sperm donor), biology (in the studying of animal behavior), and so on. (Derived from the academy website.)

In the context of this chapter, I use the word "sibling" to refer to horizontal relationships between the participants of a specific group.

Sibling witnessing has two unique characteristics that distinguish it from witnessing in individual psychoanalytic psychotherapy. The first is that witnessing is offered regarding injustice or wrongdoing in the group "here and now", and it occurs publicly, in the presence of "real others". This publicness serves two functions at the same time. One is the "witnessing of witnessing", that is, the witness witnesses other witnesses, and the second function allows witnesses a multiplicity of voices. The diverse voices that witness trauma from different perspectives provide, in my view, a "multifaceted" reparative experience of past experiences in areas in which the trauma has not been witnessed.

I believe that the witnessing group members offer to each other is perceived as more "experience-near" to the protagonist's authentic experience, since their relationship is one of "group equals", and it is sometimes even more powerful due to the lack of a financial aspect to their relationship. For example, in his many studies of groups, Yalom discovered that the group members' words to each other were remembered as more constitutive moments than the conductor's words (Yalom, 2006). It is understandable since participants' words are probably perceived as more neutral, since they do not derive from the "conductor's" role but are provided as part of participants' free flow of associations.

The second characteristic of sibling witnessing is that this witnessing takes place as protest against authority figures, other group members, or against the group as a whole in the past, present, or both. Such sibling witnessing demands a courageous action on the part of the witness, who is required to rise against the occurrences in the group reality, express his voice, and offer his testimony despite the risk and price involved. Thus, sibling witnessing in the group not only allows recognition of wrongdoings and confirmation and validation of injustices that have occurred but necessarily involves transition from a passive listener stance to a "live presence" (Alvarez, 2005) facing the symbolic group "siblings", and thus involves a risk to the witness's own status.

Back to the aforementioned session

Following Omer's words, I said to the group:

> "Ben" in Rina's dream can represent any of the group members for each one of us, here. He represents fears and parts that we don't want to see in ourselves and prefer to get rid of, this time, by rejecting Avi and kicking him out of the group circle. Omer, you have risked yourself to defend Avi and thus allowed all of us to connect to areas that we tried not to face.

"It's true", Hadas said quietly.

> Omer, until you mentioned it, I didn't remember your abandonment. I was angry only with Avi. I couldn't face what you, Avi, represent for me, which is avoidance of intimacy, deviancy, and loneliness. I felt like I couldn't "digest" you, but actually I could not accept our resemblance. I wanted you to disappear. I could see how you sabotage relationships, how you reject others or run away when people try to come closer. I'm just like you, I don't let anyone in or near, but it's easier to hate that about you.

Rina continued Hadas's words and said to Avi:

> you really are that boy in my dream. Your presence is difficult for me because of the attention you draw from the conductor and group, just like my younger brother, who gets all the support from my parents because he cannot stay out of trouble throughout his whole life. But now I realize that I, too, want to have such support and attention. I want to know how to speak up in the group, instead of waiting for others to ask me. You always say that you're intimidated by others, like I am, but in the group you're not afraid of fighting and saying what's on your mind, and I'm paralyzed even by watching that. I'm simply jealous of you.

Discussion

Rina's dream revealed an important group theme related to experiences of rejection, abandonment, and jealousy in the group. In the beginning of the session, the participants attacked Avi and grouped against him. They tried to get rid of him, along with all that he represented for them, all that they could not tolerate in their encounter with themselves in a relationship. Omer's standing up against the group was a constitutive moment, one that, in my view, demonstrates sibling witnessing in a group.

This mobilization of dormant and paralyzed areas of the psyche does not only save the witness who gives his testimony before the group – using words or through the traumatic repetition – but saves all the participants in the current scene, in which victims are no longer sacrificed on the altar of repression.

In the subsequent sessions, Omer, who used to "fall asleep" every time the group attacked Avi for his deviations, said that he experienced similar paralysis when his parents kicked his sister out of their house because of her extrovert, rebellious, and deviant behavior. He said that he did nothing to stop them and said nothing to her defense. Two years after she was kicked out of their house, his sister started doing drugs and their relationship cut off for good.

"I was there and I chose not to see it", Omer said about a month after the session in which he defended Avi.

> I didn't try to do anything, I didn't realize the danger she was in, and I didn't rise to protect her from my parents. They sent her to a sure death and I was a silent witness. To this very day, I'm ashamed of my silence and I cannot find peace. Here, too, I dissociated and fell asleep when you all tried to kick Avi out from the group. Here, too, I remained outside the situation until I couldn't take it anymore. . . . Now, I'm no longer willing to stay silent.

Omer rose against the group to protect Avi from becoming a group scapegoat and being rejected by the group, and, in that action, he emerged from the paralysis and passivity Avi's situation had put him in, which resembled the paralysis he had experienced in the past regarding his sister. While Omer was not the one who kicked his sister out of their house, his passive position and inaction made him feel guilty for abandoning her, guilt that persisted many years later.

Avi was a single 50-year-old man, who hasn't had an intimate relationship for many years and avoided social interaction in general. He described consistent experiences of rejection by his family, his alienated relationship with his mother, and the complete breaking off of his relationships with his siblings in a monotonous, detached tone. "She cancels on me without caring at all, and every time I try to engage, she makes me feel like I don't belong in the family", he told in a cold voice.

It seems that in the group, Avi repeated his mother's patterns by canceling and being absent from sessions every time the group members engaged with him. As long as he managed to remain emotionally distant from the participants, he would come regularly, but in moments in which his shield cracked and group members' words penetrated his external envelope, he would run away and disappear. I understood this as intense fear of intimacy due to his fear of getting hurt in intimate relationships given his life story, and as an act of identification with the aggressor, as part of which he enacted in the group the role of his abandoning mother, and experienced rejection through the participants' reactions in a painful role reversal. Avi desperately sought the participants' witnessing of the severe rejection he experienced from his mother throughout his life, but instead, enacted that rejection repeatedly by disappearing in reaction to participants' engagement with him.

Until Omer rose against the group, the group itself became the "rejecting mother" and thus recreated Avi's family situation, which became intolerable due to the long period he occupied the role of the rejected. The group experienced my defending of Avi in two ways: as protection of the weak who cannot take care of himself (a child) and, alternately, as my favoring him over the others (the favorite child) – which aroused in them feelings of jealousy and rage at him.

All my previous attempts to make the group share responsibility for the occurrences and interpret the attack on Avi as a desire to sacrifice him due to a wish to project onto him their intolerable parts of "self" failed. However, Omer's rising to Avi's defense and testimony on his behalf in the group "here and now" led to a shift: Omer chose to rise against the group position; it was as if he rose against the mother who rejected Avi or who, in his history, rejected his sister. He was no longer willing to shut his eyes and cooperate with the injustice that was happening. In this act, Omer recognized the injustice Avi had experienced in the group, while taking on himself the risk involved in rising against a group consensus that sees Avi as a "problematic, deviant boy" that needs to be expelled.

In this act, Omer protected Avi from the group's attack and asked himself and others to take personal responsibility and own their projected materials. In the session I have described, Avi reexperienced a traumatic experience of family rejection, but this time there was an opportunity to create an alternate reality in which "sibling witnessing" allowed siblings to protect each other. Later in that session, Avi stopped being aggressive. His body language relaxed, the tone of his voice softened, and it seemed that he was letting himself be soothed in the group matrix that created for him a new experience of "sibling witnessing".

People tend to unconsciously re-enact relationships, mostly traumatic ones, that originally occurred in a different time and place (Hopper, 2003). The vignettes described in this chapter show a process in which the group as a whole and each of its members relived traumatic past experiences and got caught in their intense fear of rejection. The desire to belong and to be included is, without a doubt, one of our deepest wishes and drives, and it is closely tied with rejection, exclusion, and abandonment anxieties, so that the very definition of belongingness necessarily includes in it those who do not belong.

The discussion of the vignette demonstrates a process in which the group freed itself from a position that sacrifices its members as "scapegoats" using the "sibling witnessing" group function. As one can see, sibling witnessing is an active act, and the witness (another group member) is required to choose it even at the cost of self-risk, as Omer chose in the session. I would like to argue that the witnessing process in groups is "semi-controlled", since reactions to group occurrences arise spontaneously and unconsciously. In addition, the sibling witnessing function is not gradual, as in individual therapy, and it involves witnessing that results from multiple simultaneous identifications, as opposed to the alternate identifications of individual therapy. This state of affairs makes the group a "semi-secure" space (Berman, 2015) and requires special alertness from the group therapist, due to the multiple roles that are unconsciously "enacted" in the drama that is being relived in the group.

Whereas in individual therapy the therapist has more control of the pace in which he reveals his otherness, which is impossible in group therapy, in the analytic group, some participants express otherness and some express identification with victimized self-states or with witnessing states; in other words, witnessing meets otherness as well as concordant identification.

In conclusion, this chapter showed how the therapeutic group holds the "aggressor-victim" drama along with the protagonist when all participants play a role in the enacted drama. The repetition involves destructive processes that constitute an inseparable part of the group reality. The group creates a situation in which the protagonist's trauma is repeated in the group "here and now" and other participants play active roles in it. These roles are not strange to the participants; they are "played" in accordance with their own personal experiences of trauma and victimhood. Therefore, when the group "succeeds" in sacrificing its "scapegoat", all the group members suffer from this action: they all realize that they can be the next in turn and this realization undermines their trust and security. In contrast, sibling witnessing is an ethical position that not only recognizes injustices and validates past wrongdoings, but necessarily involves stepping out from a passive listener's position towards a "live presence" (Alvarez, 2005) that rises against present injustices. Sibling witnessing is an expression of one's psychological development through the relationship with the siblings and not necessarily with authority figures. This position of "I am my brother's keeper" regarding the authority or other participants, from a position of "symbolic group siblings" and at the risk of endangering the witness's own status, constitutes an "Act of Freedom" (Symington, 1983) for all the group participants.

References

Alvarez, A. (2005). *Live presence.* Translated by Ella Golan. Israel: Bookworm (In Hebrew).

Berger, M. (2017). 'Thy brother's keeper': Witnessing as a moral presence in group analysis and beyond. A response to Farhad Dalal's Foulkes lecture. *Group Analysis*, 45(4): 459–471.

Berman, A. (2015). *What is the group entity in group therapy: Group analytic therapy in the land of milk and honey.* Israel: Kiryat Bialik-Ach (In Hebrew).

Berman, A. (2017). *Post-traumatic victimhood: A therapeutic-psychoanalytic perspective. Victimhood, vengefulness and the culture of forgiveness.* Israel: Kiryat Bialik-Ach (In Hebrew).

Bromberg, P.M. (2011). *Awakening the dreamer.* New York: Routledge.

Celan, P. (2001). *Selected poems and prose.* Translated by John Felstiner. New York: Norton and Company.

Foulkes, S.H. (1948). *Introduction to Group Analysis.* London: Karnac; New York: W.W. Norton.

Foulkes, S.H. & Antony, E.J. (1957). *Group psychoterapy: The psychoanalytic approach.* London: Maresfield Reprints.

Friedman, R. (2013). Individual or group therapy? Indications for optimal therapy. *Group Analysis*, 46: 164–170.

Hooper, E. (2003). *The social unconscious.* London: Jessica Kingsley Publishers.

Laub, D. (2008). *"Testimony". Crises of witnessing in literature, psychoanalysis and history.* Israel: Tel-Aviv (In Hebrew).

Mitchell, S.A. (1997). *Influence and autonomy in psychoanalysis.* Hillsdale, NJ: Analytic Press.

Nitsun, M. (1996). *The anti-group. Destructive forces in the group and their creative potential.* London: Routledge.

Symington, N. (1983). Act of freedom. *International Review of Psyho Analysis*, 10: 283–291.

Yalom, I. & Lescz, M. (2006). *Group therapy: Theory and practice.* Jerusalem: Kineret & Magnes (In Hebrew).

2.5 Healing traumatic scars

New sibling relationships in therapeutic settings

Ivan Urlić

"The unconscious is homeland, the consciousness is exile."

(*E. Cioran* p. 110)

1. Introduction

In this chapter I will take into consideration the manifold aspects of human traumatic experiences. They appear on conscious and unconscious levels since the beginning of one's existence, perhaps even before that. These experiences stimulate looking for a secure base and for the establishment of trustful relationships. In that frame of reference the importance of the quality of attachment, and even more of attunement of the relationship between mother/motherly environment and a child, is of fundamental importance and value. There resides the basic element of survival and further development. The psychoanalytic elaborations of the features of the early phases of these experiences are essential for the understanding of lifelong shaping of styles of living and reacting. The regulation of these processes is shaped by the vertical law of the father and the horizontal law of the mother, according to the traditional views on parental roles and family ties.

On that developmental line, according to Juliet Mitchell (2013, 2017), one of the most important elements is the human prohibition of violence and incest in the frame of reference of the law of the mother, which forbids the murderous wishes of the small child, especially towards his/her siblings. From one side, the law of the mother is perceived as directed towards some wounds and damaging perceptions and feelings that can be revived in certain new traumatic circumstances. Their long shadows can reappear in life and, if unconscious, influence on psychic well-balanced functioning in a decompensating way, stimulating inappropriate aggressive feelings and reactions.

Having in mind the law of the mother, the group leader/conductor can modify his/her interventions during the group process, enabling not only conscious traumatic experiences to be elaborated, but even the repetition of the unconscious traumatic experiences to enter consciousness of them and to be worked through. The horizontal axis of the law of the mother, with its prohibition of

DOI: 10.4324/9781003220060-17

violent behaviour and incest between siblings, can enable development of the reparative work of mourning (Mitchell, 2013; Berman, in this book). Thus liberated mental features and energy could then be redirected towards sublimation and the new creativity. In that way, mutual empathic encounters in the therapeutic groups, identifications and counter-identifications in action creating the richer matrix and liberating experiences, bring the law of the mother to its most valuable position in uncovering traumatic experiences during the psychotherapeutic process, especially in the frame of reference of group analysis.

In psychotherapy (individual and group) people come with their wounds and scars from more or less dysfunctional families and relationships. That represents the main source of relations disorders (Friedman, 2004), which are at a basis of the person's vulnerability, mostly even throughout life. This vulnerability requires protection and a sense of security. In particular, I will first look at this vulnerability that one carries within oneself despite the forbidden violence in relationships.

2. On being alone as one of the sources of vulnerability

During the course of life we are constantly stimulated by the myriad of impulses, but only some leave deep traces in our mind, influencing and changing our mindset (Urlić, 2012). One of these moments in my experience was the world science and technology exposition in Tsukuba, Japan, in 1985. There I was confronted with three technological advancements that were symbolising the new scientific achievements that will represent the basic directions that will influence human life at the threshold of the new millennium. One of them was the huge wall where the foetus was presented in the mother's womb at the beginning of the last month of pregnancy. Using MRI the human foetus was presented strengthening his fists leaving the thumb free and pushing the thumb into the mouth. After 10–20 seconds the cheek muscles started to contract and after taking the thumb out of the mouth the foetus was expulsing the amniotic fluid. After 20–30 seconds the whole activity was repeated. Being free-floating in the amniotic fluid, after some time the foetus was changing his position, but the exercise of thumb–mouth continued incessantly. My fascination with that insight into the living ambience of the physical mother–child symbiosis was enormous. The child was preparing for the first and most important activity immediately after birth – nipple sucking.

The other two exhibits were the artificial cultivation of plants that through addition of hormones and nutritional compounds it was possible to regulate the growing speed of plants, and one piano that was playing without musician in a virtuoso style. The message was clearly predictive: science was preparing our future in a spectacular way, creating new possibilities in researching roots and functioning of the human organism, modifying the life generally and predicting the future life intertwined with robotisation. Confronted with these achievements I was leaving EXPO fascinated by the new world dominated by technological achievements. My emotions were left in turmoil. The world of emotions and human relationships was left in a shadow of the technology. However, at the same time was it the announcement that for traditional closeness and warmth in relationships the space will be more and more restricted?

Ten years later there was the IAGP congress in Buenos Aires. It started with the rite of Pachamama performed by three Native Americans. They, as special guests of the congress, could enter freely in any part of the congress activity. The last morning, sitting with many other participants that were asking the older Native American from the Andes different questions, I asked him for his impressions while assisting our congress. Pleased to encounter that kind of interest he answered that he was an illiterate person coming from his tribe. In his childhood there were no schools. But, he was very curious; he was listening to what the elders were talking about, was looking at the animals, nature, stars, winds, light, . . . and these were his teachers: his natural environment. Listening to very knowledgeable people from the whole world talking about mostly such simple topics that anyone in his village would know to answer, he was astonished why such simple everyday expressions of life that are going on in front of everyone's senses were discussed.

Regarding the question of siblings, as puppies in the nest siblings are fighting for favors, care and protection. That is the source of rivalries and the fight for survival, not only physical but spiritual as well. Not all progeny units develop self-awareness, self-confidence and pervasiveness to fight for their way in life. The law of the mother introduces the equilibrium in these inborn instincts with forbidding killing and incest, the elimination of the competitor, the harmonisation of relationships and distribution in general. In that sense, by fading role of the father's law in the family in contemporary society, the role of the law of the mother is gaining in importance.

As the threshold of the new millennium started to show that the gap between rational and emotional sides in human beings had to be taken into consideration time and time again, it was something like human destiny that should be elaborated much more in depth. Obviously, the era of wars as means of regulating human interests and controversies was, generally speaking, overcome – at least insofar as in a traditional way. Human aggression, violent impulses, disrespectful behaviour will have to be reconsidered in the perspective of threats to planet Earth globally, and down to the private worlds of each individual, be they external or internal in nature.

Stretched between two poles that represent one of the main sources of human vulnerability, these dilemmas are accompanying human beings since birth.

The Romanian–French philosopher E. Cioran was writing on misfortune of being born: "When we were born, we lost as much as we will lose when we will die. Everything"(2013, p. 54). Working as psychiatrist, group analyst, psychoanalytic psychotherapist and in forensic psychiatry I could hear parents being shocked by the curses of their children on why they brought them into this world, and vice versa. These members of the new generation, "millennials", usually male but not only, were abandoning themselves to misuse of alcohol, drugs, or gambling and promiscuity. Thinking about great vulnerability and feelings of uncertainty and fear, and following the understanding of very accurate scientists regarding our first steps in life, it is obvious that along these developmental lines there are unlimited possibilities of damage, arrest or distortion of the further maturational processes to occur.

Winnicott (1976) writes that there is nothing new about the idea of a journey from dependence to independence. Each human being must start on that journey, and many arrive somewhere not far from this destination, and arrive at independence with a built-in social sense. In that sense the newborn starting from absolute dependence through relative dependence makes his/her way towards independence, which is never absolute. "The healthy individual does not become isolated, but becomes related to the environment in such a way that the individual and the environment can be said to be interdependent" (p. 84).

There are scientists who think that human vulnerability is due to the fact that we enter this world much too early (Laplanche, Pontalis, 1973), as the most immature creatures in the living world. The accurate observers of beginning of life like M. Klein posited the foundations of human life in the first six months after birth, dividing that period in two positions, paranoid-schizoid and depressive. The neo-Kleinians extended the exchange of these positions along the whole life course, that evoke the high and low tides of the sea, day and night, and so on, the everlasting change requesting continuous adaptation.

To better understand the first and decisive developmental phases of a child M. Mahler, Pine, Bergman (1975), studying symbiotic features and differentiation processes from the phenomenological side, described (1) the phase of normal autism (first month of life), (2) the phase of normal symbiosis (further 4–5 months) and (3) the third phase of separation – individuation (ending by the end of the third year of life). It is subdivided in sub-phases of differentiating ("cuing"), practicing ("hatching"), rapprochement (characterised by fear of loss of object and love, and castration anxiety, crisis of approaching, prototype of the everlasting fight against fusion or isolation), and subphase towards object constancy. The basic assumption is that the biological and psychological birth of a person don't coincide in time. The biological birth is a well-defined event, while psychological birth is an intrapsychic process that is slowly evolving. In that way the human development and maturation is evolving, changing phases until certain maturation is attained. On that way the horizontal and the vertical axes intersect on different levels affecting individual experience, a specific substance that represents the context that explains the facts of one's own time. Writing about challenges of the uncertainties along the developmental line I expressed the belief that it might be possible to find a shelter in sincere exchanges with interlocutors, near or distant, thinking on general interest where each person represents a node of the web of relationships according to Foulkes's group-analytic theory. But, with the development of globalisation, this question didn't become less complex (Urlić, 2011).

3. On being reduced to loneliness: accumulation of the traumatic experiences

Suggesting that one of the best inclusions in the social tissue of a person is finding the place inside the relational web of one's generation, I would like to underscore the vulnerability that can distort or arrest the maturational processes.

The case of Davor and his group

When we encountered Davor for the first time he was in his seventeenth year, the only child living with his divorced mother and her new partner. He was a hypersensitive youngster, trying to cultivate good relationships with his schoolmates and was actively avoiding any conflict with them. He had a girlfriend that he liked very much, but his main obstacle, as he was expressing himself, for that relation to deepen was his reticence, causing his withdrawal. During psychotherapeutic preparation for the group therapy he confessed his shameful phantasies of not being sure whether there were some homosexual tendencies in his mind. Obviously, he was in an identity crisis and was trying to overcome it by the avoiding behaviour and social withdrawal.

He was well received by the heterogenous group of younger persons. The group understood that some efforts should be made in order to solidify his male identity and accept his hypersensitivity as a special personal quality. In the group he was received as a sibling, the younger brother, and for some time Davor was calmed down. The group was playing the role of the good-enough mother, and in my role as a conductor I felt I was serving on double levels, as a conductor in the vertical sense and through a motherly channel as an empathic and protecting figure. Obviously, my countertransference was mirroring not only the group but the newcomer's double roles. Somehow, he was becoming the 'cherished child of the group'.

Davor was supported by the group in his decision to go in another city and to enroll in the Military Police Academy. It was for him a rather risky decision that he couldn't bear up and before the end of the first year he returned home very upset, disturbed by obsessive thoughts about his homosexual tendencies he was fighting with. The relationship with his girlfriend was discontinued and his feelings of shame were overwhelming. Since that period he was treated as having psychotic disturbance in its first phase. His traumatic experiences were overwhelming for him, and after almost ten years of medical treatment, psychosocial support and new therapy group experience, he attained the critical level of distancing his fears and obsessional thoughts in an active way and started to build up a new connection with a young women. His ambivalence and doubts started to lessen and he could critically watch his previous traumatic experiences. Even the new sibling relationships from the group experience could be reevaluated and he could use these mutual identifications in a more productive way. That evolution enabled him to reduce his loneliness, so characteristic for many psychologically disturbed persons.

During therapeutic phases with numerous oscillations of regressive and progressive levels of functioning, I found the concepts of M. Mahler very well orienting and influential in the assessment of the course of therapeutic interventions and support. In these phases understanding of the new sibling relationships of other group members suffering from psychotic or "near psychotic" disturbances (Marcus, 1992) was very helpful.

Working clinically with severely disturbed persons with psychotic decompensations or psychotic personality structures, my feeling and understanding of the existential loneliness of these persons was intra-psychically and socially devastating, requiring the "motherly channel" of communication at the beginning, or until the patient could attain a level of integration mature enough to be able to properly differentiate objects, resolve the need for symbiotic relationship and react against it (Štrkalj-Ivezić, Urlić, 2015). Only then could the sibling relationships level be attained, fostered and protected by the conductor and the whole group. The children's rivalry could be then sublimated in adult-level achievement if possible, with some positive envy in the form of identification and differentiation. After developing the capacity of differentiation in a stable form, he could pass on the level of "practicing" – usually first inside his group and, then, very slowly – outside it. Finding the courage to propose to the female person to get together as a couple he had to share first with his therapist. I was feeling as the motherly channel was enabling through time to protect the precarious feeling of self-confidence to resist his doubts, and the sharing with the group was the long-awaited applauded confirmation of his new achievement by his new siblings.

Pope John Paul I caused great resonance when he declared that "God is the mother". In that sense the horizontal axis meets the vertical one in an attempt to harmonise requirements of both axes to act in coordination. The conductor of the therapeutic group should earn that position in spite of the idealistic tone that this requirement might evoke. The levels of the very regressive patients are revealing such vulnerability, such low level of the threshold of frustration, that the conductor has to be very cautious regarding these special needs of very regressive patients or touching the very precarious layers repressed in unconscious or preconscious, and threatening to break into the area of consciousness. The Scottish artist Douglas Gordon at one exhibition in London exposed a list of enumerating fears along the pillar connecting two floors of the exhibition halls. The last two fears were the fear of everything and the fear of nothing. The very vulnerable persons do live in a special world and are not always able to control their aggressive impulses towards others or themselves, not being confident in the protective role of internal parental figures, motherly in their essence.

Choosing such delicate therapeutic relationships as psychotic, borderline, narcissistic and similar personality structures as clinical examples is partly due to my long professional experience, as well as to the psychoanalytically formed understanding of human psychological and social development and its variations, distortions, arrests, regressions and so on. The aforementioned point of view can be useful in assessment of levels of functioning not only of individuals but also of couples, families and groups of different sizes and orientations, regulating closeness and distance not only regarding the personality structure of the patients/persons but also of the mood in which the individual or group is at a given time.

4. Law of the father versus law of the mother: needs and achievements revisited

Writing about social synapses, the narcissism of differences and of the culture of forgiveness (Urlić, 2011), I found interesting what psychologist Sherry Turkle (2008) from MIT was writing about the attack of contemporary life with its accelerated rhythms especially ruining family life. The result looks like the appearance of a new type of persons in the epoch of internet and global mobility that she is proposing to call the epoch of "homo mobilis". According to the traditional terminology, until now it was distinguished *Homo habilis*, *Homo erectus* and *Homo sapiens*. Nowadays it is possible to see the creation of a modern Ulysses who is distancing evermore from the shores of his culture and community and is bound to explore new spaces. Siebert (2002) was summing up that tendency, considering that contemporary man is suffering from "lack of hearth", which is evermore present. Following considerations of Havel, Gore (2007) writes that it could be said that our synapses are signaling that social community is assembled of individuals who are much less connected among them through emotional threads, respect and cultural characteristics, and that we are guided by personal interests. The human being is under attack of egoism that instead of protecting him results in the insecurity of in an ever faster race, which paradoxically is aiming to diminish uncertainty and find security.

As a forensic psychiatrist I am encountering ever more legal cases regarding heritage, refutation of a will, because descendants are not satisfied with the decision of the testator. It is noticeable that in many cases it is not the material value that is in question, or greediness, but measuring who is more appreciated and loved in a family, especially by parents. It appears to be obvious that among siblings there is a kind of revival of the rivalry of who of brothers and sisters was more loved, or of envy that some other sibling was better loved than he/she used to be.

The case of Ana and her group

Ana is high school professor of foreign languages and the eldest of three children, having a younger sister and brother. She was complaining that her father was aiming at having a son and unless the third child was a son there would have been six or seven siblings, knowing the character of her father.

She introduced herself as a very independent personality, proud of her rational thinking. She organises her life around her profession, friends and some artistic hobbies in one small house nearby her parents' home. Her relationships with men were very cautious and until then she didn't unfold any such relationship to some deeper level. Very proud of her independent style of life she was as well proud of functioning among her siblings as a consultant of her/their father. She described her mother as a rather pale personality, existing in the shadow of her husband, and with whom Ana could not identify. Being in the middle of her thirties she wanted to explore in a deeper way why she was so diffident in establishing closer emphatic links with friends, especially with male ones. Obviously, to

Ana it was important to control her relationships on account of spontaneity and cordiality. Her phantasies were elaborated through her drawings and oil paintings.

At a certain point I was considering that the group might be a more adequate ambience for her than the individual therapy, for elaboration of her family experiences. She accepted my suggestion to join the psychotherapeutic group rather reluctantly.

Even the group was cautious in establishing relationships with her. Slowly but steadily Ana was entering communications with other group members, but the intellectual style was always dominating over the emotional possibility to express herself. It was after a year of group psychotherapy that Ana could confess that she was constantly amazed by the warmth in the atmosphere of the therapeutic group ("her group here") that she never felt in her family, not even for festivities. Finally, she could compare her stiffness in comparison with older group members, thinking how the lack of warmth in her family was damaging her internal world and was supporting envious feelings and rivalry among her siblings. She was amazed how with all her rational efforts she was not able to free her feelings and phantasies in relating with her family members, friends and colleagues.

Listening to this uncovering of Ana's newly discovered emotional capacity and new perspective of relating with her environment I was recollecting the visit to the Ryoanji temple in Kyoto, Japan. The temple is famous for its rock and sand garden. In that garden there is no position from which you can see all entire rocks changing the position of looking at them. There were always some rocks that you could see better, while some others remained more covered by some others. The message is obvious, only with sight, that is, reasonably or with restricted senses, is it possible to see, to feel, to understand in depth the elements from the worlds we are submerged to, either external or internal ones. In Ana's case, like in almost all completed therapies, the mature, comprehensive experiences of life events could be approached and elaborated on in a more complete way. The new siblings – the other group members – could be felt in a much more sincere and close way and the law of the mother could be relinquished, passing on its role to the free exchange with new and possibly with some old siblings. The "musée interieur" (according to A. Malraux) was obviously "reset" through new sibling relationship and different transferential/countertransferential experiences, enabling new integrations in lieu of previously established ones.

5. Some concluding remarks

It is said that to raise a child the whole village is needed. On the other hand, it looks like the biggest challenges of today are not free time and boredom but stress and insecurity. It seems like the same kind of essential needs we as human beings are confronted with from the beginning until the end of our lives. The law of the mother should guarantee safety and integrity in somatic and spiritual aspects, supported by the law of the father or conjoint in action since the emergence of a triadic situation and the possibility to better communicate by language. The Lacanian elaboration might help in a deeper understanding of the process.

Giraldo (2012), in his book *The Dialogues in and of the Group*, tries to explain what happens "in the venerable halls of language". When the word becomes concrete (consciousness!),

> it does not represent, and the anxiety in the group is a signal that the Real, not reality, is here in the group. Reality is what we construct with our imaginary and symbolic dimensions. Reality exists. We can talk about it. We share it. The real is what exists. . . . It is outside human reality as constructed by language. (p. 36)

And, he continues:

> Once the mother has brought the child into the semantic universe, the desire of the child must go through the requirements of the symbolic system to attain satisfaction. The child will enter into language to "figure out" in some way the desire of the mother, the first other that also becomes the Other. The child, thus, in its relation with this first mother gains access to her own desire. Her demand or request becomes now the inconscious way to get to her own desire (p. 40).

On the other side, what brings patients into our consulting rooms reflects the essential problem of attachment insecurity, writes Valerie Whiffen (2003). She says that insecurity disrupts key relationships and creates emotional distress and psychopathology from the insecurely attached individual. If attachment insecurity is at the heart of the problems our patients bring to us, then to change it we first must understand how it develops.

In my opinion, and not just mine, that represents one of the main sources of relations disorders that are at a basis of the person's vulnerability, mostly even throughout life. The sibling trauma, who's prototype is described in the Bible as the murder of Abel by Kain (Berger, 2010; Ashuach, 2012), represents the threat that the law of the mother is preventing by forbidding it. In that way, the sibling jealousy is finding some limitation (as was described in Ana's clinical example).

The corrective emotional experiences, if offered in an appropriate way, especially respecting the neurotic or psychotic type of the basic personality structure of an individual, or looking at the atmosphere of the group-as-a-whole in some given phase, could be a much more effective therapeutic tool for thinking on sibling experiences and their revival in a here-and-now situation. The dilemma of the conductor defends on his/her assessment of whether there is in action the level of corrective emotional experience on the triangular or the symbiotic level to deal with regarding the actual therapeutic elaborations.

P.S.

The actual global impact we have to deal with is represented by the COVID-19 pandemic, which is confronting the whole world with an unexpected problem.

The new public health situation puts the world into a kind of a cage where no compliance on the international level can be found. One of the dominating psychological dynamics of an attempt to coordinate actions on the global level seems to sink on the rocks of delusion in confrontation with the hopes that there will be some institution that will act as a leader or coordinator. The spreading impression in different cultures is that after more than a year of confrontation with the virus the differentiation of the institution, world recognised as a supreme authority on that area, could still not be established. With all international networking of the scientific and political institutions and streams the certain level of consensus regarding the guarantees for security and survival in the spirit of the new age could not be found. There is still no solution found for the majority of countries to be accepted. It looks like many delusions are in action, regarding idealistic expectations of the science and its curative and protecting possibilities. It seems like the human global "family" is left without trustful parents and as siblings were left to organise themselves the best they could at a given time. Looking from the group analytic point of view, the group as a conductor might function only very temporarily, provided that participants are functioning at a mature enough level. Obviously this is not the case regarding the institutions that govern this world. So, for the time being the globe remains in an atmosphere of spreading health danger and growing anxiety, but not only due to the threat of viruses but also with the ever clearer evidence that the survival question on the globe is a very questionable issue. Obviously siblings, like any group, can't function without defined structure and recognisable boundaries that are recognised and respected by all participants.

References

Ashuach, S. (2012): Am I My Brother's Keeper? The Analytic Group as a Space for Re-enacting and Treating Sibling Trauma. *Group Analysis*, 45(2):155–167

Berger, M. (2010): "Am I My Brother's Keeper?" Vengefulness as a Link Towards Reconnecting. In: I. Urlić, M. Berger, A. Berman (eds): *Victimhood, Vengefulness, and the Culture of Forgiveness*. New York, Novascience Publishers, Inc.

Cioran, E.M. (2013): *O nedaći biti rođen (Croatian)* (About the Misfortune of Being Born). Naklada Jesenski i Turk, Zagreb, Croatia

Friedman, R. (2004): Where to Look? Supervising Group Analysis – A Relations Disorder Perspective. *Lecture at the EGATIN Conference in Split (Croatia)*, The IIGA and the Israel Conference on Group Supervision

Giraldo, M. (2012): *The Dialogues in and of the Group. Lacanian Perspectives on the Psychoanalytic Group*. London: Karnac Books Ltd.

Gore, A. (2007): *The Assault on Reason*. New York: The Penguin Press

Laplanche, J., Pontalis, J.B. (1973): *The Language of Psycho-analysis*. London: The Hogarth Press

Mahler, M.S., Pine, F., Bergman, A. (1975): *The Psychological Birth of the Human Infant. Simbiosis and Individuation*. New York: Basic Books

Marcus, E.R. (1992): *Psychosis and Near Psychosis. Ego Function, Symbol Structure, Traitment*. New York: Springer-Verlag New York Inc.

Mitchell, J. (2013): The Law of the Mother: Sibling Trauma and the Brotherhood of War. *Canadian Journal of Psychoanalysis*, 21(1):145–159

Mitchell, J. (2017): *Lecture 1: The Sibling Trauma; Lecture 2: From the Sibling Trauma to the Law of the Mother*, Cambridge

Siebert, R. (2002): Prefazione. In: G. LoVerso, G. LoCoco (eds): *La psiche mafiosa. Storie di casi clinici e collaboratori di giustizia (Ital.)*. Milano: Franco Angeli

Štrkalj-Ivezić, S., Urlić, I. (2015): The Capacity to Use the Group as a Corrective Symbiotic Object in Group Analytic Psychotherapy for Patients with Psychosis. *Group Analysis*, 48(3):315–331

Turkle, S. (2008): *Homo Mobilis*. London: The Economist Newspaper Ltd.

Urlić, I. (2011): Les synapses sociaux, le narcissisme des différences, et la culture du pardon. In: D. Kalogeropoulos, W. Szafran, C.-Y. Baum (eds): *Les défis de la précarité. Psychanalyse et problèmes sociaux (French)*. Bruxelles – Fernelmont: E.M.E.&InterCommunications

Urlić, I. (2012): *Hundred Billion of Neurons, But Where is the Mind? The Brain Plasticity and the Group-analytic Approach to Groups*. Response by Ivan Urlić to the lecture of Catherina Mela, IAGP congress, Cartagena de Indias, Colombia

Whiffen, V.E. (2003): What Attachment Theory Can Offer Marital and Family Therapists. In: S.M. Johnson, V.E. Whiffen (eds): *Attachment Processes in Couple and Family Therapy*. New York: The Guilford Press

Winnicott, D.W. (1976): 3(ed). From Dependence Towards Independence in the Development of the Individual. In: *The Maturational Processes and the Facilitating Environment*. London: The Hogarth Press.

The Law of the Mother

3.1 The Law of the Mother and Its Expression in Group Relations Conferences and Organizations

Smadar Ashuach and Simi Talmi

A four-year-old boy, who has an eight-year-old brother, walked up to their father and said, grumpily, "I'm very angry at you!" The astonished father asked why.

His son replied, "Because you married mom, and now I don't have anyone to marry!" He then began to cry bitterly. Left with no other option, the boy said to himself, "Fine, I won't be a dad. I'll be just a brother."

One of the open issues in psychoanalytic thinking, which is a key theoretical source of the systemic psychoanalytic/psychodynamic approach, lies in the almost complete absence of references to sibling relationships and their impact on a sibling's inner world and psychological development.

This chapter shows how observing and gaining insight into the horizontal axis of sibling relationships and the law of the mother contribute to the understanding of processes that take place in group relations conferences, organizations, and society at large.

Group Relations Conferences

Group relations conferences based on the Tavistock model are designed to enable participants to explore leadership, authority, and roles and learn about them from experience. Learning in these conferences deepens our understanding of the conscious and unconscious processes that affect the individual within a group, the value of the group experience, and the evolving organizational culture or design. The group relations approach stems from the encounter between open systems theory and psychoanalysis (Stokoe, 2010).

Open Systems Theory

The open systems theory is based on work by Kurt Lewin (1997) on field theory and Bertalanffy's 1969 book *General System Theory*. These studies assume that, like biological organisms, any organization can be analyzed in terms of an open system, which has been defined as

> a system that can survive only by exchanging materials with its environment. The organization imports raw materials, converts them into

DOI: 10.4324/9781003220060-19

> end-products by carrying out various processes on them, utilizes some of these products for its own needs, and exports the rest by exchanging it, directly or indirectly, for additional raw materials and other resources it needs. These processes of import-conversion-export are the work the organization has to perform in order to survive. Organizations differ from one another by the various kinds of materials they import, by the processes they use for achieving conversion, and by the end-products they export. . . .
>
> Individuals and groups can also be considered as open systems, requiring exchange processes with their environment for survival. Open systems theory assumes that the individual, the small or larger group, and the whole organization demonstrate, in increasing levels of complexity, the same basic structural principle. Each one can be described in terms of internal world, external environment, and boundary function responsible for the activities connecting the two.
>
> (OFEK, 2008)

Key concepts of the theory of open systems are boundary, primary task, authority, and role.

Group Psychoanalysis

Psychoanalytic theory assumes the existence of the unconscious as a central motive in the behavior of the individual person. Group psychoanalysis is an advancement started by Wilfred Bion (1961) during his experiences with groups. Bion developed a theory about group behavior that is based on Freud's *Group Psychology and the Analysis of the Ego* (1921) and Kleinian psychoanalytic concepts (1952). Bion's main idea was that each group behaves as if two groups existed at the same time. One is the work group, which is prepared for a particular task (in a group relations conference, this group might be aiming to explore interpersonal relationships). The work group strives to fulfill its task rationally. The other group, called the basic assumption group, is the set of assumptions motivated by irrational, unconscious fantasies and primitive anxiety, limiting the effectiveness of the group as a whole.

In a group relations conference, one can learn how to take authority and use it, which roles one assumes, and how one influences, and is influenced by, others. Emphasis is placed on emergent organizational dynamics, the irrational forces that operate against the work task, the organizational vision, and the developing relationships and relatedness between groups. The conference also emphasizes the social and political forces that subconsciously influence our expectations and our assumptions about authority and leadership.

The psychoanalytic approach lies on the vertical axis, which regulates authority relationships and addresses the dynamics of the conference through the prism of the Oedipal configuration, object relations (Klein, 1952), and archaic initial anxieties and fantasies that arise within groups. There is no reference to the horizontal axis, to the relationships between siblings.

Sibling Relationships

Among current psychoanalytic approaches, the horizontal axis of sibling relationships remains an underexplored and seldom addressed aspect of an individual's inner world. Even when sibling relationships are addressed, they are usually discussed merely as a displacement of parent–child relationships. This approach is particularly intriguing because children tend to spend more time with their siblings than with their parents. Moreover, the relationship with one's siblings lasts longer.

We agree with those who argue that Freud does not completely ignore the subject of siblings in his writings. In his canonical 1921 work *Group Psychology and the Analysis of the Ego*, Freud describes the relationship between sons and their fathers; a son's identification with his father, who is the leader; and a son's affinity with his brothers. The siblings resolve the competitiveness, hostility, and envy between them through the mechanism of reaction formation, in which hostility and envy turn into a relationship of powerful fraternal identification. But Freud did not explore sibling relationships any further.

Perhaps the reason for Freud's almost complete disregard of sibling relationships in psychoanalysis involves the universal fantasy of exclusivity, the narcissistic desire to be the only child. Support for this hypothesis comes from Freud's discussion (1917) of three blows that humanity has suffered throughout its development:

> The first was when they [humans] learnt that our earth was not the center of the universe but only a tiny fragment of a cosmic system of scarcely imaginable vastness. This is associated in our minds with the name of Copernicus, though something similar had already been asserted by Alexandrian science. The second blow fell when biological research destroyed man's supposedly privileged place in creation and proved his descent from the animal kingdom and his ineradicable animal nature. This revaluation has been accomplished in our own days by Darwin, Wallace, and their predecessors, though not without the most violent contemporary opposition. But human megalomania will have suffered its third and most wounding blow from the psychological research of the present time which seeks to prove to the ego that it is not even master in its own house, but must content itself with scanty information of what is going on unconsciously in its mind.
>
> (Freud, 1917)

We suggest that the awareness of the existence of siblings – of others who are like me – is analogous to the Copernican revolution: a grave narcissistic injury to the fantasy of being the one and only, singular and exclusive. Psychoanalysis may have unconsciously colluded with this universal narcissistic wish and the injury that its relinquishment entails, resulting in the marginalization of siblings in psychoanalytic discourse.

It is our contention that this narcissistic wish, while it may vary in intensity, perhaps precedes the Oedipal fantasy developmentally.

The past two decades have demonstrated a growing interest in sibling relationships, in their significance and unique impact on psychological development beginning early in life, as either actual or imaginary primary objects. Juliet Mitchell (2003, 2006, 2018), one of the leading analysts exploring this field, views the birth of a sibling (both actual and imagined) as a psychological trauma.

The trauma is an emotional experience that is charged with feelings of hatred, envy, competition, and murderous rage alongside attraction, desire, sexuality, love, and greed. Mitchell (2006, 2018) perceives the horizontal sibling axis as independent and not merely derived from a child-parent relationship. In her view, the psyche develops through vertical and horizontal relationships that intersect and are interchanged in unconscious psychological life, much like the dynamic relationships between Klein's positions (the schizoid-paranoid position and depressive position) (1952). The vertical axis involves generational differences, hierarchic distinctions, totemism, and the taboo on patricide and incest; that is, the law of the father. The horizontal axis is based on our relationships with others who are in a position similar to our own (such as siblings, colleagues, and peers). Time and again, this axis brings us face to face with the loss of our status as the exalted baby and the trauma of the transition from being "*the* baby" to being "*a* baby." The horizontal axis involves the necessary acceptance of oneself as an ordinary person. This acceptance does not mean that the individual is not unique; rather, it means that all brothers and sisters are both ordinary and unique. The transformation of the self is gradual and endless. Its failure is manifested as distress, disturbance, or madness in an antisocial child. Such an emotionally charged relationship leads Mitchell (2018) to propose the law of the mother as a function that seeks to regulate, contain, and organize the emotional intensity in sibling relationships and protect children from the potential of real or symbolic fratricide or incest. This parental function does not necessarily reference the mother's gender identity.

We suggest that the theory of sibling trauma and the law of the mother as described by Mitchell (2006, 2018) can enrich our understanding of the processes that take place in group relations conferences, in organizations, and in society at large.

Examples of the Collapse of the Law of the Mother in Group Relations Conferences

An International Group Relations Conference

In February 2020, at the beginning of the COVID-19 global pandemic, the last (to our knowledge) international group relations conference was held. The Ofek Group Relations Conference began when the world's first restrictions were instituted to help mitigate the spread of the virus. A week before the conference, people arriving from China were banned from entering Israel, so two attendees from China had to cancel their participation. Calls came in from Israeli participants seeking to confirm that no attendees could spread the disease. The conference team decided to operate according to the guidelines released by the Israeli Ministry of Health. Thus, on the opening morning of the conference, a participant from Singapore, who was not subject to quarantine, was permitted to attend, but the participant's presence raised the anxiety level both within the conference team and among the other attendees.

The question that dominated the conference from the beginning was whether the group was protected adequately from the coronavirus. Could the conference directorate actually safeguard the staff and participants? The issue of protection from infection went through several incarnations during the conference.

Once the conference started, one of the participants became a "virus" himself, constantly attacking the thinking, interfering with the participants' ability to learn, and paralyzing communication. The conference, titled "Between Inside and Outside: Navigating Authority and Leadership," dealt with issues of identity – interior and exterior – both in general and specific to each participant, with the pandemic looming in the background and highlighting these issues.

In retrospect, the dynamics of sibling relationships and the law of the mother can explain what happened at the conference. The "virus" participant represented the offending "sibling," and the group struggled to determine whether there was a "mother" to protect her other "children." The question that the participants and staff asked at the conference was whether the conference and its director could make sure that no one would harm anyone else. For example, in one of the groups, a participant ("X") said there was someone in the conference that X would like to have removed. The declaration stemmed from participant X's distress, but the staff report described a confrontation between the consultants about whether the director was protecting the participants and could ensure that X would not hurt anyone.

Slowly, it became clear that the staff and participants needed a statement of protection stating that no sibling would murder or hurt another sibling. We understand that unconsciously X was "sent" by the conference to announce that the law of the mother was in danger of collapse. This conduct in a group relations conference is extreme and comes as a reaction to the beginning of the pandemic, which in itself represents violence between siblings and the need for a guardian parent – the need for the law of mother.

A German-Israeli Conference (PCCA)

German-Israeli Partners in Confronting Collective Atrocities (PCCA) is an organization designed to provide opportunities for participants to explore how the full range of feelings and fantasies about "German-ness," "Israeli-ness," "Jewish-ness," "Palestinian-ness," and "Other-ness" influences relations within and between the different groups . . . and how they affect and influence perceptions of the future.

(http://p-cca.org/timeline/)

The following example is taken from a PCCA conference in 2019.

Three consultants – two women and one man – were scheduled to participate in a large group of the conference. Normally, when a session is about to begin, two of the consultants are already seated, and the third, who is charged with timekeeping, closes the door. At this session, however, only one consultant was seated; just as the timekeeper was closing the door, the third consultant rushed in, and he and the timekeeper sat down together.

The session began with a story told by one of the German participants, the son of Nazi parents. The father had owned three special knives and a watch that were very important to him and had given these heirlooms to this son (the youngest one in the family). One day, the son (who perhaps felt guilty that his father had chosen him to keep the family treasures) decided to give the knives to his older brother. The older brother noticed that one of the knives bore a swastika and said that he wanted to remove the swastika from the knife. The younger brother objected fiercely. The older brother could not decide whether to have the swastika removed or not.

What was going on? The three consultants had come into the room in apparent disarray, an incident that suggested that something was awry among the consultants. The classic Oedipal, vertical axis–oriented interpretation would probably be that the three knives are the three consultants, whose interpretations are sometimes experienced by the participants as knife stabbings or as the cruel watch, which stops participants in mid-sentence at the end of the session.

On the horizontal axis, in terms of the sibling dynamics, we have a father who gave the things that were most precious to him to his youngest son, favoring him over his siblings. When the older brother finds out, the first thing he wants to do is erase this legacy, to *erase the name of the father*. The father failed to uphold the function of the law of the mother, which is not limited to the actual mother, in terms of maintaining and regulating inter-sibling dynamics. The father failed to handle the competition and hostility between the siblings, favoring the younger one over the older one. Hence, the knives can imply a "saber dance" and a potential struggle between the sibling-members (Germans against Israelis, Israelis against Israelis, Germans against Germans, right wingers against left wingers in each nation, Eastern Europe against Western Europe, eastern Germany against western Germany, and so on). The watch might stand for the participants' wish to have someone there to protect them from a potential fratricide or incest between sibling-members. This interpretation does not favor one axis over the other but, rather, acts as an invitation to think about both axes – the vertical and the horizontal – as a way of obtaining a more complex and multidimensional picture of the overall dynamics.

Examples of the Collapse of the Law of the Mother and Its Impact on Israeli Society

The Law of the Mother as Manifested in the Position of the Leader

In a press interview in 1976, which appears in the documentary film "Rabin: In His Own Words" (Laufer, as cited in *The Times of Israel*, 2015), the Israeli prime minister Yitzhak Rabin called the right-wing Gush Emunim movement, which was seeking to settle the occupied territories, "a cancer in the tissue of Israel's democratic society." The same Rabin who had once supported and aided the establishment of the settlements was now sowing the seeds of rupture in Israeli society.

With due caution, we would like to turn our attention to 1983, seven years after Rabin's statement, when Israel witnessed a fratricide stemming from ideological differences. Emil Grunzweig, an activist with a peace movement, was murdered during a rally when an Israeli right-wing demonstrator threw a grenade into the crowd.

Did Rabin's inflammatory words, which turned brother against brother, pave the way for, and legitimize, this murder? Did Rabin fail to uphold the law of the mother, an important responsibility of his role as the nation's leader? In 1995, Rabin himself was assassinated by an Israeli – one of the "sons." In the context of the law of the mother, the division in the country between the left and right wings led to a split between brothers and eventually to murder. It seems that Rabin was murdered by those brothers who felt that he had abandoned them, and they took revenge on him.

The leader can also be the state itself. At the time of its establishment, the State of Israel distributed its resources, mainly land and water sources, in a way that favored kibbutzim and other cooperative settlements. With natural resources now dwindling in Israel, protests have arisen against the past discrimination, pitting various groups – "siblings" – against each other. For example, Kibbutz Nir David is situated on the banks of a stream to which the kibbutz demands exclusive rights, while the members of the public are asking for equal access. The original sin is the failure of the law of the mother.

Sibling Relationships and the Law of the Mother in the Kibbutz

In the early days of the Zionist movement, kibbutzim were established based on the socialist doctrine of common ownership and equality and were run as shared communes. The cornerstone of the educational theory that the kibbutz movement created and applied was the minimization of the negative effects of the Oedipal complex on the sexual investment of the parent (Liebermann, 2018; Rolnik, 2007). This investment was transferred to the group of sibling-children by having all children sleep in designated "children's houses," away from the bed of the parental couple. The nannies and the group of children were offered as alternative significant figures who would protect the child from Oedipal wishes and sexual impulses toward the parental couple. The group's siblings were perceived as safe figures, as a refuge from the perils of Oedipal wishes.

Sexuality was viewed only as directed at the parents, to the extent that, in addition to having the children sleep in a communal house rather than at home with their parents, the kibbutzim also created the custom of joint showers, with boys and girls showering together up to the age of eighteen. This practice sent young and adolescent boys and girls naked and exposed (both literally and figuratively) into a shared space, under the assumption that despite their hormone-struck age, the whole thing was merely "cubs at play."

The utter disregard for the significance of the horizontal axis as independently entailing sexuality, desire, and attraction and the excessive, potentially blinding focus on the Oedipal context of the vertical axis led to notions that we find completely absurd today. Moreover, we now know from the testimony of people who experienced this practice while growing up in a kibbutz that there were a great many physical and sexual assaults that were not reported or treated. The law of the mother had collapsed.

Bereaved Siblings

Israel is known for its countless wars and resulting bereavement. Long ago, the country wisely established suitable institutions for addressing this issue. The state gives bereaved parents special help and emotional and financial support for the rest of their lives. Also, bereaved parents are always mentioned in Israel's Memorial Day services.

Until recently, however, bereaved siblings went unrecognized. Only in 2008 did Israel begin to acknowledge bereaved siblings as having been emotionally affected by the loss of their brother or sister; various state institutions finally started addressing the needs and rights of this segment of the population. The centrality of the Oedipal complex and parent–child relationships had no doubt influenced Israeli policy and its disregard for the bereavement suffered by siblings.

We might add that by referencing only the child who was killed, the state failed in its role of the mother by neglecting to protect the surviving children.

The Law of the Mother in Organizations

Organizations give rise to countless spaces involving teamwork, including the hiring of new employees and the firing or promoting of some employees rather than others. The horizontal axis is challenged and stimulated, and the employees' internalizations and experiences from their sibling relationships are brought into the corporate world and are constantly resurrected and re-enacted.

The global transition from hierarchical, pyramid-like organizations to flat, matrix-type organizations, along with the growing tendency to work in collegial teams, summons a sibling dynamic. One could say that such groups are becoming "relational" organizations. This change makes it ever more relevant for us to focus on the horizontal axis of relationships, in all its complexity, as well as to recognize the possibility that managers and subordinates will develop sibling transference.

Mitchell (2003, 2006) emphasizes that sibling transference involves the powerful trauma of the annihilation of the narcissistic ego, a trauma of sameness and difference, which is revisited and reenacted, imagined and manifested in compulsive repetitive behaviors in various aspects of life.

In organizations made up of various departments, units, or professional teams, the complex dynamics of interaction between these groups can also be understood through the axis of sibling relationships.

Example

A treatment center for parent–child relationships has requested intervention following a crisis in the relationship between employees at the center. This is an organization that for years was a small center with a manager and a small number of employees, and in the last year the center has grown and more workers have joined. At a training session in the center, it was discovered that there is a WhatsApp group between the principal and the veteran employees. This discovery led to a severe crisis of confidence. The new entrants felt excluded and the old ones did not understand what the problem was and were angry at the new ones creating a crisis. With the help of the law of the mother it was possible to help the principal understand the crisis, understand the difficulty of the newcomers to fit into the team. She decided to leave the WhatsApp group, even though she felt that this group was very supportive of her, and it was possible to understand what the "mother" was gaining from the nonexistence of the law of the mother. New thinking began about the organization as a sibling organization and through this a better understanding of working at the center with families developed.

Global Example

The COVID-19 pandemic serves as an example of global sibling dynamics, exhibiting themes of comparison and competition for taking control of the virus and developing a vaccine for it while carrying out witch hunts to find culprits, infected people, and scapegoats. We view what happened in the world as a violation of the law of the mother, a failure to create order, cooperation, and responsibility among the siblings.

A more positive enactment of the law of the father and of the mother can be seen in what is referred to as the traffic-light model in Israel (a similar system has been introduced in the European Union). Cities are classified as red, orange, yellow, or green according to their level of COVID-19 infection, and the pandemic regulations for their residents are based on the city's current color. The model can be considered an integration of the law of the father, who sets the regulations, and the law of the mother, who says that not everyone is equal but everyone will receive the appropriate treatment.

Conclusions

As shown in this chapter, the horizontal relationship axis can be highly relevant to group work, group relations conferences, and organizations.

The connection between the vertical axis (Oedipal conflict) and the horizontal axis (sibling relationships) provides a complex, multidimensional view of personal, interpersonal, group, and organizational dynamics. We are not claiming that one axis is more influential than the other but, rather, that the matrix of the encounter between the two axes offers a deep, enriching picture of relationships.

We suggest that the emerging presence of siblings in psychoanalytic discourse is likely related to the development of relational approaches that put the therapist-patient relationship and mutual influence at the center of the therapeutic encounter. The horizontal connection in the therapeutic encounter, which also binds two subjects, constitutes, in our opinion, fertile ground for the development of approaches that speak of sibling relationships as affecting the growth of the inner world and the internalized image.

References

Bertalanffy, L. von (1969). *General system theory*. George Braziller.

Bion, W. (1961). *Experiences in groups and other papers*. Tavistock.

Freud, S. (1917). Introductory lectures on psycho-analysis. In J. Strachey (Ed.), *The standard edition of the complete psychological works of Sigmund Freud*, Vol. XVI (1916–1917): Introductory lectures on psycho-analysis (Part III) (pp. 241–463). Hogarth.

Freud, S. (1921). Group psychology and the analysis of the ego. In J. Strachey (Ed.), *The standard edition of the complete psychological works of Sigmund Freud*, Vol. XVIII (1920–1922). Hogarth.

Klein, M. (1952). Some theoretical conclusions regarding the emotional life of the infant. In P. Heimann, S. Isaacs, M. Klein, & J. Riviere (Eds.), *Developments in psycho-analysis*. Hogarth.

Laufer, E. (Director). (2015). *Rabin in his own words* [Film]. Kol Miney Productions.

Lewin, K. (1997). *Resolving social conflicts and field theory in social science*. American Psychological Association.

Liebermann, G. (2018). *Freud in the kibbutz: Psychoanalysis and collective education*. Carmel (Hebrew).

Mitchell, J. (2003). *Siblings: Sex and violence*. Polity.

Mitchell, J. (2006). Sibling trauma: A theoretical consideration. In P. Coles (Ed.), *Sibling relationships* (pp. 155–174). Karnac.

Mitchell, J. (2018, February 16). *Core concepts: From sibling trauma to the law of the mother* [Paper presentation]. Group Psychotherapy Conference on Sibling Relationships, Tel Aviv University, Tel Aviv, Israel.

OFEK – Organization-Person-Group. (2008). *Open systems theory* (website). Accessed April 11, 2021. www.ofek-groups.org/en/index.php?option=com_content&task=view&id=19&Itemid=39.

Partners in Confronting Collective Atrocities (PCCA). (2021). *Our conferences: The model: The primary task of the recent conference*. Accessed April 17, 2021. http://p-cca.org/timeline/

Rolnik, E.J. (2007). *Freud in Zion: History of psychoanalysis in Jewish Palestine/Israel 1918–1948*. Am Oved.

Stokoe, P. (2010). The theory and practice of the group relations conference. In C. Garland (Ed.), *The Groups book: Psychoanalytic group therapy: Principles and practice* (pp. 152–175). Karnac.

The Times of Israel Staff. (2015, September 25). In 1976 interview, Rabin likens settler idealogues to "cancer," warns of "apartheid". *The Times of Israel*. www.timesofisrael.com/in-1976-interview-rabin-likens-settlements-to-cancer-warns-of-apartheid/

3.2 Discrimination

The Dark Side of the Law

Avi Berman

When I began researching what was written on the subject of discrimination, I was surprised to find that the vast majority does not address parent–child relationships. Hundreds of articles deal with discrimination in the broad social sphere, while only a few deal with parental discrimination. Discrimination is commonly investigated in areas such as education, racism, gender, transgender, homosexuality, fiscal and economic opportunities, immigration, and so on.

The reality of social discrimination is often addressed by laws that are designed to prevent it. These laws seem to correspond with the law of the mother in the sense of preventing one privileged group from harming another. For example: Title VII of the Civil Rights Act, as amended, protects employees and job applicants from employment discrimination based on race, color, religion, sex, and national origin.

There is no doubt that dealing with discrimination in the social sphere is of great importance. However, the dearth of studies exploring discrimination in the family and the child–parent relationship suggest that there is an unspoken or even denied theme. Is it possible that most of us address discrimination in society and overlook discrimination within our families, towards us as children, to our parents and towards our children in our blind spots as parents?

Another surprise awaits us when we examine the subject of discrimination in ethology. It turns out that in the animal world known to us (including man as an animal) discrimination is extremely common, genetically dictated, and sometimes leads to siblicide. Moreover, this discrimination seems to be in line with Darwin's principle of the survival of the fittest (Sulloway, 2007). Here are two examples:

> Among African black eagles, siblicidal competition is obligate, occurring in nearly every instance. Within a few days the older of the black eagle chicks picks the younger to death. . . . Parents do not intervene in these lethal contests, as it is not in their biological interest to do so.
>
> (Mock, 2004)

> Earlier born piglets fiercely and successfully defend access to their mother's most milk-richest teats while later born piglets are half as likely to survive past the third week.
>
> (Sulloway, 2007, p. 298)

DOI: 10.4324/9781003220060-20

Even in human societies, discrimination can be extremely offensive. It turns out that by 1800, children who had not yet demonstrated their ability to survive childhood illnesses received limited treatment, to the point of expulsion and abandonment, while their older siblings were favorized for more attentive treatment. In pre-modern times to the present-day, cases of infanticide are reported, mainly in traditional societies (Boone, 1986; Voland, 1990).

In her book, Mitchell mentions an anthropological testimony given by Cicely Williams regarding children and mothers on the African Gold Coast. In many families, particularly poor ones, the mother lets go of her child when a new baby is born. She is completely invested in the new baby and in caring for it with complete devotion and love. The baby enjoys an ideal life until the next sibling is born. The child that is let go sometimes undergoes a sudden and dangerous weaning, both physically and psychologically. These children develop a typical disease due to the lack of protein (pp. 199–200). The children who are let go grow up to be enraged and bitter.

Equal treatment of children seems to depend on the personal capacity of the mother (and parents) and her economical and mental condition. As these decrease it is more likely that parents' favoritism goes for the stronger, more comfortable and more obedient child. In 39 non-Western societies, it was found that the firstborn child is more protected, more nurtured, and sometimes given privileges in inheritance, as well as powers over his younger siblings. They also bear the family name, probably because this has prevented over-allocation of family resources, to the point of losing them (Sulloway, 2007). In addition, the studies provide us with a reminder that discrimination is always linked to favoritism. Beside every discriminated child there is another who is favored, and vice versa: any favoring of one child implies that another is being discriminated against (sometimes more than one).

Investment in a family's children appears to vary according to birth order. The first and last children get more, represented by a U-shaped curve. Lindert (1977) analyzed the hours of childcare received by children, from birth to 18 years. He found that middle-born children were constantly at a disadvantage, receiving 10% less in cumulative childcare relative to firstborn or last-born siblings.

It seems that ideas of sibling equality and equity of parental investment were gradually adopted over the last 100 years, due to improvements in living conditions. Equal inheritance distribution is also typical of Western societies, which are more capable of ensuring abundance and security.

Siblings are markedly different from each other even though they share common genes and grow up with the same parents and the same family. One conclusion from this is that children elicit different responses from their parents. As a result, different relationships are created between the parents and each child (Sulloway, 2007, p. 300).

Another possible explanation for this is that the extra-familial environment, such as the peer group, is more influential than the family. The experience of the extra-familial environment can indeed differ vastly from child to child. (Harris, 1998 mentions this in one sentence. This book deals with sibling relationships and the horizontal axis devotes much more to this.)

And what is the siblings' point of view on the issue of discrimination?

Sibling relations are perceived as bearing qualities of rivalry and competition on one hand and resources and mutualism on the other. A questionnaire study of over 600 male and female high school students (intact families and with at least one sibling) explored the phenomenon of parental favoritism. About half the respondents perceived the existence of favoritism on the part of one or both of their parents. Girls more often than boys were perceptive of such favoritism. The youngest child in the family was more often the favorite of the mother and the middle child was least often a parental favorite. Parental favoritism was associated with perceived parental incompatibility. Teenagers who perceived a sibling as being favored evidenced increased angry and depressive feelings as well as identity confusion (Pollet & Hoben, 2011).

It is clear that children are harmed by discrimination. Aside from reactions of anger and depression, discriminated children seem to have lower self-esteem, feel distanced from their parents, and find it difficult to see them as important figures in their lives (Sulloway, 2007).

It seems that the attitude towards discrimination, in human society as well, is a dual one. On the one hand there is a degree of concern towards the pain and harm that is caused by discrimination, and on the other hand, favoritism and discrimination are performed without hesitation, out of economic and social needs or out of personal emotional tendencies.

It seems to me that the law of the mother, which deals with the protection of children by their mother, should deal with discrimination. This chapter is devoted to an exploration of the phenomenon of parental discrimination in terms of the law of the mother and the implications derived therein for psychotherapy.

Discrimination and the Law of the Mother

> And in process of time it came to pass, that Cain brought of the fruit of the ground an offering unto the Lord. And Abel, he also brought of the firstlings of his flock and of the fat thereof. And the Lord had respect unto Abel and to his offering: But unto Cain and to his offering he had not respect. And Cain was very wroth, and his countenance fell.
>
> (Genesis 4: 3–5)

Cain's murder of his brother Abel is a biblical reference to the horrors of siblings' murderousness, and marks it as a sin. The biblical story does not, however, address God's discrimination against Cain, which preceded the murder. The story does not explain it. However, we can understand that discrimination can evoke murderous emotions.

At first glance it seems that the law of the mother is intended to regulate such murderous wishes. The law of the mother, according to Juliet Mitchell, includes two prohibitions: the prohibition of harming siblings and the prohibition of incest. The mother warns that violating this prohibition will lead to the removal of her maternal concern. Mitchell explains the law of mother as such:

> The toddler cannot kill the mother, but it *can* and indeed sometimes does, seriously damage and even kill the baby. Murdering the baby is utterly forbidden by the Law the mother. Her demands shall operate *between* her children. . . . Her law also prohibits sexuality between the children. . . . The Law of the Mother threatens withdrawal of care while also insisting that the toddler is now a big girl or boy and must go off and play (or work) with its peers.[1]

So, the law of the mother is intended to prevent children from harming each other and ensure a transition to peer society and social affiliation on the horizontal axis. But what about discrimination? In the subjective experience of sibling relationships, the discriminating mother may cause the favored sibling to create (sometimes unknowingly) an abusive experience for the discriminated sibling and evoke feelings of envy, jealousy, anger, and revenge. The law of the mother and parental discrimination seem diametrically opposed. Discrimination is a clear and blatant violation of the law of the mother.

Yet, surprisingly, the wording of the law, as cited earlier, does not include a parallel and complementary obligation on the part of the mother to take care of all her children when they *are* fulfilling their part. In other words, the mother threatens her children that she will withdraw her love if they violate the law, but she does not guarantee her love for her children when they do obey it. The law of the mother does not protect children from parental discrimination.

Juliet Mitchell's answer to this asymmetry is that the mother law is based on the assumption of an "all-loving mother." That is, the law of the mother, in its spirit and essence, deals with the protection of all children. If so, I suggest that the meaning of the mother law is similar to that of Winnicott's concept of the "good enough mother" (1956, 1965). Both good-enough motherhood as well as the law of the mother cannot be taken for granted. Both deal with possibility and intention rather than a description of realistic motherhood. The law of the mother is dependent upon its beneficent application. Otherwise, it seems that differences between siblings as human beings, their order of birth, their sex, the decreased capabilities of their aging parents over time – all of these create differences that evoke (sometimes unconsciously) harmful parental favoring and discriminatory behaviors.

It is important to note that sibling trauma and discrimination are completely different events. Sibling trauma is presented by Mitchell as a universal and inevitable event. The child loses his experience of uniqueness in the face of the birth of a new brother. Instead, he experiences replaceability. The painful experience of being replaceable is one aspect of the sibling trauma. Yet, despite the child's fear of abandonment the toddler is going to realize that he/she is still taken care of. The law of the mother organizes the sibling trauma and enables it to turn into *a rite of passage* so that the toddler who is no longer the baby can become the social child, together with her classmates, playmates or work-peers, sexual partners, and brothers-in-arms. Sending the toddler into the social world that has always surrounded her may be a life-affirming possibility, even if it is one that entails a threat to the subject's sense of uniqueness and omnipotence. Therefore, most of us eventually understand and accept the universality and inevitability of our replaceability and the personal achievement of being included in the social aspect of our lives.

Discrimination is not included in sibling trauma. On the contrary: it might be experienced as a betrayal. The toddler feels that she fulfilled her part in the deal (the law), then finds herself denied equal rights in return. In the absence of this parental protection, sibling relations may regress to the primary position of murderous desires and experiences of being obliterated. In such places, sibling trauma may manifest as depression and/or vengefulness, and eventually as the breakup of relationships. Maybe we should take into account that on a larger social scale, discrimination and favoritism among siblings may deteriorate into civil wars.

It seems to me that the intention of the good enough mother should refer to the possibility of discrimination. Addressing maternal discrimination can be based first and foremost on acknowledging it and its abusive effect. I suggest that, good enough parenthood listens to the protest of the child who feels discriminated against and shows tolerance for his protesting behavior, as long as it does not violate the mother's law. Beyond that, it seems to me that the comparison among siblings can be contained and tolerated if it is based on an alternating favoritism. Acknowledging discrimination by parents may create a familial environment in which negotiation and reparation is possible. Every sibling yearns for moments in which he is favored, moments in which the maternal preoccupation of infancy is revived. But these moments of favoritism are possible only if they are transient and alternating, similar to the social agreement on celebrating birthdays, where each receives his or her day in the spotlight.

Here we come to what I think might be the contribution of psychotherapy. Psychotherapy cannot cure sibling trauma, but it can help encourage personal development. It seems to me that this processing includes two necessary principles. One is the forming of a space for mourning the losses involved in the sibling trauma and its verbal expression in discourse. The second principle deals with the creation of a space in which experiences of discrimination may be transformed into inclusion of mutual replaceability. In the next section I will expand on these ideas.

From Discrimination to Mutual Replaceability: Notes on Psychotherapy

Ron is a lawyer. He is over 50 years old and has been in individual psychotherapy for three years. Recently he lost his only sister after her long struggle as a cancer patient. Ron was his mother's favorite. When he was born, his only sister was four years old. As soon as he was born, she was forsaken by her mother, losing her love, save for sudden expressions of affection or care that came and went unexpectedly.

In talking about his work, I found out that he deals with inheritances, among other things, and I suggested a connection between his early experience of sibling relations and his work. The subject immediately connected him to difficult moments in his practice. He told me:

> You have no idea what I see here. I saw a mother who told her third child, whom she excluded from the inheritance: "I never wanted you." I saw two sisters who lost their part in the inheritance because their mother favored her son, their brother. I've seen brothers who begged their elder brother, who was awarded the entire family property in the village, to sell one of the houses and give them the proceeds. He answered, coldly: "This is what mom and dad intended and thus it shall be." The relationship between them is dead and if they could ever exact their revenge upon him, they will. When I can, I influence things. Often, however, it's a lost cause.

Then he added, "When my sister passed away, I said to her husband: 'You don't have to worry. You'll get everything you deserve. We are going to love each other here and respect her wishes.'" That was Ron's resolution of being favored as a child and his personal moral choice in light of the disastrous relationships he encountered in his work.

Ron had been a different person till he was 30. However, at that point in his life, something happened that transformed his social relations though he did not understand its causes.

The event took place on a month-long boat cruise he had taken with a group of six people. He was a skipper and professionally skilled. There was a large gap, however, between his interpersonal skills and his professional abilities. The members of the group gradually came to see Ron as an arrogant, egocentric person, and soon became ambivalent towards getting closer to him. Ron knew that, in the past, people had drifted away from him without telling him why – or he could not remember why. In the confined circumstances of the cruise, however, he was forced to hear them out. It was a long and difficult conversation one quiet evening at a beautiful bay in Greece. They told him that he seemed to be reluctant to help, he was not encouraging and on the other hand considered himself to have the best ideas, he was cast as the "haughty Mr. know-it-all." One woman reminded him that he did not bother to thank her for helping him use technology he was unfamiliar with to call his family members. Someone else told him that he was having a hard time listening to Ron's criticism when everyone was doing their part. He couldn't sleep that night and felt lonely on the boat. Some years later, in therapy, we understood together that he had a kind of panic attack disguised as sea-sickness. Only one lone woman approached him and mediated between what he had been told and his capacity to take it in. This woman had been one of his fiercest critics in that conversation. Unlike the other people present, she chose to talk to him afterwards without going back on her critique. Listening to her immediately led him to change his behavior and meticulously apply what he had been told. By the end of the cruise, he had become more sociable, more humble, and eventually found out that he enjoyed reciprocity. He stayed in touch with that woman, Naomi. Today, she is his wife.

In the early stages of treatment, Ron did not connect important attitudes and decisions in his life to his sibling relationships as a child. His life was mostly good and stable. He was married and the father of two children. He was successful in his work as a lawyer and a partner in a thriving firm. He and his partners were business-oriented and learned to be aggressive in negotiations. One of their methods was to issue legal restraining orders on the business activities of their rivals. They would stop their operational activities through court verdicts to get better terms from them. They didn't mind the suffering they caused. Gradually he began to feel antagonism towards his work accompanied by a sense of meaninglessness and emptiness. As the bond with his sister grew stronger, he learned from her that her childhood with their parents was completely different than his. She felt overlooked by their mother, while he was treated as the diamond in the family crown. His father was a cautious and avoidant figure and was overshadowed by his mother's dominance. Her self-esteem was badly damaged and had recovered slowly since she left home and got married. Now she is a schoolteacher, divorced and the mother of three children. She had attributed every achievement in her life to her decision to stay away from their parents and their mother in particular. Despite all this she was still taking care of her parents in their aging needs. Ron understood from her that she probably had a different mother than his own. When he turned to his mother with questions about it, she did not find anything wrong with her behavior. For her part, his sister was just a complaining daughter. For the first time in his life, Ron responded to this and accused his mother of discriminating against his sister. His mother denied it. As she saw it, she loved her children. His profound understanding of the injustice his sister had suffered affected his professional orientation. Once a confrontational and harsh attorney, he became a talkative, congenial person. He discovered his professional creativity and took pleasure in it.

When Ron noticed my attitude towards his sibling relationship, there was a change in his transference to me. Thus far, he had listened to me as a professional consultant and treated me with respectable and indifferent distance. My reference to his sister's experience of discrimination, aroused an emotional closeness to me. In his experience I became a protective father who cared for his children in the sense of the law of the mother. Signs of identification appeared for the first time. Mostly he adopted my attention regarding replaceability and reciprocity.

Psychotherapy can be a place where mutual replaceability is experienced and mourning is processed. Concerning the mourning process, it seems to me that individual therapy contributes more to the patient than group therapy, while group therapy offers a special contribution regarding experiencing sibling trauma and a possible transformation towards mutual replaceability.

When Ron told me about the encounter he experienced on the cruise, I referred to it as a group therapy session, even though it was not a therapy group in the professional-formal sense of the term. Some of the crucial insights Ron needed to have had to wait for his personal therapy that began years later. Indeed, I would like to open my approach to the case from the point of view of group analysis. From a group analytic point of view, belonging is a component of mental health and the relationships formed between group participants are of therapeutic quality (Foulkes, 1948 [1983]). Group therapy unfolds sibling relationships in the room and allows participants to participate in relevant reconstructions of them in their lives and derive insights from them.

According to Mitchell (2006), on the horizontal axis, which is created following the child's deportation to the social world, natural groups are formed. In a group analytic sense these groups provide their participants with a sense of belonging and sustain spontaneous healing processes within them. Ron found himself within such a group on the cruise. In the difficult encounter that developed following his behavior, he was offered to give up his aspirations for favored status and belong to a mutual relationship, or to preserve it and stay out of their company. He chose the first option. He stopped claiming the crown, learned to acknowledge the contributions of his teammates and to thank them. He offered his help and gradually began to talk about himself. I suggested to Ron a connection between being his mother's favorite and his difficulty in belonging to a group of people who did not obey his mother's preferences. I told him that within the group formed on the cruise he had undergone an experience of being replaceable. He was actually experiencing late sibling trauma.

In my view, implementing the mother's law is not solely the mother's job. Just as women can strictly adhere to the law of the father, when they enlist to keep the vertical axis around them, so can men, therapists, and siblings themselves internalize and implement the law of the mother.

May I add that in group therapy, the replaceability of each member is experienced as a partial consolation. The experience of replaceability is presented consciously and unconsciously as a common denominator that unites those who belong: all members have undergone a unique and yet universal sibling trauma. In its most rehabilitating form, sibling trauma undergoes a transformation from being a fateful blow of deprivation to sharing a universal existential experience of sibling vulnerability that may stir empathy and compassion. Moreover, belonging encourages alternating contributions. The unique contributions of each individual are rewarded with recognition and empowerment. Something of the grandiose uniqueness of having been, once, the only loved child is experienced once again in a partial, fleeting, alternating manner. Unlike the natural group of Ron's cruises, in group analysis all these processes are differentiated and spoken with the help of a conductor. Moreover, in group analysis the group conductor, together with the group participants, can conform to the law of the mother. We may assume that this combination of belonging and challenge cultivates ego-strength and increases the capacity for containing tension and tolerating differences.

I suggest that the transformation between discriminatory-favoring experiences to the possibility of reciprocal replaceability also occurs in individual therapy, even though therapists may not notice this. As an individual therapist and psychoanalyst, I have noticed that many patients restore in therapy the initial bond of the mother–child dyad. The therapist and patient create a dyad of exclusivity dedicated to the needs of the patient. Until a certain moment no one else exists in the patient's experience. And then suddenly the patient refers to small changes in the room and realizes that someone was here before him. Then it occurs to her that someone else is going to come when he goes away. "I'm just a name on your list," an insulted patient in his second year of treatment tells me. Or another patient dreams that she arrives at her hour and finds that I am in a group supervision session. In her dream, I give her a small smile of acquaintance and invite her to join. She feels isolated and paralyzed. I suggest understanding these events as a recurrence of the sibling trauma that has not been brought to treatment so far. The spontaneous moments in which the patient notices the existence of other people in the therapist's world signal, in my opinion, his emerging capability to wean himself from the exclusive therapeutic dyad that has been essential to her so far and her ability to deal with his sibling trauma.

According to Mitchell, even under these benevolent conditions, recovery from sibling trauma involves mourning the loss of dyadic mother–child bond. Mourning the loss of the possibility of receiving full support for the wished-for uniqueness of mother–child dyad, mourning the differences that cannot be changed and the psychic injuries of parental discriminations. Mourning processes may digest the pain of loss and injustice and transform it into acceptance of mutuality, replacing anger with sorrow. This allows for the release of energies that were hitherto held in anger and depression.

Ron opened up to mourning processes. His mourning for the loss of exclusivity in his relationship with his mother was not experienced in treatment simply as such. Ron mourned above all the discrimination his sister suffered. He became a partner in her sibling trauma. When he first heard about her illness, his grief deepened. He felt that the opportunity for sibling love was taken away from him as discrimination against his sister and the disavowed tension between them kept them apart. During the treatment, many childhood memories arose. His interpersonal relations were filled with tenderness. Ron and his sister enjoyed a time of sibling honeymoon.

In Conclusion

It seems that discrimination and favorizing may free-float almost unnoticed, under our radar, while being perceived by its victims as injustice and evoking feelings of depression, disappointment, anger, and revenge. Parental discrimination can export into the horizontal axis precisely these feelings and resonate them on a social scale. Indeed, it seems that most of the social conflicts we are familiar with include an element of anger over discrimination. If indeed "everything starts at home" then our modest contribution as therapists may focus on the recognition of parental-discrimination and creating a therapeutic approach to it. It seems to me that the law of the mother should include an explicit reference to the possibility of discrimination and the need to curb it. Discrimination and favoritism may not be totally avoided. The solution appropriate to the law of the mother may focus on the constant alternation of favoritism and discrimination and reconciliation with mutual replaceability.

Note

1 A citation from Mitchell's lecture in a psychotherapy conference at Tel Aviv University on February 16, 2018.

References

Boone, J. L. (1986). "Parental Investment and the Elite Family Structure in Preindustrial States: A Case Study of Late Medieval-early Modern Portuguese Genealogies." *American Anthropologist* **88**: 859–878.

Foulkes, S. H. (1948 [1983]). *Introduction to Group Analytic Psychotherapy*. London: Karnac.

Harris, J. R. (1998). *The Nurture Assumption: Why Children Turn Out the Way They Do*? New York, Free Press.

Lindert, P. H. (1977). "Sibling Position and Achievement." *The Journal of Human Rsources* **12**: 198–219.

Mitchell, J. (2006). "Sibling Trauma: A Theoretical Consideration." In *Sibling Relationships*, ed. P. Cole. London, Karnac: 155–174.

Mock, D. W. (2004). *More Than Kin and Less Than Kind: The Evolution of Family Conflict*. Combridge, MA, Harvard University Press.

Pollet, T. V. and Hoben, A. D. (2011). "An Evolutionary Perspective on Siblings: Rivals and Resources." In *The Oxford Handbook of Evolutionary Family Psychology*, eds. C. Salmon and T. K. Shackleford. Oxford, Oxford University Press: 128–148.

Sulloway, F. J. (2007). "Birth Order and Sibling Competition." In *The Oxford Handbook of Evolutionary Psychology*, eds. R. I. M. Dunbar and B. Louise. Oxford and New York, Oxford University Press: 297–313.

Voland, E. (1990). "Differential Reproductive Success Within the Kummhorn Population (Germany, 18th and 19th Centuries)." *Behavioral Ecology and Sociobiology* **26**: 54–72.

Winnicott, D. W. (1965). "Ego Distortion in Terms of True and False Self." In *The Maturational Processes and the Facilitating Environment: Studies in the Theory of Emotional Development*. London, Hogarth Press & The Institute of Psychoanalysis.

Winnicott, D. W. (1956 [1992]). "Primary Maternal Preoccupation." In *Through Pediatrics to Psychoanalysis*. New York, Basic Books: 300–305.

3.3 Snitches – a rupture in "sibling" relationships

*Martin Mahler and Liat Warhaftig-Aran**

Introduction

In this chapter, we want to shed light on political snitching.

We will mention snitching in communist Czechoslovakia during the past century, but our argument is that its characteristics are universal in all totalitarian regimes. Snitching is a complex phenomenon: on the one hand, it expresses personalized aggressive and perverted aspects of social relationships, but, on the other hand, it can be also be viewed as an impersonal attribute of large-scale societal, often (post)traumatic functioning. It can be viewed as a relational pathology on both individual and collective levels. We were driven to discuss this subject partially due to our own experiences with snitching:

Martin: When I was 19 years old, I arranged a private meeting with an important dissident in a small café in Prague, to introduce myself.

A few days after, my father confronted me: it turned out that he was well informed about my meeting with that dissident. My father even knew some details from that meeting! Gradually, I came to realize that the meeting was wiretapped by the secret police and that my father was warned about it. Even now, I do not know why he was protected by another informer (in reality, my father was also persecuted because of his anti-regime behavior) and who that "guardian angel" was. This remained a family taboo until my father passed away a few years ago. This experience put the brakes on my enthusiasm for underground activity for a long period of time.

My father strongly asked me not to put other members of our family, him included, in bigger danger "than necessary". I was confused about my father's role in this incident: was he both persecuted and protected by the regime? After the fall of communism, I was relieved to not find his name in the registry of informers. Like many other intellectuals, he probably had to find a way to negotiate with the secret police; so did I enter this "arena" uninvited? Either way, I felt humiliated and a little paranoid because of the almighty presence of the snitches and, of course, this intensified the loyalty conflict with my father.

Liat: I grew up in a religious Jewish family and society. My experience of religion was one of many rules that required obedience, and their violation involved threat of being punished by God. My painful experience of being

DOI: 10.4324/9781003220060-21

observed by big superego as a child was one of the reasons I was attracted to the subject of snitching. Also, I remember an incident in which as an adolescent, I snitched to my mother that my brother violated a punishment of hers. My mother forgave him, since she thought that he was punished enough. I cannot recall my experience back then, but today I feel relief that my snitching was not rewarded. Except for a few memories of this sort, my relationships with my siblings and friends were my shelter throughout all my childhood years. In incidents in which I found myself confronted with destructive envy or evil in my close friends, I felt much more betrayed than when authority figures engaged in similar behaviors. The question of the sources of love and hate in "sibling relationships" brings me to our next discussion of snitching.

The definition of snitching

Political snitching is a part of hierarchically organized violent acts intended to prevent anti-regime activities. We must differentiate between snitching and whistleblowing: A whistleblower acts with good will, without personal profit. Usually, he is an employee who draws attention to illegitimate, unethical, or lawless practices that are approved by his superiors. These practices contradict public well-being and there are no internal mechanisms in place to regulate them.

Criminal informants are people who provide incriminating information about other people to law enforcement authorities in exchange for leniency for their own role in an unlawful act. There is also a fourth type of snitching, that is, civilian snitching, in which non-criminal individuals are asked to provide information to law enforcement authorities if they witness breaking of the law (for example, people who do not pay their taxes).

It is difficult to distinguish clearly between various motives for snitching, as the following example shows:

Liat: In a therapeutic group that I conduct, two newcomers recently joined the group. They were both dominant and charismatic and it seemed that they easily found their place in the group. Even though they knew the group rules, they used to take cigarette breaks together before the group meetings. It was brought to my knowledge during one of the group meetings by one of the old timer members of the group. He argued for the adherence to the group rules, which he cared for. I knew that he wanted to protect the group, but at the same time, I felt that his unconditional status of dominance in the group was challenged by the new male group member, who also "took" the new lady. To my understanding, jealousy and wishes for revenge were mixed with the desire to protect the group. I reminded the group's rules again and proposed the group to explore this pairing as a communication of experiences that were threatening and therefore were not verbally formulated in the group discourse.

Therefore, we propose as an essential rule to differentiate snitching from whistleblowing or civilian informing, based on the question whether the snitching is used by the leader to isolate and punish the opponents and enforce "one truth" in a group or society, or the conductor uses whistleblowing to support and encourage various opinions.

Snitching in Czechoslovakia

Martin: I grew up in former communist Czechoslovakia, where many people were voluntarily or forcefully engaged in snitching. It is likely that without them, the totalitarian regime could not have lasted for such a long time. The atmosphere of persecution paralyzed most of the political and intellectual protests and anti-regime activities. It is estimated that about 150,000 citizens operated as snitches in communist Czechoslovakia, under the orders of the secret police. In addition, there were the one and a half million members of the communist party who were expected to collaborate with the police, if needed. Both organizations, the secret police, and the communist party, had special hierarchies for snitching. The first structure consisted of an upper floor of the residents directing the agents who commanded the informers (or the confidents) and special subgroup of the candidates of informing and of the owners of conferred flats, while the snitching "pyramid" of the communist party was partly based on house confidents and street committees. Of course, these two organizations were interconnected and supported each other. The recruitment of snitches was a sophisticated procedure. Preferably, they were recruited deliberately. In the long-term history of the secret police, 20–25% of the snitches were successfully recruited from random parts of the population. At a minimum, every tenth person was ready to collaborate with the secret police. Some of the snitches enjoyed their work, while others collaborated only because of fear. However, even the snitches' elite was not safe from possible persecution. All snitches could eventually come to share their victim's fate: they, too, could be watched. To validate the usefulness of their activity, they were ready to form even false accusations against their victims. Naturally, they supported the system that guaranteed them impunity. The only and risky defense against their engagement was to talk publicly and to be de-conspired. Education that legitimized snitching had begun much earlier than the recruitment by the police, as early as in elementary and high schools. There were methods to "break the character" of young people.

Martin: In the late eighties, when my daughter attended elementary school, the teacher – especially at times she had been absent from the classroom – delegated to her favorite kids the task of watching their classmates and recording the names of those of them who were undisciplined. These "sinners" were consequently punished, while the little snitches were praised by the teacher. When I protested this method, the teacher did not understand my objections. She believed that this method only supported children's sense of responsibility. She was unaware of how this practice destroyed peer solidarity.

A friend of mine had told me, in pain, of his moral failure when he was 17. One girl from his class had had a love affair with a dissident and attended anti-regime concerts. One day, the school director unexpectedly entered the class along with a few inspectors and asked the students to sign a petition to expel this girl from the school. No one was permitted to leave the room and the students who objected to signing were immediately considered as supporters of dissidents. Except for one student, all 30 frightened students obeyed the director's command. The punished girl committed suicide soon afterwards. Of course, this had harmful moral consequences for many students. Some of them felt broken for the rest of their lives, but some adopted cynical attitudes to underestimate their personal involvement. None of their parents protested this violence; it was too risky. Typically, they justified their passivity as a "reasonable" choice and criticized that rebellious girl.

In 1989, the communist regime fell. Its fall raised questions also about recovery from the experience of snitching. The part of archives of the secret police was intentionally destroyed. However, many documents survived up to this day. It turned out that the registered confidents and agents included some successful politicians, intellectuals, and businessmen of the present era. Most of them, when confronted, denied their responsibility and downplayed their secret collaboration. Only rarely did snitches apologize before their past victims. We believe that when the democratic authorities do not advance moral or juridical punishment of past snitching, its working through is inhibited. The so-called "law on compulsory vetting of persons" that prevents snitches from infiltrating power structures in democratic societies is often violated. Too often snitches' crimes are forgotten and the distinction between them and their "objects" is blurred. These un-mourned experiences remain in society like seeds of future pathology.

A psychoanalytic view of snitching

The psychology of siblings is one possible model for understanding the dynamics of snitching, although we are aware of its limitations. Snitching represents much more complex social-psychological phenomenon that cannot be understood from a family matrix point of view. Still, we believe that a peer perspective allows the exploration of snitching as relational pathology that is based mainly but not solely on horizontally disturbed, traumatizing experiences. Juliet Mitchell (2003) proposed that siblings' experiences do not result primarily from Oedipal and castration complexes, but from earlier matrices. She formulated "the law of the mother", which prohibits violence and incest between siblings and is directed against obliteration of differences. In her view, horizontal prohibitions of sexuality and aggression are weaker than their vertical equivalents (there are reports that incest taboo is violated more frequently between siblings than between parents and children). It seems to us that snitching can be viewed as an expression of peer conflicts, when the "law of the mother" fails. Mitchell highlighted the crucial role of the mother in supporting the development of healthy relationships between siblings. Then we could understand snitching as a failure of the protective and benign roles of authorities that, instead, come to represent the dominance of rather cruel, sadistic elements in psyche.

Let us remember a pleasurable and exciting sadomasochistic fantasy that was mentioned in Freud's "A Child Is Being Beaten" (1919) paper, which involves the idea of someone else (i.e., a hated rival sibling) being beaten by a parent, while the fantasizing person can believe that he is the unique object of the parent's love. Can we recognize similar psychic organization when it comes to snitching? We assume that the snitch can also deflect aggression aimed primarily at parental authority and peers (and the associated fear of punishment) to the "objects" he watches.

Obviously, voyeurism plays an important role in snitching. The watching eyes and listening ears are symbols of aggressive penetration into others' homes. In the 18th-century underworld slang, in which the word "nose" was used to refer to a snitch – perhaps because a snitch is nosy. In Hebrew, the word (originating in Yiddish) that is used to refer to a snitch is "stinker", that is, a person who stinks. Then, snitching is mainly associated with sensing the smells of other people. This brings us to anal terminology and the associated versions of sexuality and aggression. Privacy is not valued as developmental achievement, but it is equal with threatening, envied space where otherness is placed.

Lewis Aron (1996) described the dialectics between the wish to know and be known by the other and the equally present wish to remain unknown. Snitching involves perverted knowing the other without permission and its misuse. Paradoxically, snitching can also be seen – at least in some cases – as a perverted attempt at intimacy. Sometimes, snitches become personally engaged with their "objects" and lose their stance. Their hatred can be partially transformed into love. In the Czech film "Bonds" (2010), the tragedy of a snitch who falls in love with his "object", a young woman, shows that perverted intimacy cannot be easily transformed into natural closeness. The desperate snitch feels isolated and ends up committing suicide. In the German film "The Lives of Others" (2006), the snitch identifies with the drama of the people he watches. He finds new meaning in secretly protecting them and sharing their lives, instead of remaining alienated.

The group analytic view of snitching

There are no references to snitching in group analytic literature, perhaps because, historically, Foulkes paid little attention to aggression in small groups and was ambivalent regarding the value of the large group concept and methodology. Weinberg and Schneider (2003) discuss the group analytic view about aggression in societies: as related to survival anxiety (fears of injury and death and fear of psychic annihilation), competition, envy, and the death instinct (Nitsun, 2006) to dependence on leaders (Shaked in Scneider and Weinberg, 2003) and as embedded in the context of collective post-traumas (Hopper, 2003). Sheila Thompson, Patrick de Mare, and Robin Piper wrote about "Coinonia" (1991). They proposed that frustrated wild libido in society generates hatred between people and groups and to a regression to mindlessness, that is, to an absence of reason and individual thought.

We found that psychoanalytic explanations of snitching are limited since they derived from individual psychology. At the same time, group analytic models are beneficial for small groups and are limited in explaining societies. We were driven to formulate a more specific model for snitching that takes into account how it emerged in totalitarian regimes and we found in Václav Havel's essays one of the most authentic explanatory models of this dynamic.

Living in a lie and living in a truth

Havel was the president of former Czechoslovakia and later the Czech Republic. During the communist era, he was one of the leaders of dissident initiatives in this country, including Charter 77, and spent five years in prison. He is known worldwide as a humanist and a symbol of opposition against communist violence.

In his essay "Power of the Powerless" (1991 [2018]), Havel proposed that people are driven by conflicting motives – either to "live in a lie", that is, to lose one's moral integrity and adopt collective preferences, such as profane materialism and pragmatism – or to "live in truth", which guarantees preservation of personal dignity and free thought/behavior.

Havel claimed that communist regimes in the Soviet bloc had unique characteristics that were different from previous dictatorial regimes. One of them was central place of utopian ideology. This ideology dominated everyday life and had even the quality of a delusional dictating power. It gained an autonomous status of a pseudo-reality, a kind of collective fantasy that was superior to individual experiences. This ideology built a bridge between power and reality and created coherence between the communist system and ordinary people. The majority of the people submitted to "the rules of game" and agreed to "live in a lie" in exchange for personal safety and peace.

However, according to Havel, society's acceptance of communist ideology did not result only from anxiety, but he believed that it was easier for some people to submit to a collective identity than to struggle to develop their own truths. This universal tendency could explain how ordinary people who were victims of the totalitarian ideological system also found themselves participating voluntarily in the perpetuation of "living in a lie".

Therefore, betrayal of truth and pretense were immanent parts of everyday life in Czechoslovakia and other Soviet countries. This was the "road to perdition", since it unavoidably led to self-alienation: individual identity was sacrificed for the sake of the so-called system identity.

Since this regime was based on obedience to the ideological discipline, it could not tolerate free search for truth. When truth and individual freedom were expressed, they immediately received political value and represented an unpredictable threat to the totalitarian stability.

The following example from Havel's essay can shed light on the role played by ideology in everyday practices in the 1980s of the previous century:

> The manager of a fruit-and-vegetable shop put on his display, between onions and carrots, a poster with the slogan: "Workers of the world,

> unite!" . . . Was he genuinely enthusiastic about the idea of unity among the workers of the world? . . . I think that it can safely be assumed that the large majority of shopkeepers never thought of the slogans that they put in their displays. . . . He put them all on the display simply because this is what has been done for many years. . . . If he were to refuse, he could be accused of disloyalty. He did it to guarantee himself a relatively peaceful life "in harmony with society". . . . Let us take note: if the greengrocer had been instructed to display the slogan "I am afraid and therefore I am unquestioningly obedient", he would have been ashamed and embarrassed. Ideology became a façade to hide this.

Havel stressed that one shopkeeper's slogan on his display was meaningless, but the massive participation of the population created an illusion of collective compliance with communist ideology. It was not necessary to believe those mystifications, but to live as if believing them. The ideology occupied the place of emotions and honest motives, which were considered as subjective truth, and therefore dangerous. The citizens' fear from persecution and the communist leaders wishes to gain power and control were concealed under dogmatic untouchable ideology.

Snitching served as an instrument of power and communication of lies and half-truths between and against the members of society. The practical role of the snitches was to register and destroy all seeds of free thought. The continued existence of the communist regime crucially depended on loyalty to these mystifications. People who excluded themselves from the collective "game", such as the dissidents and other people, were viewed as abnormal and provocative.

The possibility to "live in truth" was in the hands of each person, according to Havel. He emphasized that dissidents were not necessarily politically active; they mainly acted as free-minded citizens. The access to truth was not granted to or owned by a limited social or political group; it remained as a potential present in all society, including the leading structures. This is a good place to mention Winnicott's idea about a minimal 30% mature persons and 20% indeterminates (living in a "grey zone") that are necessary in every society to maintain collective freedom. Winnicott suggests that this minimal percentage should hold democratic machinery and compensate for open or hidden anti-socials (Winnicott, 1986, p. 245). Hidden anti-social individuals are identified with authority without their self-discovery. They are like a "frame without sense of the picture", obeying with no thought and fostering conditions for dictators. Snitches often belong to this category. Havel put forward the idea that people are pushed to live in lies also because they are able to adapt to such conditions.

Hopper's (2003) concept of incohesion seems to fit, to some extent, to the situation of Czechoslovakian society after World War II and during the communist era. According to Hopper, incohesion is characteristic of post-traumatic societies. People who experienced fear of annihilation, losses, and abandonment are likely to form groups that are characterized by unconscious defensive processes of "aggregation" – in reaction to fission and fragmentation – or by "massification" – in reaction to fusion and confusion, and by oscillations between the two. In massification, society is identified with an idea of oneness and homogeneity, which helps to obliterate differences and the heterogeneity of voices. In aggregation, individuals are split and isolated, living in small social "bubbles". Perhaps we can recognize both manifestations of incohesion in communist Czechoslovakia: collective pretense externally, and an aggregated, more individualized way of private living. Massification was encouraged by the communist regime and it was evident mainly on the public level, while aggregation existed in the separate "bubbles" apart from public life. We propose that snitching worked in the service of massification and facilitated the homogenization of various aggregated parts of society.

Havel stressed the impersonal character of a vast range of totalitarian activities – snitching included – and their ritualization: these activities had to be done to keep the automatism of the totalitarian regime in motion. The main aim of this automatism was to reproduce itself and to expand outward and inward. The citizens were not important as individuals but as anonymous particles that co-created the panorama of totalitarian continuity. This continuity depended on the collaboration of the majority of the population. The invasion of snitches into private areas and their violation of the boundaries between public and private was only one example of the omnipresent control and ideological "sterilization" of the society. Snitching can also be viewed as an expression of an expanding totalitarian power that did not respect any boundaries. Without the existence of democratic regulation, this power had no limits to stop expanding.

Much social and psychological energy was needed to delay the moment in which communist ideology unavoidably lost its vividness and influence and turned into an empty construct. When World War II ended, the war-like mentality in middle Europe did not diminish. On the contrary, it was idealized, kept alive, and fueled new communist enthusiasm. The generations born after World War II were raised listening to heroic war stories. War and military narratives invited the offspring to identify with a post-traumatic ethos. The political term "cold war" was coined to address the conflict between the communist "camp" and capitalist Western countries. Snitching became a part of this war-like scenery, where the continuous threat of external or internal enemies was articulated. This scenery was not always linked to a real threat – rather, it was constantly fed by a military or paramilitary rhetoric. Snitches were identified with "peace warriors", who protected the society from internal foes. At least some of them did their job believing in their righteousness.

Nevertheless, the snitches were also people who were potentially exposed to a conflict between an individual search for a true identity and a desire to merge with a mass identity. Obviously, they were primarily driven to eradicate signs of free thought in society. However, in due time, at least some of them reconnected to repressed seeds of truth. Following Foulkes' (1948) idea of "mirror reactions" in small groups, we propose that these can be expressed also in the broader context of society. The facing of dissidents as mirrors of their own projected parts may have re-awoken in the snitches their own loyalty conflict with the regime; their witnessing of the dissidents' courage could have also provoked envy and fear. Both experiences, anger and envy of the dissidents, may have strengthened their adherence to the war-like discipline.

De Mare, Piper, and Thompson (1991) share Havel's hopeful view on transformation of traumatized societies, but they stressed that profound discourse is necessary to change a mindless society into a thinking society. As group analysts, they also claimed that a discourse is essential for the recovery of siblings' relationships in society. We believe that snitching represents not only a symptom of mindless society but also a breach in trust between individuals in society, which deserves exploration as well.

We propose that the prohibition to be in touch with one's core truths creates alienation in society, as well. Bollas (1992) suggests that in perverted relationships, the other is pushed away and hated because he represents life, passion, and genuineness instead of using the other as a container.

Snitches not only documented the dissidents' unfaithfulness to ideology but voluntarily made up fictions about the dissidents' alleged burglaries, addictions, pornography, and sexual deviations. We suggest that snitching was used also as an instrument to attack relationships that entailed a potential for truth and passion.

Discussion

In this chapter, we invited snitches to leave their place behind the curtain and tried to formulate a few introductory hypotheses about their functioning. This engagement on our part involved ambivalent feelings of curiosity, post-traumatic memories, and acknowledgment of the potential for hatred in societies.

We attempted to use psychoanalytical models and group analytic explanations to understand snitching, but we found them both as limited. Psychoanalytic explanations tend to use familial models that can partly explain individual cases of perverted snitching, but they are not sufficient to explain snitching in large societies. We showed that snitching can be approached as an asymmetrical relational process between two or more persons accompanied with specific pathology of hatred, often dissociated from love. This perverted violence could be explored on the continuum with other anti-social expressions, for instance bullying, harassing, mobbing, or stalking.

Group analysts explore aggression often via large groups that are conducted in institutes and conferences, but they pay less attention to the exploration of aggression in societies.

We believe that every society has a potential for auto-destruction. Havel gives us authentic socio-historical and philosophical reflections of hatred working in the communist society, including the phenomenon of snitching. He emphasized the role of utopian ideology in totalitarian regimes. We propose that ideological or political snitching was the regime's instrument to make sure that any attempt for free thought would be attacked. We suggest that snitches' activity was driven also to attack relationships representing vividness, passion, and honesty, which were considered as dangerous to the regime. Always it was aimed to de-differentiating between public and private zones. Maybe certain neglect on Havel's part of disturbed social relationships can help explain his policy of avoiding punishment of former snitches.

We also propose that "mirrors reactions" exist between groups in society and not only in small groups, and that snitches may have felt envy when observing dissidents' courage to seek a truthful life. The snitches' envy when looking in the mirror could explain their willingness to collaborate with their authorities and their investment in their work.

Bion (1974) highlighted truth as an aspect of mental health, and a universal conflict as to being in touch with one's emotional truth, an idea that we find as meaningful. We perceive psychoanalysis and group analysis as spaces that foster candid communication between patient and himself, between patient and other members of the group including a conductor and an analyst. We are aware that not all people can take part in psychoanalytic treatments and in analytic groups, still we see our work as a humble contribution to "life with a truth".

References

Aron, L. (1996). *A Meeting of Minds: Mutuality in Psychoanalysis*. Hillsdale, NJ: The Analytic Press.

Bion, W.R. (1974). *Bion's Brazilian Lectures: Book 1*. Rio de Janeiro: Imago Editera Ltd.

Bollas, C. (1992). Violent innocence. In: *Being a Character: Psychoanalysis and Self Experience*. London: Routledge.

Bonds (2010). Director Radim Spacek.

De Mare, P., Piper, R. and Thompson, S. (1991). *Koinonia: From Hate, Through Dialogue, to Culture in the Large Group*. London: Karnac Books.

Foulkes, S.H. (1948). *Introduction to Group Analytic Psychotherapy*. London: Karnac, 1983.

Freud, S. (1919). A child is being beaten a contribution to the study of the origin of sexual perversions. In: *The Standard Edition of the Complete Psychological Works of Sigmund*. London: Hogarth Press.

Freud, Volume XVII (1917–1919): An Infantile Neurosis and Other Works (pp. 175–204).

Havel, V. (1991 [2018]). The power of the powerless. In: Paul Wilson (trans.; ed.), *Open Letters: Selected Writings: 1965–1990*. New York: Vintage Classics.

Hopper, E. (2003). Aspects of aggression in large groups characterised by (ba) I:A/M. In: S. Schneider and H. Weinberg (eds.), *The Large Group Revisited: The Herd, Primal Horde, Crowds and Masses* (pp. 58–72). London: Jessica Kingsley Publishers.

The Lives of Others. (2006). Director Florian Henckel Von Donnersmarck.

Mitchell, J. (2003). *Siblings: Sex and Violence*. London: Polity Press.

Nitsun, M. (2006). *The Anti-Group: Destructive Forces in the Group and Their Creative Potential*. London: Routledge.

Weinberg, H. and Schneider, S. (2003). *The Large Group Revisited: The Herd, Primal Horde, Crowds and Masses*. London: Jessica Kingsley Publishers.

Winnicott, D.W., Winnicott, C., Shepherd, R. and Davies, M. (1986). *Home Is Where We Start From: Essays by a Psychoanalyst*. New York: Norton.

3.4 "Law of the mother" – its impact on love and hate between siblings and in society

Gila Ofer

Yet am I justified in wisdom's eyes.
For even had it been some child of mine,
Or husband mouldering in death's decay,
I had not wrought this deed despite the State.
What is the law I call in aid? 'Tis thus
I argue. Had it been a husband dead
I might have wed another, and have borne
Another child, to take the dead child's place.
But, now my sire and mother both are dead,
No second brother can be born for me.

Antigone by Sophocles, in Tr. F. Storr. Cambridge, MA (1912): Harvard University Press

(Antigone is torn between her love for her brother, who she feels deserves burial, and his declared status as a traitor, who therefore must be treated as one. She chooses to openly honor her brother by burying him. This means that she too will die, as in burying her brother she has violated the law of Creon, the King.)

Years ago, Juliet Mitchell conceptualized lateral relations between siblings along an autonomous horizontal axis, but this axis interacts with the vertical parent–child axis. Everyone who engages in group analysis is in need of this material, but in psychoanalysis, in individual treatment, there is no analysis without the appearance of prominent elements related to siblings, be they younger siblings, twins, older siblings, or being a single child.

It is important to note that although psychoanalysis has indeed seldom referred to the issue of siblings, the Bible, as well as Greek and Shakespearean tragedies, have dealt abundantly with the issue (*Antigone*, *King Lear*, *As You Like It*, etc.).

Professionally, we all tend to refer to the dynamics of brothers and sisters as stemming from the Oedipal triangle. But, in fact, we miss a great deal of important information if we disregard transferences related to siblings.

In this chapter I focus on several aspects:

1 The location and focus of the law of the mother as I see it
2 Examples of the absence of the law of the mother in the Bible

DOI: 10.4324/9781003220060-22

3 Clinical vignettes of complex cases of the law of the mother in individual psychotherapy, and in group analysis
4 The significance of the law of the mother in society in general

In the essay "From the Sibling Trauma to the Law of the Mother" Mitchell emphasizes that it is not only siblings who are absent from psychoanalysis, the mother is too. One can say that the mother, since Melanie Klein, is not so much absent, but she is present as an object, an object for the child that becomes an inner object, but not as a subject. Mitchell adds a particularly important role for the mother: a mother who connects to reality in general, and to social reality in particular. The law of the mother is related to this. If the mother does not lay down the law of the mother, she causes division, denial, and dissociation from the social aspect. In a similar manner, psychoanalysis has recreated this situation by ignoring the issue of siblings and the law of the mother, and thus there are few direct references to siblings in theory and case descriptions.

I conjecture that part of the extensive avoidance of the issue of siblings in psychoanalysis over many years is related to one-person psychology. In this respect, group analysis and relational psychoanalysis, with their emphasis on the shared construction of the unconscious and treatment processes, have to a large degree changed the picture. But the issue of siblings remains in the background, along with the law of the mother. To summarize Mitchell's law from her paper (2018):

> The law of the mother originates as a source of authority that sharply distinguishes between the mother and the toddler; the toddler is not identical to the mother. It cannot give birth to children. This is the vertical axis that enables a transition to the horizontal axis, which is also the social axis. The law of the mother organizes the sibling trauma and enables the infant to grow into the social. It forbids the infant from murdering its sibling and similarly forbids sexuality between siblings.

This law is rooted in the motherly attitude of love towards each child. Each child is special and equivalent; and this implies that each child is unique and equal at the same time. This is also the law that consecrates differences between parents and infants, and it precedes the law of the father, which is related to the Oedipal complex.

Ultimately this law facilitates the expression of the need to be special and unique (everyone is similar to everyone else only in a partial sense) with the need for intimacy and trust. It is a law and therefore, along with the law of the father, is embedded in the unconscious.

The vertical axis is indirectly reminiscent of Benjamin's essay "Father and Daughter: Identification with a Difference" (1991). In this essay Benjamin indeed refers first and foremost to fathers and daughters, describing the need for identificatory love, complete identification with the father or the mother before maturation and passage into the Oedipal stage of object love, of heterosexual love. In other words, both male and female infants must feel that they are exactly like the mother in order to develop and acquire the ability to love 'the other'. Mitchell, too, argues that full identification with the mother happens and is necessary as a first stage before the infant understands that he is different from the mother, and before the transition to acceptance of the sibling and the law of the mother on the horizontal axis.

Ogden too refers to this pre-Oedipal stage in his essay about the Oedipal transitions in female development (1987). He refers to the importance of the pre-Oedipal stage but conceptualizes it through Oedipal thinking and identification of the mother with her father, and not through the direct link of the mother with the lineage of motherhood. Interestingly, the two essays I mention here attempt to deal with female development.

Mitchell is a renowned feminist, and the conceptualization of the law of the mother as preserving the uniqueness of each sibling (along with the emphasis on a social and sharing direction) is anchored, I believe, in her thinking as a mother, philosopher, and feminist. But when numerous feminists attacked psychoanalysis as reflecting a patriarchal society, she herself argued that the law of the mother does not support the patriarchal society; rather, it reflects society with the law of the mother, in depth and with courage (Mitchell, 2013). Out of this feminist thinking she added the law of the mother *as a necessary pillar* of her theory, alongside the law of the father, and in this she added another important strain of feminism to psychoanalysis, along with feminists such as Chodorow, Benjamin, Chasseguet-Smirgel, Kristeva, and others. She also anchors the mother not only as an object (as Benjamin argued, 1991) but also as a subject, with authority, intentions, and desires of her own.

The application of the law of the mother is a gradual process of negotiation in which the infant discovers and creates social aspect. This description is reminiscent of the transitional space of which Winnicott wrote (1969). This process carries the risk of losing uniqueness and omnipotence if it is carried out in a severe and disempowering manner. However, I believe that the process of accepting the law of the mother among siblings is identical to that described by Winnicott in his essay "The Use of an Object and Relating through Identification" (1969).

Winnicott describes the process that occurs between mother and baby, and I argue that this process also takes place among siblings, due to the law of the mother. It is a process of concurrent love and hate, in which one 'the subject-sibling' must discover the other sibling, one through his destruction, and the ability of 'the other', in this case 'the sibling', not to be destroyed. Thus, the destruction of the sibling object removes him from the omnipotent control of the subject-sibling.

The sibling object develops an autonomy and life of its own because it has survived and contributes to its own subjectivity. This is a mutual process, of course, between the two siblings, such as I have seen between my children when they were little (and to some extent today as well), when they would get into serious fights and struggle with each other, and finally emerge from the process hugging and loving each other. To quote Winnicott:

> This is a position that can be arrived at by the individual in the early stages of emotional growth only through the actual survival of cathected objects that are at the same time in the process of becoming destroyed because real, becoming real because destroyed.
>
> (1969)

While psychoanalysis ignored the law of the mother and the sibling trauma, the Bible certainly did not. There are numerous sibling stories to be found in the Bible, and here I will mention two cases in which it seems the law of the mother was not upheld. In the first case, one brother murders the other, and in the second case a brother has sex with his sister. In both cases the mother is not mentioned, and one can conclude that the law of the mother was not put into practice. The results are disastrous in both cases.

The case of Cain, a farmer, and Abel, a shepherd, is the well-known biblical, archetypical story (Genesis 4:1–16). They both submit their offerings to the Lord, who accepts Abel's but rejects Cain's. Cain is consumed by jealousy and kills Abel. In this story the mother, Eve, is mentioned only at their birth; after this she is not mentioned at all. She is not an authority figure and the absence of a mother encapsulates the Lord's discriminatory attitude toward the two brothers. The law of the mother – which guarantees the brothers' difference and separateness but also makes possible their joining, uniqueness versus sharing – is not implemented and a murder is committed.

The second case is the story of Amnon and Tamar (2 Samuel 13:1). Amnon desires his (half) sister and attempts to seduce her. When he fails to do so, he pretends to be ill and asks his father, King David, to send Tamar to him so that she can prepare delicacies for him and feed him. David orders her to do so and when she obeys, Amnon rapes her. After the rape, his passion turns to hatred and he throws her out of his room. David hears of this and is angry at Amnon but does not punish him. Amnon is killed two years later by Absalom, Tamar's brother. Tamar herself is not mentioned anymore and apparently never recovered from the incident.

As in the story of Cain and Abel, here too the absence of a mother is prominent. The father, David, thoughtlessly is an accomplice to the act, then later does not punish Amnon, and he certainly does not support Tamar. The absence of the mother also signifies the absence of the law that forbids incest among siblings, and the absence of the law that forbids murder of siblings.

Examples from individual psychoanalysis

Here I present cases in which the mother herself experienced a trauma that prevented her from applying the law of the mother, and as a consequence a distorted version of the law of the mother prevailed among her children.

Dana has been in analysis for several years. Both of her parents are Holocaust survivors. Her father lived among the partisans, and her mother is the only member of her family who survived when she managed to escape the death march. Both parents and two older brothers were killed during the march. Dana's brother was born in 1947, two years after the end of the war, while Dana's mother was, apparently, still suffering from the effects of the war and death. Dana herself is four years younger than her brother. The mother appears to be a depressed, withdrawn woman, surrounded by barriers, which makes it impossible to communicate with her. Dana's brother had no boundaries and was ousted from school on a daily basis; he was aggressive and could not adjust to any framework. His parents had no idea how to control him. The only way to communicate with him was through the father, through strict discipline, and corporal punishment. At a young age he was sent to a kibbutz where he grew up until he left for the army. Dana herself was a 'good girl', disciplined, and did not appear to be in need of anything. However, when she was away from home with friends, she felt compelled to go back home every couple of hours to make sure that her mother was alright. She always said that the only thing that her mother knew how to do was to provide a warm meal and a clean house. Dana, as a child, adolescent, and woman, grew up knowing how to serve others, as can be seen in her current chosen profession. She was consumed by guilt for the beatings suffered by her brother and for his expulsion from home. Dana's brother became a failed entrepreneur who borrowed money from friends and lost it. He lives in a lavish apartment but barely manages to get by and pay alimony to his ex-wife. At the same time, Dana works for a living, providing for herself as well her husband. When Dana was fifty years old her mother became ill. She wrote a will, while she still alive, leaving the apartment to both children. Dana immediately and unthinkingly relinquished her share of the apartment to her brother. When I asked her to reflect on why she did this, she pounced on me angrily saying that other than herself there was no one to take care of her brother and that otherwise he would be homeless: "Would you desert your brother?" she said. I will not go into the details regarding the process in which we engaged, but as expected, the brother sold the apartment after their mother died without ever moving into it. Two years later there was not a penny left from the proceeds.

The story of Dana and her brother can be viewed from various angles. But it is also possible to say that since Dana's mother was absent as a mother to both siblings, this absence prevented the law of the mother from being fully internalized: that is – the mother gives birth to children and the siblings have equal but separate standing in the social order. Dana was left with the need to stand in for the mother in order to safeguard her brother's life and uniqueness. He did not become part of the social order and she could not be there as a sister but rather as an alternate mother. The way she saw it was that if she had not given him the apartment, it was equivalent to abandoning him and leaving him to die.

Karen is another case: her mother, also an Auschwitz survivor, grew up without a mother and her entire family was destroyed in the Holocaust. The mother related to Karen as a twin forming a complete symbiotic relationship to satisfy her needs. But when Karen's younger brother was born, three years after her, he contracted a grave illness and the mother, who was unable to take care of both children, sent Karen to live with her cousin for several months. After the brother recovered Karen returned home and needed to take her place again, but she was still greatly affected by the harsh separation from her mother. Her feeling that the mother preferred her brother intensified, unless she was symbiotically connected with the mother. Today, Karen has a profession and is successful, while her brother has been trying to establish a freelance business for years and is getting into deeper and deeper financial trouble. When their mother died, Karen's brother asked Karen to give up a significant part of her inheritance for him. Karen agreed immediately. Here, too, when I asked her why, and if she could explain this, she grew angry at me and said: "Would you have deserted your brother? He could have collapsed without this." From her point of view, not giving him the money was like murdering him.

I argue that the mother was unable to function as a mother with motherly authority. Instead, she turned Karen into her clone and passed a distorted version of the law of the mother on to both Karen and her brother. You, Karen, must be a mother to your brother; you are not his sibling, you are his mother. In other words, the vertical axis that distinguishes mother from daughter was not preserved here, neither was the horizontal axis, which preserves siblinghood in a manner that allows each sibling to be unique along with owning social responsibility and trust. A symbiotic mother or an absent one cannot pass on the motherly attitude and therefore cannot pass on the law of the mother in its entirety. In both cases the brother as well as the sister were affected by the fact that the law of the mother was not transmitted and internalized by them. It is also possible that there were additional factors, such as gender differences, involved in both cases and contributed to the partial functioning of the brother and the sister taking the role of caretaker or life saver.

Example from group analysis

Lili was referred to me at her request. She had spent about two years in individual therapy and decided, contrary to the opinion of her therapist, to terminate individual therapy and enter group therapy. At the intake interview, she stated that her reason for wanting to join the group was a bewildering recollection occasioned by a dream, that she was ostracized by her classmates throughout sixth grade. She could not remember the reason for being ostracized, nor had she talked to anyone about it since. In addition, she said that she lost her job and did not know exactly why, and added "anyway, I did not like my colleagues and my boss was too bossy". She related that her mother adored her sister but was emotionally indifferent to her, Lily. The mother abandoned her at an early age, but took her sister with her, for reasons that were unclear to her. She also had little knowledge of why her mother eventually came back with her sister. Lili ended up avoiding any kind of relationship with both her sister and her mother for years, refusing any attempt on the part of friends and family to reunite them. Lili seemed to be a highly intelligent woman, somewhat aggressive, with little capacity for self-reflection.

Immediately upon joining the group, Lili assumed a dominant position. Anyone who chose to share anything was bombarded by a barrage of questions. She never seemed to run out of interpretations or the inclination to offer them. It was clear that these interpretative interventions were her way of overcoming her fear of being ignored by the group. The group itself, which had been somewhat listless before her arrival, snapped into liveliness. They accepted her at first with enthusiasm. Whenever Lili spoke, the group would fall silent. Some members could not hide their admiration. In others, her dominance evoked much resistance and they saw her behavior as condescending. This affected me and more than once I felt paralyzed. I felt as if she was looking at the members and even me as children. The members who were angry with her did not spare her their opinion. They did not mince their words. I could tell that she was deeply offended by this and offered the following group intervention:

> It is not easy for you to accept someone new into the group. Some of you are silent because you are swallowing your anger at me for bringing someone new into the group and letting her control the group. Since you can't take it out on me, you're angry at Lili, who has no trouble speaking her mind.

That same night, she sent me a text, thanking me for defending her. From that session on, however, her domineering behavior grew more and more pronounced. She shared nothing about herself, while handing out a multitude of interpretations to anyone else. The other members commented on this, but her response was "I'm not keeping any of you from talking". Something about her tone became more and more arrogant. She occasionally criticized me, claiming that I offered someone the wrong interpretation. She also complained that I talked too little. When I said that my silence makes her relive her experience of being abandoned, she laughed and said that I "can't touch" her. "You can only touch the others here, but not me". The hint of sadomasochism in her words worried me. I felt that she was challenging me and did not accept me as overseeing the group. I was concerned both for her and for the group. In one of the sessions, she did mention being ostracized many years ago, and it was like murdering her; but her tone was distant and void of emotion. I said to her:

> You're trying to show us that you don't care about this harsh ostracism. It is a terrible punishment and you have no idea why it happened to you. Maybe you even prefer not knowing, because you are afraid that it might hurt too much. But your face tells us that you're hurting. Maybe you're afraid that this group will also cast you out.

She fell silent and withdrew. I thought that she felt accused. She soon resumed her onslaught of condemning questions, accusations, and interpretations against anyone who shared anything personal.

One day, when another member shared some problematic feelings he had concerning his daughter, she suddenly blurted out that she also had something to share with the group. She told us that she threw her son from her first marriage (which ended many years ago) out of the house, and he has not spoken to her for over a year. She threw him out because her current partner told her that he could not stand having her son around. The group was struck dumb. Most members brought attention to her son's pain at having been abandoned.

I turned to the group and said:

> Lili's son is certainly having a difficult time. But she herself is torn between wanting the love of her husband and that of her son. In driving your son out, Lili, you were actually repeating in your distress what your mother had done to you. More than this, what you picked up from your mother is that it is impossible to love two loved ones at the same time – each in a unique way.

I was quite anxious in saying this, as I did not know how she would take it. In the following session, I was glad to hear that she had contacted her son. Things were still very fragile, but they were back on speaking terms. That was the last time she used the group to work on her own personal issues.

A month went by and Lili kept throwing endless questions at anyone who shared anything in the group. Her dominance seemed to dwarf the other members. In one of the sessions, another member Ruthie, snapped at her: "Cut it out, Lili, we are sick and tired of you bossing us around, again and again, and you won't even give us enough time to answer you!"

Lili turned red and mercilessly went on the offensive: "Who even asked you, anyway? What right do you have, telling me what to do? You're so narcissistic, so self-absorbed, you can't respect me! Fatty!"

I intercepted saying: "There is so much anger here now because you feel that only one of you can survive; as if the other is being rejected, murdered".

Lili started lashing out in such a way that I could no longer reason with her. She retorted:

> I don't want to listen to you. What do you think you're doing? Going about shoving things in my face. Sitting there thinking all the time, creasing your forehead, trying to figure things out, you usually end up not getting anything. You have no idea what you're doing! What kind of therapist are you? And there are people sitting here, who used to be your patients? And they have this direct line to you that I don't even see. I can be a better therapist than you! I can't stand you people – and you most of all!

She rose from her chair and said that she would mail me a check for her unpaid sessions. The group members were in shock. We were almost at the end of the session. She saw them outside and burst out, "Well done, you ostracized me just like I've been ostracized before".

Naturally, I was left feeling very uneasy. My further attempts to reach out to her outside the group setting were unsuccessful. In the following sessions, group members talked about how she was actually re-enacting her childhood experience, and seemed unable to change.

Being or staying in a group for Lili was like reviving the primordial pain where her mother was more absent than present. She could not give both her children the feeling of being loved in a unique way. Therefore, Lili would not accept me as a conductor/mother, and could not be part of the group, the social world where more than one person can coexist. She was only able to survive by fighting or dominating and 'murdering' the others in her psychic life. She was able to feel her uniqueness in a distorted way and avoid and deny her feelings of rejection and abandonment. This, however, prevented her from experiencing acceptance and support when these were offered by the group. She ended up leaving the group without accomplishing true change.

A look at society as a whole

Mitchell emphasizes that the law of the mother comes with the transition from omnipotent narcissism to the social child (more or less at the age of two, two and a half years). If it does not occur, then sibling murder or incest, whether symbolic or physical, may take place. Sibling murders are prominent in mobster movies, such as *The Godfather*. There, the law of the father reigns and the mother is absent, and we see how the younger brother murders his brother after he did not comply assiduously with the law of the father.

We see that entire societies in coping with their identity do so from a narcissistic, omnipotent place in order to differentiate them from the Other, but only through mass murder or rape. A few examples in which this can be seen are: Hitler who had to be different from others, from other brothers, by killing millions of others, Jews, homosexuals, cripples; the struggle between the various branches of Islam, which continues to this day with ISIS at its apex, leads to the murder of everyone who is suspected of being an Other and does not obey the law of being identical; in Burma, the horrifying massacre of the Rovinga; and things that happen in my own country, such as the deportation of refugees, separation of Ethiopian Jews in ultra-orthodox schools, and more. All of these are societies that are organized around the law of the father and not around the law of the mother as defined by Mitchell. In fact, it is no wonder that figures such as Michelle Obama are so popular. The search for mothers can bring about the law of the mother.

We see that entire societies are defined by the law of the father in a way that accentuates the absence of the law of the mother and also characterizes the massification defense (Hopper, 2003a) – we are all the same and identical in our thinking – or alternately, a majority that hides behind the aggregation defense (Hopper, 2003b) – each to his own – which prevents healthy siblinghood.

In conclusion: the influence of feminism on psychoanalytical theory has enriched it and added numerous areas that are not related only to the development of girls. The questions: are the sibling trauma and the law of the mother theoretical concepts that must be developed and treated in depth? Some will argue that previous theories cover the development of the child at this age and therefore it is doubtful whether these concepts are in fact needed. I believe that according to what I have presented in this chapter, Mitchell's innovations, including the vertical axis of the mother and the horizontal axis in psychoanalytical theory and group analysis, are important concepts. They are necessary for understanding broad intrapersonal, interpersonal, and social processes. Without these concepts we overlook additional significant aspects that can help us understand normal processes and cope with destructive ones.

References

Benjamin, J. (1991). Father and Daughter: Identification with Difference – Contribution to Gender Heterodoxy. *Psychoanalytic Dialogue*, 1(3): 277–299.

Coppola, F.F. (1972). *The Godfather* (Movie). USA.

Hopper, E. (2003a). *The Social Unconscious: Selected Papers*. London: Jessica Kingsley.

Hopper, E. (2003b). *Traumatic Experience in the Unconscious Life of Groups: The Fourth Basic Assumption: Incohesion: Aggregation/Massification*. London: Jessica Kingsley.

Mitchell, J. (2013). The Law of the Mother: Sibling Trauma and the Brotherhood of War. *Canadian Journal of Psychoanalysis*, 21(1): 145–159.

Mitchell, J. (2018). Core Concepts: From Sibling Trauma to the Law of the Mother. *Paper Presentation in the Conference on: Siblings in Individual and Group Psychoanalytic Psychotherapy*. Tel-Aviv University, Israel.

Ogden, T.H. (1987). The Transitional Oedipal Relationship in Female Development. *The International Journal of Psychoanalysis*, 68: 485–498.

Sophocles. (1912). *Antigone*. Tr. F. Storr. Cambridge, MA: Harvard University Press.

Winnicott, D.W. (1969). The Use of an Object. *The International Journal of Psychoanalysis*, 50: 711–716.

The Horizontal Axis

4.1 The Tree and the Rhizome and the Horizontal Axis – Reflections on Individual and Group Therapy Following Deleuze and Guattari

Avi Berman and Limor Avrahami-Reshef

Deleuze and Guattari: The Tree and the Rhizome

The philosopher Gilles Deleuze (1925–1995) and the psychoanalyst Félix Guattari (1930–1990) began their collaboration in Paris, in the late 1960s. In 1980, they published *A Thousand Plateaus*, the second book they co-wrote and the second part of their two-volume project titled "Capitalism and Schizophrenia" (1983) (the first part was *Anti-Oedipus*, 1983). Its introduction begins with the following words: "The two of us wrote Anti-Oedipus together. Since each of us was several, there was already quite a crowd" (Deleuze and Guattari, 1987/2007, p. 3). By writing together, Deleuze and Guattari were not only able to talk about multiplicity but to actually multiply.

They created a paradigm that enables two forms of cognition (epistemology) by means of two metaphoric concepts: the tree and the rhizome. These are two possible ways of thinking, observing and experiencing, which may address both internal reality (as a reflection on how one thinks and experiences things) and external reality.

The Tree

According to Deleuze and Guattari, the notion of the tree is a metaphor for thinking in hierarchic and causational terms. Much like a tree, this type of thinking has roots and bears fruit. It has both a trunk and branches, in the sense of directionality, derivation, causes and effects. Such thinking is grounded in a hierarchy of concepts and order and is characterized by well-defined boundaries and distinct causality. This view is manifest in scientific and causational thinking. In postmodern thinking, the tree metaphor is considered the "modern," more classic option – the one that necessitates an alternative.

As a metaphor, the "tree" stands for a clear, stable and hierarchic constellation, which has a distinct source and which moves in a single direction – both spatially (from the bottom to the top) – from the depths of its roots to the height of its canopy, and from top to bottom (from the leaves to the roots) and temporally (from the past to the future). Memory is of the utmost importance. Things

DOI: 10.4324/9781003220060-24

that happened in the past offer meaning and context to the present. There are causes and effects and this allows one to examine and evaluate the past as well as to predict the future.

This hierarchy establishes different sectors and classes including meanings of "high" and "low". From the point of view of human relations, the hierarchy explained through the metaphor of the tree includes power relations, administrative hierarchy and control and surveillance mechanisms. Within the framework of such control mechanisms, the tree model entails the establishment of entire organizations (which can be called "branches") devoted to these aims, such as the military or the police, as we experience them in our daily lives. Thus, the tree represents both the temporal unfolding of genealogy and the structural organization of nodes and relations, as the *only* points between which lines of movement and change can be drawn.

Tree thinking is linear. It enables a clear relationship between two points, a relationship that can be precisely located on a vertical axis, from which one can create branching principles. Tree thinking is manifest in the media as popular majoritarian opinion, which is based on fixed and definite identities that compete with one another within a distinct territory. Tree language, like tree thinking, is necessary for many forms of communication.

Because it stresses the aspects of time and depth, the tree modality can be associated with the classic psychoanalytic meaning of consciousness and unconsciousness, explicit and implicit layers or even the realm of the readily known and the realm of the secret that must be uncovered. The past depends on memory and documentation. The relation to the future entails intentions and plans that are based on the past and may simultaneously involve emotions, intentions, wishes and fears.

The Rhizome

In botany a rhizome is a modified subterranean plant stem that sends out roots and shoots from its nodes. Rhizomes develop from axillary buds and grow horizontally.

The rhizome as a metaphor, represents a constant, multidirectional process of becoming, which involves multiple events and motions. The rhizome is a metaphor for a network or web, a thicket of lines, bifurcations and intersections with no end or beginning. It grows many ways simultaneously and every line can sprout new lines. In contrast with the hierarchy represented by the tree metaphor, the rhizome suggests lateral growth.

The rhizome network is nonlinear, nonhierarchic and loosely organized. It enables connectivity between any two points, without having to go through a central switching station, which determines the proportionality and hierarchy of the communication. From the perspective offered by this chapter, the rhizome is characteristic of the horizontal axis.

It represents expansion that derives from a multiplicity of truths, meanings and possibilities. It may be considered as the postmodern alternative to contemporary thought, an alternative mode of thinking through which one observes a world that is ever changing and becoming.

Rhizomatic experience has no interest in concepts, it is neither challenged by questions of identity nor preoccupied with relations to the self or the personal, to anything that is "mine." Deleuze and Guattari view the concept itself as an event, even if each event is its own specific type of event. Rhizomatic thinking reads events from a viewpoint that diminishes any self-criticism on the part of thinking. A conceptual recurrence that revolves around undifferentiating differences; a blind reflection that exists on the surface.

In order to understand the mode of action through which Deleuze and Guattari are trying to tackle the language of the rhizome, they propose that rhizomatic language is a "minor language" (1986). Such a language seeks to elude the kind of thinking that structures and applies power and such concepts as surrender and victory. Instead, it offers thinking *with* things:

> *the* axiomatic manipulates only denumerable sets, even infinite ones, whereas the minorities constitute "fuzzy", nondenumerable sets, in short "masses" multiplicities of escape and flux.
>
> (Deleuze, 2007)

According to Deleuze, rhizomatic thinking is always in a state of addition, putting together everything that is unconnectable in life. It constantly unsettles life. Rhizomatic thinking is the thinking of multiplicity, which seeks to liberate itself from "either/or," from "thinking about," offering to replace these with thinking *with* things; instead of "looking at" things, Deleuze proposes "looking the" and/or "looking with" – from the grass-level of things.

The rhizome relinquishes the need for a single, preferred direction and thus also one's reliance on a single, final authority, authority figures, hierarchy, classes. The rhizome is a kind of anarchic organization, which cannot be formulated in a fixed form or represented by a single scheme. The rhizomatic thicket is a flat, nonhierarchic model. The movement of the rhizome is not subservient to any dynastic principle. Conceptually, it contains neither preferred or overriding concepts nor any logical derivatives of thinking or imperative consequences from any other methodology. This does not mean that it is a space that is free of all influence. In the rhizome, influence may begin anywhere and reach everywhere. Such influences may seem like leadership, due to the potential influence every node can exert on the entire space. If this is indeed leadership, it is characterized by ever changing figures and initiatives.

Rhizome time is different from tree time. While the tree model contains the past-present-future axis, the rhizome only has a shared here and now. Aspects of "then and there" may be recognized as they are represented in "here and now". Rhizomatic thinking is memoryless. In fact, memory disrupts the natural movement of the rhizome.

Because the rhizome model is sprawled out and void of levels, layers past and future, orthodox psychoanalytic models of consciousness and unconsciousness do not apply in it. In the rhizome, everything is accessible. We can view its spread as indicative of being fully revealed and attribute it with transparency. Something known at a single node, is known by the entire space. Psychoanalytic notions of dissociation are equally invalidated by it. There is no splitting in the rhizome. The psychoanalytic context that may most benefit from the rhizome model is that of the constant generation of meanings and perspectives. In contemporary psychoanalytic literature, constant creation of meanings is seen as contributing to the analytic exploration, to the development of the subject and subjectivity and the expansion of possibilities (Stern, 2013).

This chapter was written during the COVID-19 pandemic. The coronavirus, which is putting our lives in danger at the moment, acts just like a rhizome, according to the botanical model of grass. Regardless of its starting point, its spreads out in all directions, replicating additional points of origin. With its flat sprawl, it reaches everywhere. Each of its branches bifurcates into more branches. It acknowledges no vertical height differences: its spread is blind to social class. It forces its particular time dimension on global human reality. The "here and now" joins the "then and there", and the presence of danger and attempts to deal with it have become a shared experience. The virus is as void of secrets as it is void of class differences. It and its consequences are ubiquitously revealed. However, our encounter with it may be very rich with the meanings it generates, including the text being written at this very moment.

At this point, we wish to note that our writing in this chapter is mostly tree-like. We define concepts in the conventional manner and we draw conclusions and derive applications from assumptions. Rhizomatic writing is featured later, in our clinical vignettes.

Tree and Rhizome – Vertical and Horizontal

The tension created between the tree and the rhizome is interesting to explore and experiment with. This tension is created through the attempted interaction between them. According to Deleuze, the tension between the tree and the rhizome generates an active process of breaking down the form and preserving existing material. Because each of them is a complete alternative to the other, the transition from one to the other is tantamount to breaking down and reassembling the understanding of what is happening. This can be seen as a process of pulling on loose ends until they unravel and then reweaving them. Rhizomatic thinking is capable of observing tree thinking without being subservient to its rules. Moreover, rhizomatic thinking notices the limitations of tree thinking and chooses a different *modus operandi*.

The tree and the rhizome appear as botanical metaphors, grounded in the observation of the outside world and its association with models of thinking. For example, the roots of the trees and the threads of fungal webs maintain an empowering tree-rhizome relationship, which offers mutual support for their individual growth and spread. In our view, this is an example of mutual enrichment.

Human relations can be described in tree and rhizome terms. It seems that the vertical and horizontal axes can also engage in mutual observation and mutual influence. Alongside this, we can assume that the horizontal axis and the vertical axis can engage in such interrelations. For example, a family (for the sake of the example, we will consider a good-enough one) includes both the vertical and the horizontal axes. Parent–child relations can be mutually empowering. By carefully upholding the law of the mother (Mitchell, 2006) and its derivatives (the vertical axis), the parents are supporting sibling relations. Sibling relations (the horizontal axis) help the parents. Moreover, the perspectives of sibling relations and parent–child relations may complement each other and contribute to the mutual understanding of each family member in their process of becoming. Later in the chapter, we suggest that group analysis may follow this paradigm of interrelations of the two axes for therapeutic purposes.

Observing, for a moment, the reality arounds us, we see that, much like the rhizome, the internet can also be described in rhizomatic terms. Social networks simultaneously involve both a dense branching-off and a constant inclusion of contributions and contributors from every direction.

It is interesting to notice how the COVID rhizome has created a human rhysomatic response. In this human rhysomatic response, a shared method of coping emerged, in which accumulated knowledge (including pseudo-knowledge and hearsay) came from everywhere and reached everywhere without – or despite – the interventions of professional authorities.

The Significance of "The Tree and the Rhizome" to Individual and Group Therapy

Deleuze and Guattari argue that there is a relationship between the presence of the other in the world and the rhizome and they address the multiplicity that begins in the individual. The other is, first of all, the existence of another possible world. This possible world has a reality of its own. They propose viewing the other not as an other, a stranger, but as the revelation of further possibilities in the world, which have been hidden from us and uncovered by the other (Deleuze, 1987/2007).

We suggest that the notions of "the tree and the rhizome" can be applied to psychotherapy. The other and all others are the rhizome – the horizontal axis. We propose that, much like the curative power inherent in the vertical axis, which involves doctor–patient or mother–infant relations, the horizontal axis of sibling relations also has an inherent curative force, because both parent–child relations and sibling relations entail a curative capacity. The horizontal axis represents the rhizomatic expansion of sibling relations. From this, one can derive therapeutic rhizomatic structures. The therapeutic group can be described in precisely such terms. However, we will later argue that the therapeutic dyad, which contains only two people, may itself be rhizomatic.

We propose that therapy can entail shifts between tree-like and rhizomatic-like states of being. The shift to rhizomatic thinking involves the effort to contain not-knowing, an effort which may open a space for re-exploration and for unraveling familiar and known concepts. This opens a new and surprising potential for change and for life's movement.

Both the therapist and the patient can shift from a rhizomatic state of being, which involves not-knowing and a multiplicity of experiences and contexts, to insights that can be verbally formulated and communicated. In such moments, formless experience is given personal "tree like" meaning, which can serve as a leverage point. It can strike root and generate meanings and conclusions, like the branches of the tree. Just as in life, tree thinking is vital to us because it serves our attempt to hold on to our temporary knowledge and communicate it. Perhaps the balancing of these two worlds and the containment of the tension between them is a developmental achievement in itself. The capacity to live in uncertainty through our attempts to create concepts and understanding brings us, if only for a moment, to a safe harbor, which inevitably fades and becomes unraveled again, *ad infinitum*. It is important to stress that the shifts between the tree and the rhizome involve considerable mental effort and that, in a sense, they are the essence of the therapeutic endeavor according to the model hereby proposed.

The therapist can contribute to the creation of rhizomatic space by unraveling the model in which she is the one who knows and joining the emerging movement of shared exploration. Still, in one's tree-like role, the therapist's position remains unique in terms of their responsibility to benefit the patient and their obligation to serve as an observer.

Individual Therapy

Orthodox individual therapy was conceived, for the most part, as having a tree-like meaning. It entails both hierarchy and designated roles: the therapist is charged with benefitting the patient; they are the guardian, the setter of boundaries and the interpreter. Note how the notion of therapy changes when we shift to rhizomatic thinking. The latter may create a new space in which therapist and patient form a rhizome together. It should be stressed that we are in no way proposing a therapeutic technique that is strictly rhizomatic. The therapist remains responsible for directing whatever happens in therapy to the benefit of the patient. In so doing, they are maintaining their tree-like role in a manner that both parties have agreed to in advance.

It seems that, today, psychoanalytic conceptualization is moving in this direction. We will now offer a brief review of several psychoanalytic notions (most of them contemporary) that, taken together, depict the therapeutic encounter as rhizomatic. Sullivan (1953) suggested that human experience takes place within the "interpersonal field." The mind is not separately located in each individual's skull; rather, it is essentially interpersonal, arising from interactions with other minds (Mitchell, 2000). The therapist is not an external observer; they are inevitably a participant-observer. To the same extent, the patient can also learn to become an observer, both in themselves and in the interpersonal field they inhabit. Sullivan, followed by Mitchell, propose that throughout the therapy, both therapist and patient learn to become participating-observers in the here and now of each session and in the course of the entire therapy. We argue that becoming such participating-observers, who make equal contributions, which are both distinct and shared, is a rhizomatic event. The notion of interpersonal emotional inter-penetrability, as formulated by Mitchell, refers to the multidirectionality of interpersonal emotional permeability: additionally, the notion of enactment seems to acknowledge the unconscious creation of therapeutic events that uncover material that had been blocked and unknowable for both parties. The orientation toward such companionship can be part of the therapist's professional world (Grossmark, 2016).

In his book *Experiences in Groups*, Bion (1961) has shown that we are trapped in fixed "basic assumptions," which essentially involve an escape from truth and a search for illusion: the search for a savior-leader who knows and/or a struggle to flee which essentially destroys the individual attempt to know and the expectation for the arrival of a messiah (which also involves expectations from the therapist as a vertical figure). All these allow group members to escape a state of not-knowing and an inability to tolerate frustration and to embrace basic assumptions that are grounded in previous experience and thus generate new learning (Bion, 1961, p. 53). Giving up the savior, the leader, the knowing therapist – these are tantamount to suspending tree thinking and making space for rhizomatic being.

So far, we have addressed the rhizomatic axis in interpersonal terms. It is easy to make sense of its nonhierarchic multiplicity in terms of different people and their interrelations. However, the notion of the rhizome can give rise to additional relevant meanings. The rhizome is also an intrapersonal occurrence, such as the constant unfolding of meanings in each of our individual minds (Stern, 2013). Rhizomatic occurrences can also be unconscious. Moreover, the unconscious itself may be co-constructed shared (Gerson, 2004).

Bion talks about "being without memory or desire" and seeks to attain a state of open wondering, which requires the capacity to tolerate frustration and think without knowing until an idea or a concept is born. According to this approach, change takes place when one experiences an unsaturated mindset, that is, a preconception (the search for meaning within a space of exploration; Bion, 1970). This notion was embraced by thinkers who further developed the field theory (the Barangers, Ferro, Civitarese, Stern). The field is rhizomatic. The shared unconscious fantasy that is created in the field belongs to the rhizome and develops through it. The field generates meanings that enhances therapeutic contribution. Consider the following vignette as an illustration:

> Dan, a 44-year-old man, is divorced and father to a 11-year-old son. He works as a programmer at a tech company. He has been in analysis (with Avi Berman) for five years. He turned to psychotherapy following his prolonged difficulty in maintaining a productive relationship with his superiors at work.

Toward the end of one session, Dan seemed embarrassed. He said that he was afraid that he had been sweating and might have left sweat stains on the couch. Initially, the analyst contemplated this as an expression of a regression to anal infancy, probably to his feeling of being rejected as an infant during toilet training. In previous sessions, Dan had brought up certain memories from his childhood which suggested that his toilet training was too strict or began too early. Towards the end of the session, Dan sighed. Despite the reasonable traditional understanding he had reached, the analyst felt there was something else in the patient's experience. Somehow, he felt that the sigh expressed some extra effort that Dan put in during this particular session. The analyst said that maybe he felt that the session was *strenuous* and that is why he had been sweating so much. Dan confirmed this immediately, but there was no time left to explore the meaning of this effort.

When contemplating this brief exchange, it occurred to the analyst that there was another profound meaning to what was said in this session. The Hebrew word for "strenuous," *me'umatz* has an additional meaning; quite remarkably, it also means "adopted." In the following session, when Dan mentioned his sigh, the analyst pointed out this double meaning: "you felt strenuous/adopted in that session." A long silence followed. Then, Dan said: "Yes. Both meanings are true. Throughout my childhood, I was ashamed of my parents. These immigrants, who never read a book, suddenly managed a little better and moved to a much better neighborhood. I was ashamed and worried. I became a spy – going to my new friends' houses to learn how to behave. I envied them and hated them. (He pauses . . .) and I also wanted them to adopt me."

For several sessions, he only talked about his socially disguised behavior and his plea for acceptance. He said that he never felt at ease, even in the presence of his friends: "I always play the normal guy, as if I am like them, as if I am on my way to becoming one of them, having a home, a wife and a child. I always speak to an audience." Within the field that was created by both of them, the analyst also encountered similar-yet-different memories from his own childhood, that brought him closer to understanding the patient past and present experiences. At a certain moment, the analyst suggested that maybe he (the analyst) himself had become an audience for him including ongoing feelings of fear, envy and longing to belong, as memories, emotions and meanings emerged in the sessions following the analysis of the double meaning of "strenuous-adopted."

We suggest that the homonym "strenuous/adopted" was used within a rhizomatic field, created by therapist and patient as partners. It does not matter at all, in our opinion, who said it and who was the first to notice its double meaning. Once it was there, it created additional value for each of them. In this case, the discourse that followed the understanding of the double meaning facilitated connection between the patient's dissociative self-state and childhood memories about experiences of inferiority and the effort to hide them.

Group Therapy

In a group, a new member shares that she is living with her partner, a woman. Another member, a 70-year-old man, reacts to this: "as a straight person, I think that all the gays and the lesbians are perverts." This same member once shared that he has a son with whom he had not been in contact for over a decade – and that a relative had suggested that his son might be gay. However, from within the resonance in the group and in the context of rhizomatic thinking, other members voice additional perspectives and different views: one member talks about how her older brother would beat her every time he felt that she was not chaste enough. A Muslim member said that had it been his son, he would have preferred that he never set foot in his home village, because he would have ended up being murdered. A woman of color talks about her experience of being different during her school years:

> No one approached me, they kept whispering behind my back. The cleaning guy, a migrant worker from Sudan, he talked to me. During breaktime, he would invite me to his room and offer me tea. But I wanted *them* to want me. I was completely alone for a whole year. I never spoke in class. I was a shadow.

And she adds: "a black shadow."

The conductor thinks to himself that being different and feeling shame are so multifaceted and that the group has unfolded many layers. At least for the present moment, it is possible to stay with all these voices, without judging them, with each voice finding its place in the shared space. Following these thoughts, the conductor proposes that the group is preoccupied with experiences of difference and exclusion, presented through the life stories of its members.

Following this intervention, another member, who only recently joined the group and who has been rather silent in the sessions so far, speaks up:

> I never imagined that I would be saying this here. Definitely not in the next year or two. It is the hardest thing in the world to share that I was admitted to a psychiatric hospital. I was an honors student doing a degree in medicine. Right before the final exams of the first year, I got these terrible panic attacks. My roommate had gone to stay with his parents. I was all alone. I started imagining things. . . . I still can't talk about that. I ended up jumping out the window. I was running from something. Luckily, it was just a first story window. At the hospital, they also gave me a psychiatric diagnosis.

Following these words, the group discourse shifts in a different direction. Members talk about overcoming shame. The affect changes from shame and vulnerability to anger. One member addresses the conductor:

> I keep suspecting that you're looking down on us. Not that you've said anything condescending here, but it looks like you have never had to endure any hardships, or that you don't consider us as partners you can share these experiences with.

Group discourse is rhizomatic. What each member says gives rise to what others will say. The directions of the discourse emerge spontaneously and are not determined by any authority. It is emotional resonance (Foulkes, 1948) that activates the growth of the rhizome in the group. It appears that the group's therapeutic value is grounded in the ability to move from the realm of secrets and silence to the realm of words and sharing. Talking is the grass growing. It stems from what just emerged and affects what will emerge next. We propose that belonging to the rhizome and becoming part of it again have a curative impact on group members.

In the rhizomatic state, both conductor and members exist within a rhizome where the views of any one person are not favored over those of any other and even excludes the possibility that an authority will decide in favor of one view or another. The importance of multiplicity and the embracing of a minoritarian position can facilitate an expanding group discourse that can contain a multiplicity of views and move away from racist views. For as long as a member chooses to stay part of the group, they belong to a society that enables multiplicity. In addition, if members are able to move between tree and rhizome points of view in the group, they may be able to recognize in themselves rigid, fixated tree aspects that do not sufficiently belong to its environment and cannot be included in its surrounding rhizomatic space. Such insight may lead members to try and move towards the new and unfamiliar. The 70-year-old member in the preceding vignette was able to use this quality of the space to realize how his views have been pushing people in his life away from him. Eventually, he was able to observe the rhizomatic multiplicity of views that was present in the session and to understand that his view was only one of many.

The therapist should address the members' expectation from him to become an exclusive authority, in order to facilitate them to share the responsibility and look for authority within themselves. Both conductor and participants may contribute to "tree thinking" in the group. Tree thinking can draw conclusions from information and speak the language of insight and recapitulation, causes and effects. Meanings can be formulated verbally in a way that momentarily halts the rhizomatic flux and comes together to form a definition or a conceptualization. "Loneliness," "shame," "difference" and "anger" help members to give meaning to their experiences and immediately come back to the discourse.

One can also contemplate the theoretical transition performed by Bion and Foulkes, two of the key founders and theoreticians of group therapy, as a transition from a tree-based approach to a rhizome-based one. The shift from the world of the dyad to that of the group necessitated the shift to rhizomatic thinking, which facilitated the creation of new ideas, while maintaining the conceptual and practical framework of psychoanalysis. Foulkes and Bion, each from his own unique position, invite the therapist to inhabit a position that actively unravels existing knowledge and explores the process that is emerging in the here and now.

We suggest that Wilfred Bion's notion of avoiding memory and desire stresses the present moment, the "here and now" and the shared reality. As he put it: "instead of trying to bring a brilliant, intelligent, knowledgeable light to bear on obscure problems, I suggest we bring to bear a diminution of the 'light' – a penetrating beam of darkness: a reciprocal of the searchlight" (1974, p. 20). In this sense, Bion's recommendation is a rhizomatic one: it favors focusing on what is becoming over the vertical exploration of the past. It views the yearning for a "knowing" and authoritative vertical figure as an illusion that hinders development. Bion unravels conventional concepts such as the transition from "unconscious to conscious" and shifts from a causational analytic inquiry to explorations in O, an exploration which requires the capacity of rhizomatic thinking to break concepts down and dwell in not knowing.

Siegfried Heinrich Foulkes began the establishment of radical concepts, some of which crucially departed from the classical theories of the 1950s. In his 1948 book *Introduction to Group Analytic Psychotherapy*, he argued that thinking and psychic development took place in interpersonal, rather than intra-psychic, space. Foulkes stresses that "everything is in the matrix" and argues that one should not use concepts that precede the matrix in one's explorations – a statement that unravels the boundary between I and we (Foulkes, 1973). Thus, as a conductor, the group analyst aims "*to replace submission by cooperation of equals among equal terms . . . without giving up the courage to lead*" (Foulkes, 1984, p. 65; emphasis added).

It is important to highlight the similarity and the connection between Deleuze and Guattari's notion of the rhizome and Foulkes' notion of the matrix. Foulkes proposed that we should view the individual as a junction point in a fabric of interpersonal communication. In his view, human existence is, first and foremost, interpersonal and social. Foulkes termed the fabric of communication between individuals in a group the "matrix". In fact, the matrix determines the meaning and the importance of any event. The sum total of communication and interpretation, both verbal and nonverbal, is based on it (Foulkes, 1946/1990). This total field is the fabric of communication that emerges at a given moment and it is both the only way one can learn about the here and now and the closest thing to the truth (Foulkes and Anthony, 1957). We propose that Foulkes' matrix can be viewed as a form of rhizome. It is the same fabric (matrix) that teaches us how the social dimension impacts our individual thinking and being.

> It seems difficult for many at the present time to accept the idea that what is called "the mind" consists of interacting processes between a number of closely linked persons, commonly called a group. . . . When a group of people, by which for our purposes I mean a small number of persons, form intimate relationships, they create a new phenomenon, namely, the total field of mental happenings between them all.
>
> (Foulkes, 1973)

According to Foulkes, whatever happens in an individual's psychology is determined by their "total state," meaning, the social web that surrounds them. This means that one can no longer view mental disorders as localized disruptions contained within the individual psyche, but as located in the total field of interpersonal interaction – the group matrix.

Weaving together and unraveling are interrelated actions, which stem from Foulkes' unique contribution. As we see it, for Foulkes, the action of unraveling focuses on the seams: between "I" and "We," between internal reality and social reality and between the personal and the other. Whatever is inside comes trickling out and vice versa; the "I" trickles into the "We" and vice versa; the personal stems from the social as well.

Conclusion

In the group, the tree and the rhizome alternate as states of being, each with its unique contribution. These two worldviews serve us as a paradigm for examining group-analytic psychotherapy. In our view, these notions of the tree and the rhizome should be present, as alternating options, in the conductor's therapeutic outlook; they should be accessible in the conductor's mind and readily available for flexible application.

References

Bion, W.R. (1961). *Experiences in Groups*. London: Tavistock.

Bion, W.R. (1970). *Attention and Interpretation*. London: Tavistock Publications.

Bion, W.R. (1974). *Bion's Brazilian Lectures 2*. Rio de Janeiro: Imago Editora, 1990.

Deleuze, G. and Guattari, F. (1983). *Anti-Oedipus: Capitalism and Schizophrenia*. Tr. R. Hurley. Minneapolis: University of Minnesota Press.

Deleuze, G. and Guattari, F. (1987/2007). *A Thousand Plateaus: Capitalism and Schizophrenia*. Tr. B. Massumi. Minneapolis: University of Minnesota Press, 2007.

Foulkes, S.H. (1946). On Group Analysis. In *Selected Papers: Psychoanalysis and Group Analysis* (pp. 127–136). London: Karnac, 1990.

Foulkes, S.H. (1948). *Introduction to Group Analytic Psychotherapy*. London: Karnac, 1983.

Foulkes, S.H. (1973). The Group as Matrix of the Individual's Mental Life. In E. Foulkes (ed.), *Selected Papers*. London: Karnac Books, 1990.

Foulkes, S.H. (1984). *Therapeutic Group Analysis*. London: Karnac.

Foulkes, S.H. and Anthony, E.J. (1957). *Group Psychotherapy: The Psychoanalytic Approach*. Harmondsworth: Penguin.

Gerson, S. (2004). The Relational Unconscious. *The Psychoanalytic Quarterly*, 73(1):63–98.

Grossmark, R. (2016). Psychoanalytic Companioning. *Psychoanalytic Dialogues*, 26:698–712

Mitchell, S.A. (2000). *Relationality: From Attachment to Intersubjectivity*. Hillsdale, NJ: The Analytic Press, Inc.

Mitchell, J. (2006). Sibling Trauma: A Theoretical Consideration. In P. Cole (ed.), *Sibling Relationships* (pp. 155–174). London: Karnac.

Stern, D. (2013). Field Theory in Psychoanalysis, Part I: Hurry Stack Sullivan and Madleine and Willy Baranger. *Psychoanalytic Dialogues*, 23(5):487–501.

Sullivan, H.S. (1953). *The Interpersonal Theory of Psychiatry*. New York: Norton.

4.2 Traversing the Axes

The Intersection of Parental and Sibling Relations in the Film *The Return*, by Andrey Zvyagintsev

Rina Dudai

> And Adam knew Eve his wife; and she conceived and bare Cain, and said, I have gotten a man from the LORD. And she again bare his brother Abel. And Abel was a keeper of sheep, but Cain was a tiller of the ground. And in process of time it came to pass, that Cain brought of the fruit of the ground an offering unto the LORD. And Abel, he also brought of the firstlings of his flock and of the fat thereof. And the LORD had respect unto Abel and to his offering: But unto Cain and to his offering he had not respect. And Cain was very wroth, and his countenance fell. And the LORD said unto Cain, Why art thou wroth? and why is thy countenance fallen? If thou doest well, shalt thou not be accepted? and if thou doest not well, sin lithe at the door. And unto thee shall be his desire, and thou shalt rule over him. And Cain talked with Abel his brother: and it came to pass, when they were in the field, that Cain rose up against Abel his brother, and slew him.
>
> [King James translation; Chapter 4, 1–8][1]

The Book of Genesis begins with the story of how the universe was created. It moves on to the conception of Adam and Eve, the world's first couple; the tale of the primal sin and the banishment from the Garden of Eden; and the establishment of the first family with the birth of Cain and Abel. After giving an account of these firsts, Chapter 4 embarks on a tale of the first interpersonal relationship, which culminates in a vague description of the world's first murder, in which one brother kills the other. Genesis, while surveying the origins of the foundations of humanity, skips entirely over parenthood: there is no mention whatsoever of paternal or maternal relations between the first parents and their children. The book engages, not with patricide or the murder of a child, but rather with the murder of a sibling. Much later in the book, in Chapter 22, the tale of the binding of Isaac relates the trial of faith in which God commands Abraham to kill his own son, but is stopped at the last moment by the miraculous appearance of the ram. The murder of a son or a father does not occur in the entire Book of Genesis; but that of a sibling is front and center.

Greek mythology, on the other hand, tells the story of patricide via the myth of Oedipus Rex, in which the son murders his father and consummates a sexual relationship with his mother. Freud chose to base his theory of the formation of the psyche on the Greek myth rather than on the Biblical text, placing the Oedipal

DOI: 10.4324/9781003220060-25

conflict – the murderous rivalry between son and father, and its resolution via an internalization of the parental figures by the child – as central to the development and structure of the psyche.[2] Psychoanalytical trends since Freud have at times been intrigued by relations between siblings, but as a theoretical model for the constitution of identity and the structure of the psyche, the theme of sibling relations has evolved slowly and is far younger than Freud's Oedipal model.

Theories giving significant weight to the interpersonal relations and behavioral patterns of sibling relations as independent of parental ones only began to emerge towards the end of the previous century.[3] The theme gained traction with the publication of Juliet Mitchell's book *Siblings* in 2003.[4] In the book, Mitchell claims that by focusing solely on the Oedipal relationship, psychoanalysis had ignored the significance of sibling relations in the formation of the subject, and goes on to set out an alternative conceptual framework that takes into account sibling relationships as a "horizontal axis" alongside the intergenerational Oedipal framework signified by the "vertical axis."[5] Mitchell also introduced the concept of the "law of the mother" which, in contrast to Lacan's singular "law of the father", emphasizes the serial dimension of the sibling relationship. The role of the Mother, according to Mitchell, is to acknowledge the seriality inherent in the appearance of siblings, which requires a distinction between them and a vitalization of their presence in relation to each other.

In this chapter, I will continue along the path indicated by Mitchell and further explore the relationship between the two axes – the vertical intergenerational axis and the horizontal sibling axis – and the dynamic ways they intersect, through an analysis of the film *The Return*, directed by Andrey Zvyagintsev (2003). By tracing the reciprocal relationships between parent–child relationships and those forged between siblings, I will show how the axes influence and are influenced by each other and weave together an integrated whole, opening up new spaces for discourse. The connections and transitions created by the intersections of the axes do not necessarily fit into rigid generalizations and cannot be strictly conceptualized; they are, rather, dependent on idiosyncratic situations that color the relationships in a less disciplined manner. Shining a light on these poetic spaces allows me to demonstrate an evolution of the psyche that develops through conflictual interactions as they fluctuate between intimacy and distance, attraction and repulsion, with no clear-cut final resolution. The sibling model will be investigated as a complex web of relationships in which one finds not just a rivalry over birthright, as in the story of Genesis, but also delicate touches of reciprocal support and a process of identity formation that mirrors – or opposes – the sibling's identity.[6]

The Return (2003)

The film *The Return* tells the story of two brothers, 14-year-old Andrei and 12-year-old Ivan (Vanya), who grew up with their mother and unexpectedly found themselves on a journey with a father who has appeared out of nowhere at their home after having been inexplicably gone for 12 years. The road trip takes place over a period of seven days and takes the trio through cities, ports, and unpaved roads, finally culminating on a deserted island. Throughout the trip, the father attempts to reclaim his paternity over the boys, and is portrayed from the perspective of the children as a stern, authoritarian, and at times even violent and threatening figure. The older brother seems to react with awe toward his newly found father, doing everything he can to win his approval. In contrast, Ivan repeatedly confronts the father and refuses to trust him. Their confrontation escalates as the film progresses, and climaxes in a dramatic scene in which Ivan climbs to the top of a tall watchtower and threatens to jump to his death. It is, however, ultimately the father himself who inadvertently falls and dies while attempting to climb the tower in order to reach his son. After the death of the father, the brothers carry his body to the boat and row it back to the mainland. While they are transferring their bags to the car, the boat with the corpse is carried off by the tide and sinks to the depths of the sea as the boys watch, helpless.[7]

The Vertical Axis: The Relationship between the Father and the Sons

From the moment the father appears at the family home, Ivan suspects him of being an imposter: his first reaction, after seeing his father asleep on their mother's bed, is to run up to the attic to open a chest, extracting from it an old illustrated bible that holds an old family photograph of the parents with their two sons. Andrei joins him, and together they verify their father's identity: "It's him," they agree. Nevertheless, Ivan continues throughout the film to struggle against the father's heavy-handed attempts at domination. He stubbornly ignores his recurring demands to call him "Papa" asking Andrei at one point "How do we even know he's our father?" The father, stung by his failed attempt to impose his will on his son, becomes violent towards Ivan, initiating a vicious circle of terror and hostility between them. The conflict comes to a head in one of the most excruciating scenes in the film, in which, just when the father seems to be on the verge of exploding into a rage after the boys come back late from a fishing outing, Ivan believes the father is about to kill Andrei with an axe. In order to protect him, Ivan takes out a knife he had previously stolen from his father and attacks him:

> Stop! Touch him and I'll kill you. Stay back! I could love you if you were different, but you are terrible! I hate you! Stop torturing us! You are nobody! You got it? Nobody!

The father responds to this outbreak in a surprisingly heartfelt emotional transformation, in which he turns softly, even gently, to Ivan and says "you are my son." The boy, confused by the father's metamorphosis, continues to yell but breaks down in tears, casts the knife aside and runs away, towards the watchtower. The father calls to him, referring to him by the nickname used by the mother – "Vanya" – and chases after him. Trying to rescue Ivan from his suicidal intentions by climbing the rickety tower, the father grasps onto a rotting plank that detaches from the structure, and he, not the boy, falls and dies; paradoxically, at precisely the same moment when his paternity is finally accepted. The story echoes the Oedipal model, even if it does not adhere to it accurately. The distance between the father's random fall from the tower and patricide is not great: the transformation of patricide into an accidental death can be interpreted as a realization of Ivan's death wish for his father.

Only at the end of the film, when the boat holding the father's corpse is carried away by the tide and sinks into the depths of the sea, Ivan cries out to his father: "Papa, Papa, Papa" – the word he adamantly refused to utter while his father was alive – thereby acknowledging his fatherhood. The camera's framing of the dead father's corpse in the boat echoes the image of the boys' first encounter with him, asleep on their mother's bed.[8] The father's disappearance into the watery depths comes full circle, as he sinks back down into the depths of oblivion and is thus transported back into the realm of the symbolic: a dead father is always a symbolic one.

After the boat with the corpse is claimed by the sea, Andrei turns to the car and takes the father's place at the wheel. Ivan, in Andrei's old spot on the passenger side, takes down the sunshield only to discover an old photograph hidden in it: a mirror image of the photograph the boys look at in the attic at the beginning of the film. The two photos are almost identical, but the first includes the father, while the newly discovered photo does not. The photograph shows the mother holding baby Ivan in her arms and Andrei sitting beside them on the father's motorcycle. The motorcycle serves here as a metonymic representation of the father, making present the father's absence and returning us to Ivan's ambivalence of his real identity. In the end, after all traces of the father are gone, one is left to wonder: was he even real? The father's resounding absence at the start of the film and at its end signifies the transitional state found between a concrete and a symbolic father and, in this sense, serves as a creative metaphorical solution for the moment at which the brothers separate from their father.

Andrei starts the car and backs away from the beach. The camera remains, following the tire tracks left behind and lingering to gaze at the serene water from which all memory of the events has been erased – only to return, as a ghost, in the series of photographs projected in the film's coda – and we hear the car shift into gear and drive away.

The Horizontal Axis: Sibling Relations

At the beginning of the film, even before the father appears, the relationship between the brothers is saturated with envy and competition. The opening scene shows a group of boys jumping from the top of a tower into a lake. The two brothers are part of the group, but while Andrei, the eldest, jumps nonchalantly into the water, Ivan is seized by terror. The boys taunt him for his cowardice and then abandon him there and Ivan, paralyzed with fear and freezing in the cold, waits alone until his mother climbs up to the tower and brings him home.

During the journey with their father through unknown territory, the boys manifest opposing positions towards the father. Andrei, in his desperate attempts to please him, stands in stark contrast to Ivan's sullen, suspicious attitude. Andrei is infuriated by his brother's contrarianism, blaming him for "making trouble." At the same time, it is clear that Ivan, the "coward" from the film's first scene, is the one who dares to stand up to the father's aggressions, unafraid of the consequences, while Andrei recoils in fear from provoking his ire.

As the brothers are confronted with hardships along the way, the complex relationship between them evolves, articulated by means of minimalist, intimate codes of nonverbal dialogue; a private language through which the boys establish themselves as brothers contrary to the parental world. This language includes physical gestures (a rich variety of facial expressions and silent stares), photographing each other with a camera, and writing a journal together in order to document their trip.[9] These subtle codes shed light on the subterranean pact of survival forged between the boys; a collaboration under conditions of danger and uncertainty on which they both rely. The scene in the tent before the boys fall asleep provides us with a precious glimpse into a moment of empathy: as the sound of rain mixes with the sound of Ivan's whimpering in the dark that he wants to go home, Andrei calls him "little one" and suggests they wake up early so they can go fishing together before their father wakes up.

The shocking death of their father brings the brothers into an even closer intimacy: struck by the shadow of death, the boys find themselves together in a place of silence, a Ground Zero of language, where action is needed in place of words. They cast aside the mischief and petty arguments of youth, and instead work together in absolute coordination, led by the older brother.[10] The brothers drag the father's corpse across the island to the boat and row together, wordlessly, back to the mainland. During this journey back, the brothers undergo an accelerated process of maturation from childhood to adulthood, in which their pact of collaboration is consolidated. The sound accompanying the scene in which the boat carrying the father's corpse sinks into the water imbues the scene with a primal state: the notes hover above the water like a meditative flow of consciousness, giving the viewers the sense of a shared experience of banishment from childhood's Garden of Eden.

Intersection of Parental/Vertical and Sibling/Horizontal Relations Axes

In order to shine a light on the intersections of the horizontal and the vertical axes, of parental and sibling relations, I will address three anchors that provide a window onto the fluctuating movement *between* the axes:

1. An Incomprehensible Reality

The stretch of time captured by the film is one of crisis. The long-absent father has arrived out of the blue with no explanation; he then proceeds to take the brothers on a journey to unknown territory, a trip that changes course several times for no apparent reason. Along the way, the father engages in several obscure dealings: he stops at a port to talk with some men and exchange a heavy package with them; he digs up a mysterious chest from an abandoned shack on the island, whose contents – to the very end of the film – are not disclosed. The boys (and along with them, the viewers) are plunged into a space of incomprehensibility, in which the accepted schemes of daily life are fractured and the reality of habit can no longer provide a conceptual system of interpretation. The hour of crisis opens a window for Otherness to enter into the stable, albeit deficient, world of habit.

2. An Unattainable Reality

Alongside the uneasy sense of incomprehensibility, the film continuously evokes a melancholic aura of an unattainable world; one that briefly floats to the surface, but then immediately dives back down into the abyss of oblivion as a secret that does not reveal itself. The story demands a contention with an absence, with a yearning that will forever remain, hovering, as a remainder, a ghost that is glimpsed but then returns to its chest.

3. The Photographs in the Coda

The photographs that appear at the end of the film function as poetic testimony for the processing of grief, holding together the intersection between the two axes. This testimony adds an additional layer of observation in hindsight that is simultaneously grounded in the future. The photographs, the only trace they have of the father, are in fact the remains of the brothers' shared experience.

I would like to suggest that these three anchors link the axes and weave them into a multidimensional structure through which we observe both the father and the brothers, who are called on to mourn over something they never actually had, and will never have.

Incomprehensibility as an Intersection of the Axes

Even before the action begins, the film opens with an underwater camera surveying the sea floor. The shot floats slowly over the remains of an abandoned boat. The boat's identity is revealed only toward the end of the film, when we realize it is the same boat that sinks along with the father's corpse. The appearance of the boat at both the beginning and the end of the film, at different times and in different places, transports the entire film from the realm of the real to that of the symbolic. The linear narrative is in fact a circular one, portrayed as such even before the viewers become aware of it. With this ruse, the film signals – at its outset – a quality of mythical timelessness. Other aspects of the film reinforce this sense: the parents are nameless, referred to only as "the mother" and "the father"; explanations of specific circumstances, reasons, and purposes are not revealed. The atonal music that accompanies many of the scenes invokes an abstract sense of melancholy and loss; from which the film's title emerges: *The Return*.

Although the film is propped up by means of a strict organizational structure of the days of the week, a clear echo of the Seven Days of Creation (the film begins on Sunday, and ends on Saturday), this structure unravels in light of the sense of meaninglessness, the lack of any causality, and the utter incomprehensibility that accompany the story from the moment the father returns. The father's sudden appearance raises many questions: Why was the father away for 12 years? Why has he returned? Why does he take the boys on a road trip? Why to these specific locations, which change several times with no explanation given? Why this specific island? What is in the box the father digs up from the ground? Why does he hide the chest in the boat without mentioning it to the boys? These questions remain unanswered.[11]

Indeed, with the help of images, the film succeeds in placing us at the center of the existential question: in the incomprehensible/world that unfolds before the viewer, in what sense is the father real? In what sense does he actually exist? Or is the father, in fact, not a real father but a symbolic one, who undergoes a transformation in the brothers' consciousness on their journey from childhood to maturity – from an absent father, to a concrete one, and then again to an absent one, of whom no trace is left apart from the abandoned boat, a remainder that becomes the witness to the absence itself? And to what degree do the transitions between the axes, and their intersections, succeed in translating the experience of the brothers' coming-of-age journey, in light of a father who becomes symbolic by being internalized and leaving his mark in the brothers' psyche? The riddle acts as a symbol of the remainder that contains the secrets of the psyche and resists interpretation.

An Unattainable Reality as an Intersection of the Axes

In the film *The Return*, the treasure chest that appears twice in the film represents the *Agalma* – that hidden, unattainable yet endlessly yearned-for object.[12] The chest first appears in the beginning of the film, when the boys come home to find their father asleep in their mother's bed after 12 years of absence. The brothers run to the attic and find a chest that seems not to have been opened in many years. The chest holds an old illustrated Bible in which an old family photograph is hidden; a photograph the boys use in order to verify their father's identity. The second time the chest makes an appearance is on the island, toward the end of the film. The father, alone in an abandoned shack, digs a deep hole in the ground and unearths a large treasure chest, from which he proceeds to extract a smaller chest. He carefully brings the box to the boat without disclosing its contents to the viewers – or its very existence to the boys – and hides it in the boat. The only ones who bear witness to the existence of the chest, albeit without knowing what is inside, are the viewers. The brothers wander into the shack during their exploration of the island, but do not pay attention to the hole from which the chest was taken – although they come very close to the spot.

At the end of the film, the boat sinks to the bottom of the sea along with the father's corpse and the hidden chest. Any hopes the viewers have nourished of discovering the precious contents of the chest, perhaps providing a key for solving the enigmas of the entire story, sink along with the boat. The chest activates in the viewers the same insatiable yearning as that of the characters in the film: the yearning by the father and the brothers for a nameless lost object. We are called on to mourn the loss of something that we have never had, and will never have, whether as parents or as siblings: a loss that always hovers over us all, parents, children, siblings.

Once there is no concrete remnant of the trip – the father is gone, the boat is gone, and the chest, of which the brothers were not even aware, is gone forever – the boys become the carriers of the father's memory. The only thing left is the brothers' shared memory of the journey, comprising the beginnings of a community memory. When the camera in the prologue glides underwater over the submerged boat accompanied by atonal, water-like bubbling sounds, we are provided with the contours that allow us to create the unconscious dimension that encompasses the entire story, a darkness hovering over the deep. The father remains enigmatic, and his absence at the ending amplifies the sense of his own incomprehensibility.

The absence of the father is starkly evident in the series of photographs that seals the film. The film ends in a series of black and white photographs that provide a mise-en-abyme summary of the entire story from the reflexive perspective of the witness.

The Photographs as an Intersection of the Axes

The Return ends with a photographic slideshow, showing 25 photos projected just before the final credits. The photographs are separated from each other by a black screen, from which the images emerge as light. The slideshow is composed of two sub-series. The first series contains 21 photographs, which are part of the diegesis of the film. The other four photographs are taken from a time that is ex-diegesis, when the boys were much younger. One photo is the one found by the boys in the attic at the beginning of the film. Another is of the boys and their mother, taken at the same time, which Ivan finds in the father's car sunshield as they drive home at the end of the film.

Metaphorically, the epilogue sets up a kind of time travel, which contains two forms of Return: a return to the events of the fishing trip with the father which ends with his death, and a return to early childhood, the faraway past before their father left, of which they seem to have no memory. Since its release, numerous critiques of the film have addressed this slideshow coda of the photographs as a memorialization of ephemeral moments of happiness – the usual motivation for such photos – but not as an episode of remembrance. In his insightful essay "The Return of the Photograph: Time, Memory, and the Genre of the Photo-Film in Andrei Zvyagintsev's *The Return*,"[13] Philip Cavendish addresses the coda in a way that distinguishes it from habitual pictures taken for photo albums. Cavendish claims that the coda can be understood as a photo-diary, allowing for an analysis that makes use of concepts such as tone and impression.

Along these same lines, I would like to suggest that the series of still photographs, separated by the black screen, undermines the structure of the symbolic order and allows the real to break through and to be present in the texture that seals the film. The black spaces and the accompanying music return us to the atmosphere of incomprehensibility with which the film opens, and which lingers throughout.

The film thus ends in a return to the world of the sensual, the experiential, from which the brothers are required to extract an understanding of what happened on the island: in that liminal sphere where childhood metamorphoses into adulthood. The black spaces between the photographs, like the no-man's-land of the island, are empty spaces from which chaos bursts forth, but which also allow for growth from within the pain of loss. The film's coda extracts itself from linear, historical time and enters into the primal spheres of the psyche: the photographs can be interpreted as testimony for a "rebirth" of the father in the hearts and minds of his sons, after his death.

The photographs in the coda are seemingly a surplus, an afterthought that at first viewing sinks into the abyss of oblivion and is often not even remembered by viewers. However, on careful observation, we find that the photos are layers of memories, each layer delving deeper than the previous one. The topmost, superficial layer perceives the photos as mirroring those taken on a school trip, capturing moments of fun, laughter, and mischief. Slowly, other layers of the trip are revealed: the layer of the intimate relations between the brothers, in a photo in which Ivan lays his head on Andrei's shoulder, a photo taken on the island. Moving deeper, there are a series of pictures from the distant past: the mother, Ivan as a small child on his father's motorbike, Ivan and Andrei on the motorbike, and the final photo of the series: the father holding Ivan the baby in his arms. The father, whose absence overwhelms the film's final scene, reappears at the end of the epilogue as a present, loving father; a father in the role of a nurturing mother, more so than at any other moment in the film, even more than when he sacrifices his life in an attempt to save his child. The photos echo the law of the mother, which bends the axis of familial relations from the vertical to the horizontal, to the axis of sibling relations: they are the reservoir of the brothers' collective memory. Witnessing the tragedy of their father's fall has transformed them into the carriers of a memory that is no longer only subjective but holds the seeds of a memory held by more than one person, one that can be validated and vitalized beyond the boundaries of the story. In this sense, the slideshow becomes the brothers' "Totem and Taboo", holding them together and making them into a community.

The coda, as a poetic ruse employed by the director, holds together this double-vision through the eyes of the brothers. The father figure, which has been deeply internalized by the brothers, transforms them into carriers of the memory of a tragic event in which they both participated. The act of remembering, via the photographs that emerge from the abyss at the end of the film, is a form of mourning in which the brothers carry the memory of their parents, but also separate from them.

Notes

1 The Book of Genesis, Chapter 4, Verses 1–8, King James translation.
2 It is interesting to consider why Freud, a Jew, chose this path. See Feldman (1993): 72–88.
3 Zeligs (1974): 88; Forsythe (1991): 453–510; Yerushalmi (1991): 92; Miron (2010); Feldman (1993): 88–72; see also Netzer (2018); Ashuach (2012): 155–167.
4 Mitchell (2003). Thormann (2003).
5 Thormann (2003).
6 Many thanks to Gissi Sarig for collaborative thought process that sparked the idea for this essay.
7 While working on the film *The Return*, I learned that Vladimir Garin, the boy who gave such a touching performance as the elder brother Andrei, drowned in the Osinovetskoe lake near Saint Petersburg on June 20, 2003, and his body has not been found to this day. Garin drowned two days before the film's world premiere, which took place in Venice, and did not get to participate in the Golden Lion Awards ceremony in which the film won first prize. I dedicate this chapter to his memory.
8 The two images, in turn, echo the representation of Christ in Andrea Mantegna's famous 15th-century painting *Lamentation Over the Dead Christ*, a ruse that links these two moments together and transports them into the realm of the symbolic.
9 Other examples of this rapport can be found in a conversation the night before they embark on the journey, in which the brothers exchange good-night wishes in their own private language ("ho" says one, and the other responds "ho").
10 The boys' relationship poses a stark contrast to the myth of Cain and Abel, who competed for the price of their father – the Heavenly father, in their case; a competition that ended in fratricide.
11 The director intentionally creates this atmosphere of confusion. In an interview with the director, Zvyagintsev says: "I'm afraid there is no clue. You either perceive it, or you don't. There are things which are without answers, and there is nobody who can explain them. . . . Art is not some sort of guideline for understanding. It's a thing unto itself. The most important thing for me is the image, not the thought". – Zvyagintsev, as quoted in Gritten, David, "The director who came in from the cold," *The Daily Telegraph* (11/06/04), p. 22.
12 In his words of praise to Socrates in the "Symposium", Alcibiades referred to an "Agalma": a statue in the form of a satyr that, when opened, contains the image of the gods and that he believed to be hidden deep inside Socrates. In Seminar 8, Lacan interprets the image of the Agalma as the object Alcibiades is searching for in Socrates. Alcibiades, according to Lacan, imagines that the object of his love has a secret, yearned-for treasure – the Agalma – that comprises the entirety of the abilities and ideals he idolizes in Socrates, and dreams of appropriating for himself. In love relations, Lacan claims, one attempts to come ever closer to the thing that is beyond one's reach; the excess that cannot be expressed in words. The term "Agalma", borrowed by Lacan from Plato's "Symposium", manifests the force that drives us toward the Other.
13 Cavendish, Philip. "The Return of the Photograph: Time, Memory and the Genre of the Photo-Film in Andrey Sviagintsev's *The Return*." *Slavonic and East European Review* 91, no. 3 (2013): 465–510.

References

Ashuach, Smadar. "Am I My Brother's Keeper? The Analytic Group as a Space for Re-enacting and Treating Sibling Trauma." *Group Analysis* 45, no. 2 (2012): 155–167.

Cavendish, Philip. "The Return of the Photograph: Time, Memory and the Genre of the Photo-Film in Andrey Zviagintsev's *The Return*." *Slavonic and East European Review* 91, no. 3 (2013): 465–510.

Feldman, Yael S. "'And Rebecca Loved Jacob.' But Freud Did Not." *Jewish Studies Quarterly* 1, no. 1 (1993): 72–88.

Forsythe, Dan W. "Sibling Rivalry, Aesthetic Sensibility and Social Structure in Genesis." *Ethos* 19, no. 4 (1991): 453–510.

Gritten, David. "The Director Who Came in from the Cold." *The Daily Telegraph*, June 11, 2004, 22.

Lacan, Jacqes. *Transference: The Seminar of Jacques Lacan, Book 8*, trans. Bruce Fink. Cambridge: Polity Press, 2015: 209.

Miron, Dan. *From Continuity to Contiguity: Toward a New Jewish Literary Thinking*. Stanford, CA: Stanford University Press, 2010.

Mitchell, J. *Sibling: Sex and Violence*. Oxford: Polity Press, 2003.

Plato. *The Symposium*, trans. Seth Benardete and Allan Bloom. Chicago: University of Chicago Press, 2001: 215b.

Ruth Netzer, November 18, 2018. www.hebpsy.net/articles.asp?id=3749 (in Hebrew).

Thormann, Janet. "Review of Juliet Mitchell: 'Siblings'." *European Journal of Psychoanalysis* (2003).

Yerushalmi, Yosef Hayim. *Freud's Moses: Judaism Terminable and Interminable*. New Haven: Yale University Press, 1991: 92.

Zeligs, Dorothy. *Psychoanalysis and the Bible: A Study in Depth of Seven Leaders*. New York: Bloch, 1974: 88.

Filmography

Zvyagintsev, Andrey. *The Return*. Russia, 2003.

4.3 Power relations in psychoanalysis as conditioned by capitalist structures

Felix Guattari's critique and new horizons

Esther Rapoport and Gita Kiper

It is striking that as a therapeutic modality that attributes much importance to the frame and the physical setting in which treatments occur, psychoanalysis remains largely myopic about the impact on the therapeutic relationships of one salient aspect of the frame, namely, the monetary exchange between analyst and patient. Some literature has been produced on patients' struggles with money and payment (e.g., Eissler, 1974; Freud, 1908; Fenichel, 1938; Gedo, 1963; Krueger, 1991); significantly less has been written about analysts' struggles with the same and the impact of those on the treatments (e.g., Bandini, 2011; Dimen, 1994; Haynes & Wiener, 1996; Josephs, 2004). With few exceptions, the existing writing deals with patients' difficulties accepting the financial underpinnings of psychoanalytic relationships, while the writing on the therapists' difficulties typically touches on the clinician's discomfort and conflict, related to her or his actual financial needs. Very few authors from within the discipline have found ways to think in more general terms about the materiality of the financial structure of psychoanalysis and the objective, rather than the subjective, impact on psychoanalytic processes of the money exchange within the dyad.

Of these, Muriel Dimen stands out. In her text *Money, Love and Hate: Contradiction and Paradox in Psychoanalysis*, Dimen reflected on capitalism, and its corollary, the class society, as the only conditions in which psychoanalysis could possibly develop and thrive (Dimen, 1994). Elaborating on Masud Khan's idea that psychoanalysis owed its existence to the long process of the evolution and alienation of the individual in the West (Khan, 1972, in Dimen, 1994), she stated,

> I think of psychoanalysis as the perfect therapy for a culture of alienation, for in it you pay a stranger to recover yourself. Paradoxically, psychotherapy that is bought and sold under conditions of alienation generates a "dis-ease" in both the person who pays the stranger and the stranger who is paid, and that needs treatment too.
>
> (Dimen, 1994, pp. 81–82)

DOI: 10.4324/9781003220060-26

Indeed, it is conspicuous that psychoanalytic cultures have emerged and flourished primarily in capitalist economies, failing to take root, or attaining a marginal status, in tribal and socialist economies alike.

Guattari and Deleuze: psychoanalysis as a reactionary form of desiring-production

Lacanian psychoanalyst, philosopher and political activist Felix Guattari (1930–1992) was likely the first theoretician to conceptualize the psychoanalytic process as a subtype of the broader, more sweeping capitalist process, and one of the very few practicing psychoanalysts and psychotherapists of all times to have done so. In his best known work *Anti-Oedipus: Capitalism and Schizophrenia*, co-authored with the philosopher Gilles Deleuze,[1] Guattari framed capitalism as an encounter between two powerful flows: the deterritorializng flow, cutting individuals off of their social environments, and the equally powerful, "artificial and violent" reterritorializing flow, directed by bureaucracies of the state and other agencies seeking to create a semblance of stability within capitalist economy (Deleuze & Guattari, 1972, p. 34).

Deterritorialization releases massive quantities and uncontainable intensities of desire, which, if not reterritorialized, could be invested directly in the social field, revolutionizing the latter. That is precisely what the reterritorialzing forces work to prevent. Freudian psychoanalysis, Guattari and Deleuze argued, sought to invest the vigorous desires released as part of the deterritorialzing process of capitalism in small, close-ended and socially conservative circuits – "mommy-daddy-me" – in which they would then remain trapped, blocked from being reinvested in the social field. Reinterpreting Reich, Guattari and Deleuze suggested that the nuclear family was the basic unit of the suppression of desire. Unlike Reich, however, they considered social, not sexual, desire to be originary – it was this social desire, then, that nuclear families suppressed. Freudian psychoanalysis, through its investment in intrafamilial processes and familial metaphors, helped preserve the existing social system.

To rouse, rather than placate, social desire, a different form of analysis was necessary: schizoanalysis, in which the emphasis would be placed on the question how desire was made to desire its own extinction. Schizoanalysis was a rhysomatic (i.e., multifocal) process, whose purpose was continued release of the powers of productive machinic unconscious, capable of producing new social structures.

Even as Guattari administered his merciless critique of psychoanalysis (Freudian and, subsequently, Lacanian as well), he continued throughout his life to work as a psychoanalytic psychotherapist at the innovative psychiatric clinic La Borde. La Borde, still in operation today, is a facility jointly run by patients and "carers" (Pollack, 2011). Among the first facilities where institutional psychotherapy, as envisioned by Francois Tosquelles, was practiced, La Borde employed radical practices such as decompartmentalization of aspects of administration and constant shifting of staff's responsibilities, with the idea of disrupting the illusion of staff's sanity and thereby reducing power inequalities between patients and staff, prioritization of non-symbolic aspects of the setting and group analysis (Guattari, 1995/1992; Pollack, 2011). Patients were paid for their work and often played pivotal roles in each other's treatment, by means of the group analytic work.

The capitalism of today: not your grandfather's (or Felix Guattari's) capitalism

Guattari and Deleuze's reference point was capitalism as it looked in the late 1960s and early 1970s. In the past fifty years, capitalism itself has mutated, assuming its contemporary forms, known as late capitalism (Jameson, 2013) and neoliberalism (e.g., Chomsky, 1999; Harvey, 2005; Layton, 2020). Under the influence of the rapid changes taking place in the global economic system, the economic-material foundations of psychoanalytic treatment are also in flux.

The changes that have taken place in capitalist societies have included a qualitative change in the relationship between production and consumption, globalization of the markets and a sharp decline in the socioeconomic security of the white middle class. While at earlier stages of capitalism, manufacturers (in possession of solid capital) largely determined what would be consumed, at its current stage, marketing and erratic, shifting consumption patterns (fluid capital) drive production, leading to greater insecurity, and subsequently harsher competition, for entrepreneurs and hired employees alike. Furthermore, in the neoliberal global social order, the primary role of state governments has shifted away from responsibility for citizens' social welfare, toward responsibility for safeguarding the freedom of commerce. As industries and resources that used to be public in welfare states, including medical care, national security, education and natural resources, were gradually privatized, or alternatively outsourced to charitable nonprofits, citizens learned that there is little they can expect from any public agency – instead, it is on the individuals, and them alone, to ensure that their own and their dependents' primary needs are fulfilled. Collective abandonment of citizens by their states has triggered a range of mental-behavioral reactions, including withdrawal into amoral familism (Rodger, 2003, in Layton, 2020), motivated by the perceived need to focus on supporting one's immediate dependents, high anxiety, manifesting as either a heightened sense of personal responsibility or, alternatively, panicked flights from responsibility, and intense anger, often directed at socially marginalized groups, which are seen as taking away the increasingly scarce public resources (Layton, 2020).

While the exact form, extent and impact of neoliberal policies differ from one society to the next, some common elements can be traced. Job insecurity appears to characterize most industries, and as job competition rises, the pressures on employees to function highly in order to compete for employment rise accordingly. Importantly, high functioning is demanded under conditions of uncertainty and lack of support. In addition to professional or technical skills proper, employers typically expect workers to demonstrate advanced capacities to function under stress, be a self-starter and a team player, positivity in the face of setbacks and openness to variable work hours. In line with the neoliberal doctrine, all responsibility is displaced from public agencies and organizations onto the smallest human unit, namely, the individual – thus, it is not the responsibility of the government, or the employer, to guarantee stress-free working conditions – rather, it is the worker's responsibility to work well under pressure; nor is the employer obligated to give clear instructions – rather, it is on the worker to be a self-starter.

In couple relationships, too, demands are rising. Faced with a stressful work life and an uncertain financial future, young people look to romantic relationships for security and acceptance. But in that area of life, competition is no less cruel, and the romantic partners' varied and high expectations of each other are difficult to meet. Furthermore, as psychology and popular forms of feminism encourage individuals to subject their romantic relationships to scrutiny and to an ongoing analysis of costs and benefits (e.g., is my relationship sufficiently fair and equal? Does it meet my needs?), such relationships are increasingly thought about in impersonal terms, as quantifiable and comparable to one another: if the current relationship fails to meet one's needs, then it might need to be replaced with a different, more satisfying one (Illouz, 2007). As a result, individuals strive to function highly also as relationship partners, often under conditions of insecurity.

Late capitalism and psychoanalysis: who is topping whom?

All these changes have had a direct bearing on the structures of psychoanalysis. Today, with fewer elements of the welfare state remaining in place, both the analyst and the patient are to work exceptionally hard if they are to survive in the jungle of the increasingly unrestrained free market. Many of the patients consulting us at this time are facing the pressure to continuously function at the peak of their mental capacities in order to preserve their middle-class status. They need our help to perform under extraordinarily challenging and sometimes inhuman conditions, with the stakes of failing being terrifyingly high – in the words of the parents of one of Lynne Layton's patients, "it's [either] Yale or jail" (Layton, 2020, p. 173). The current socioeconomic crisis, precipitated by COVID-19, has exacerbated some of these pressures as well as made them more visible.

As the white middle class, still privileged by comparison to most other social groups, has to work harder to maintain its privileges – the status of white middle-class professions, including psychoanalysis, becomes more precarious – while still elitist, such professions now lack solid economic foundations. Dimen described psychoanalysts as an "anxious elite" (Ehrenreich, 1989, in Dimen, 1994, p. 79); more pertinent to our argument is this being an economically insecure elite. Even though, at present, our services appear to remain in high demand, as a guild that is largely sustained financially by out-of-pocket payments of the educated middle class, psychoanalysis cannot be more secure than its client base.

While the changing contours of global capitalism have been taking a toll on the psychoanalytic profession, necessitating changes such as more flexible frames, psychoanalytic communities cannot be described as passive victims of capitalism. Eva Illouz has reflected on ways in which the language and values of psychoanalysis and psychotherapy have been absorbed into corporate cultures, helping make them more equitable and outwardly friendlier, but at the same time masking the power abuses that lie at the core of corporation-dominated economy (Illouz, 2008). Zaretsky (2008) and Layton (2020) have both discussed the role of psychoanalysis in fostering consumerist attitudes and, more generally, in encouraging people to seek individual and often purchasable solutions to socially caused frustrations, thereby dissipating rage and reformist passions that might otherwise be directed into the social sphere. Most generally, perhaps, it would be warranted to charge our profession with helping the society tolerate socioeconomic conditions that, without our expert help, may have long ago been overturned on account of their intolerability.

Power relations in psychoanalysis as conditioned by capitalist structures

In capitalist societies, psychoanalysis and psychotherapy are among the socially encouraged ways of dealing with suffering; both are regarded as valued commodities (Goodman, 2016). Patients typically enter psychoanalysis due to suffering, with the hope that their suffering may be alleviated or that they may learn to deal with it more efficiently. The capitalist framework within which psychoanalytic relations take place situates them as economic exchanges between agents occupying binary, complementary positions. The patient is the consumer: she pays to consume the service, which may be defined as an expert-mediated encounter with emotional pain, confusion and conflict. The analyst occupies the complementary role of the service provider: she is the expert in mediating such encounters, in ways that are supposed to eventually benefit the patient. These binary positions shape the psychoanalytic arena as a built-in conflict of interests: for the process to take off, both patient and analyst need to see the analyst as benevolent, concerned about the patient, attuned to her and wishing her well, yet what would sustain the clinician financially would be for the patient to continue suffering (Hutchinson & Stadler, 1975).[2] This conflict of interests is sometimes experienced by the analyst as an internal conflict. It is also frequently played out in analytic relationships, with the patient declaring her wish to leave and the analyst attempting to interfere by interpreting this wish as premature, impulsive, self-destructive, a re-enactment of the past or otherwise hurtful to the patient. (In such negotiations, the analyst's own financial need may be invoked by the patient but never by the analyst.)

In addition, these mutually exclusive roles – patient and analyst – provide each side with a discursive framework for the construction of action and meaning, and for understanding the actions of the other side. The two positions distribute differential speech and action expectations and entitlements for the two participants, defining the mechanisms and extent of their potential mutual influence. They also place each of the participants in a differentially vulnerable position (Guilfoyle, 2006). The degree of mutual dependence and vulnerability of each member of the dyad varies as a function of multiple other factors, including their individual psychological and socioeconomic backgrounds and the regional supply and demand of psychotherapeutic services.

Psychotherapeutic relations, analytic relations among them, are paradoxically situated at the junction of intimacy and economic activity (Dimen, 1994; Kupersmidt & Silver, 2013). At this junction, monetary transactions and intimate relationships are co-produced and mutually sustaining, involving tension between intimate and impersonal relations, but also inseparably fusing these two spheres, ordinarily viewed as disparate. Viviana Zelizer and Eva Illouz have both analyzed the hybrid formations that are produced when monetary transfers coexist with intimate relations, describing them as *impersonal intimacy* (Illouz, 2008; Zelizer, 2005). According to Illouz, the commodification of the selfhood and self-realization stemming from this fusion makes it virtually impossible to distinguish the self as a bought or artificially constructed structure from the agentic self, capable of shaping and helping itself, and of engaging in deliberation and in communication with others (Illouz, 2008). For example (provided by these authors, not by Illouz), a patient who has learned to set boundaries, by identifying with and internalizing with the analyst's ability to end sessions on time, demand payment and limit contact between sessions, may then enact in her or his intimate relationships a boundaried way of relating that may be more suited to work relationships than it is to intimate ones. For some people, this may be just what they need to regain a sense of control over their lives. By and large, however, the process of "importing" the boundariedness characteristic of work relationships to personal relationships may contribute to the weakening of social ties and obligations, making those individuals who are particularly vulnerable to isolation and abandonment, such as seniors and people with disabilities, increasingly less protected from the ills of isolation.

While the artificial and organic aspects of the psychoanalytically constructed self are bound to become fused to the point of indistinguishability, between the selves of the patient and the analyst sharply delineated, binary processes of mutual objectifications take place, which make it possible and legitimate to treat the other in ways in which intimate others of a different kind could not be treated. The patient is allowed and encouraged to objectify the analyst in multiple ways: the analytic contract implies the expectation that the analyst will be experienced as figures from the patient's past, and that the analytic regression will lead the patient to wish for the analyst to gratify her early emotional needs. Departing from the conventions that dominate most other social contexts, the analytic context makes it legitimate for one of the participants to speak without listening to the other (Budick & Aronzon, 2007). On the analyst's end, the patient, unlike intimate others of other kinds, can be freely thought of, and sometimes spoken about or to, as disturbed or infantile. It is legitimate for the analyst to mediate her encounter with the patient's otherness with the help of various theories, framing the patient's utterances or behavior as part of a known (to the analyst) pattern, rather than pure intersubjective difference. She also holds the privilege to choose to limit contact with the patient to in-person sessions, a form of arbitrary boundary setting that in non-therapeutic intimate relationships would be considered unduly controlling and one-sided.

The fundamental power relation at the core of the analytic process, making inevitable a conflict and arguably setting limits on the degree of cooperativeness and solidarity that can be expected, may be conceptualized as a power relation between two financial "giants", standing behind the backs of the two participants: capital and expert knowledge. The charged power relations between these two forces are fundamental to technological and economic developments in late capitalism, and have been termed "knowledge economy" (Adler, 2001). The economic development of companies and nations increasingly depends on expert knowledge, and as a result, highly knowledge-dependent industries, such as the high tech industry, reward employees in multiple ways (Adler, 2001). Knowledge can, therefore, be a strong card, in itself constituting a form of capital. At the same time, the contradictory trend that is also operative in today's economy is the systematic de-skilling of highly skilled workers (i.e., hiring them to do work for which they are overqualified, and which in fact is far more mechanical or repetitive than the job title implies) and part-time, contingent-contract employment, which keeps experts as economically insecure as line production workers (Kennedy, 2010).

In the context of psychoanalysis, the patient may be seen as the investor, whereas the analyst is akin to the expert developer. These two types of power dominate the different "spheres" or "areas" of the analytic relations. Money is the power that sustains the process and determines some of the core aspects of the setting – for example, how many times a week the analyst and patient will meet – while other aspects of the setting, such as the possibilities of maintaining contact between the sessions, are set by the analyst, whose expertise in technical matters pertaining to the treatment method the patient is seeking. It is within the patient's capacity to end the process or to withhold payment in case of dissatisfaction.

In general, the capitalist framework of the treatment and the position of the patient as the customer shape psychoanalytic relations in a particular way. Although this may change at certain stages of the treatment, as the patient regresses and becomes increasingly emotionally dependent on the analyst, by and large, patient-as-customer typically views herself and is viewed by the analyst as entitled to define the desired treatment outcome. For example, one person may undertake a personal analysis because she is interested in establishing an intimate relationship or in getting married, while another may be seeking treatment in the hope of leaving a relationship or marriage. While psychoanalytic treatments tend to be lengthy and often change course due to unconscious factors, the patient's desire, especially if it is normative, is usually allowed to guide the process – the patients' consumer right to determine what kind of welfare they wish to purchase for themselves is respected (Saketopoulou, 2019). Even non-normative desires, such as the desire for a queer identity or gender change, are typically not directly challenged or altogether discarded; although the analyst may attempt to question such desire surreptitiously, if the patient is persistent enough, she will eventually, with the analyst's reluctant help, obtain the identity and/or embodiment of her choice (Pula, unpublished manuscript). Hence, the field of psychoanalytic clinical practice generally follows the capitalist logic, according to which the paying customer is entitled to consumer choices.

With regards to the treatment process as such, the analyst's expert knowledge imparts to her considerable power to shape that process through the "codes of knowledge" that she offers the patient. The patient has to learn the rules of the engagement – what kind of speech is expected, professional domain, into which the patient has no choice but to be socialized (Totton, 2006). Gaps in the relevant knowledge and information, which exist in psychotherapeutic relationships of various types, are typically wider in psychoanalysis, as psychoanalytic theories are complex and analysts in training are often expressly instructed to conceal or blur information for the sake of the analytic process (Herlihy & Corey, 2001; Hutchinson & Stadler, 1975).

As many writers have noted in the past, the knowledge-related power imbalance leaves the patients vulnerable in multiple ways. The patient's self-esteem and self-efficacy may deteriorate as a result of the analyst emphasizing her weaknesses over their strengths (Chaplin, 2006). Resistances may be met with "corrective" forces, directly or indirectly (Guilfoyle, 2006). Therapists and analysts may occasionally or chronically override, judge, insult, attack and patronize their patients (Totton, 2006), justifying such responses in reference to their expert knowledge and technique. Because the patients lack the expert knowledge to assess the professionalism of the analyst's interventions, they are potentially vulnerable to emotional manipulation and sexual abuse (Totton, 2006). And since patients learn to examine themselves from the expert's point of view, the analytic process has been argued by some to produce obedient subjects who are overawed by authority (Lees & Freshwater, 2006).

In conclusion, the capitalist infrastructure at the core of the psychoanalytic setting consistently inflects the analytic relationship, the process of analysis, the personal and intersubjective unconsciouses of the participants and, less directly, the society, from which patients are sampled and into which they return. The impersonal intimacy of the setting, characterized by complex and pernicious conflicts of interests and mutual objectification, is bound to produce selves that will seek to reproduce these conditions, normalizing patients and others into the capitalist order.

Answers that cannot be questioned or questions that cannot be answered?

This preliminary inquiry leaves us with more questions than answers. Among the important questions that we have not addressed is the question of group analysis: in what ways, and under what conditions, may group analysis, as a modality that fosters sociality and relies to a large extent on peer relations, be able to challenge capitalist structures and their effects, instead of reproducing them? We imagine that answers to this question would vary as a function of both the theoretical approach to group analysis and aspects of its material setting.

The editors of this volume wish to emphasize the importance of horizontal relating in psychoanalysis and group analysis, arguing that

> parent–child relationships and sibling relationships [are] two distinct developmental axes: the vertical axis represents parent–child relationships and is an abstraction of hierarchical relationships of any kind; the horizontal axis represents sibling relationships and is an abstraction of reciprocal and non-hierarchical relationships.
>
> (Berman & Ashuach, 2022, p. 2)

While in agreement with the editors that it is important to nourish both the practices and the theoretical conceptions of horizontal relating in psychotherapy, psychoanalysis and group analysis, we find the idea of tracing the horizontal to sibling relations, thereby metonymically linking horizontality and sibling ties, inherently problematic. Sibling relations are indeed different from both the dyadic and Oedipal relationships, and it is true that psychoanalytic theory has paid far more attention to the latter than to the former. However, both the sibling and the parent–child relationships exist within the same social structure, namely the nuclear family. To think of that structure as the most basic social unit is to reproduce the original bias of the Freudian and other pre-relational psychoanalytic theories, namely, that the nuclear family and the individual are originary, while all other social structures are their outgrowths and extensions. This bias obscures the understanding of the broader sociocultural and socioeconomic forces, both vertical and horizontal, that deploy the nuclear family to advance their agendas while also shaping family members' values and practices. How siblings live out their predicament is to large extent a function of the political, economic and cultural contexts within which the given family is set. Thinking of the horizontal through sibling relations may be yet another way of reinstating the nuclear family as the basic social unit and, as Guattari and Deleuze have convincingly shown, by helping keep the potentially revolutionary social desire trapped in the closed circuits of nuclear families, psychoanalysis has aided the conservative reterritorializing forces of capitalism. For group analysis to become a force of liberating social desire and rechanneling it back into the social field, the discussion of the group dynamics needs to focus on the sociopolitical forces that shape them, and familial metaphors may need to be overshadowed, or at least balanced out by, truly inclusive metaphors of horizontal relating.

Another relevant question that we have not engaged in this text is, whether and how can class solidarity be fostered between the analyst and the patient? As most analysts and patients come from middle-class backgrounds, there is a potential for class solidarity, alongside competition and power struggles.

Forming solidarity in the consulting room can be the first step to rebuilding social links, which capitalism in its contemporary form, neoliberalism, seeks to sever (Layton, 2020).

Perhaps the broader question at stake is whether or not the effects of the material arrangements at the core of the psychoanalytic setting can be transformed by addressing them on the symbolic plane? Different authors who have entertained this question have arrived at different conclusions. Muriel Dimen thought that the contradiction between money and love could at best be transcended "in a brief, utopian fashion" (Dimen, 1994, p. 98), or transformed into a paradox between love and hate. Lynne Layton, conversely, optimistically believes that "honesty about the power relations asymmetry and the money exchange for care", if practiced in the consulting room, can help preclude the enactment of these issues that usually occurs, and that treatments in which money and power are spoken about rather than bracketed can produce "social subjectivities, versus the sovereign capitalist subjectivities that mainstream psychoanalysis fosters" (L. Layton, personal communication, August 23, 2020). On our own part, we refrain from embracing either position. Our main intention here was to raise this insufficiently explored problem, pointing to capitalist structures as a limit to the possibility of horizontal relating in analysis.

Notes

1 While is it common to attribute *Anti-Oedipus* largely to Deleuze, who is viewed as the more serious writer from among the two, in practice, it was Guattari who drafted most of the text, as well as developed some of the key concepts (such as deterritorialization) on his own, sometime before his collaboration with Deleuze commenced (Herzog, 2016; Pollack, 2011).

2 In our view, this is not a radical view that might require an elaborate discussion regarding its complexities. Rather, H&S accurately describe an inevitable outcome of the financial structure of psychotherapy: psychotherapists benefit from their patients' emotional suffering, similarly to the way physicians benefit from their patients' physical suffering. We believe that professional ethics compels us to acknowledge the paradoxes and structural problems in our profession. Moreover, it compels us to engage in honest and transparent explorations of the said problems – as we try to do in this chapter.

Bibliography

Adler, P. S. (2001). Market, Hierarchy, and Trust: The Knowledge Economy and the Future of Capitalism. *Organization Science*, 12(2), 215–234.

Bandini, C. (2011). The Good Job: Financial Anxiety, Class Envy and Drudgery in Beginning a Private Analytic Practice. *Contemporary Psychoanalysis*, 47(1), 101–117.

Budick, E. M., & Aronzon, R. (2007). *Psychotherapy and the Everyday Life: A Guide for the Puzzled Consumer*. London: Karnac Books.

Chaplin, J. (2006). The Bridge Project: Radical Psychotherapy for the 21st Century. In: Totton, N. (Eds.) *The Politics of Psychotherapy: New Perspectives*. Berkshire UK: McGraw-Hill Education, Open University Press, 159–166.

Chomsky, N. (1999). *Profits Over People: Neoliberalism and Global Order*. New York: Seven Stories Press.

Deleuze, G., & Guattari, F. (1983/1972). *Anti-Oedipus: Capitalism and Schizophrenia*. Minneapolis: University of Minnesota Press.

Dimen, M. (1994). Money, Love and Hate: Contradiction and Paradox in Psychoanalysis. *Psychoanalytic Dialogues*, 4(1), 69–100.

Doherty, W. J. (1995). Bridging Psychotherapy and Moral Responsibility. *The Responsive Community*, 5(1), 41–53.

Doherty, W. J. (2008). *Soul Searching: Why Psychotherapy Must Promote Moral Responsibility*. New York: Basic Books.

Eissler, K. R. (1974). On Some Theoretical and Technical Problems Regarding the Payment of Fees for Psychoanalytic Treatment. *International Review of Psychoanalysis*, 1, 73–101.

Fenichel, O. (1938). The Drive to Amass Wealth. *Psychoanalytic Quarterly*, 7, 69–95.

Foucault, M. (2003). *Madness and Civilization*. London: Routledge.

Freud, S. (1908). Character and Anal Erotism. In: *The Standard Edition of the Complete Psychological Works of Sigmund Freud, Volume IX (1906–1908): Jensen's 'Gradiva' and Other Works*. London: Hogarth Press, 167–176.

Frosh, S. (1987). *The Politics of Psychoanalysis: An Introduction to Freudian and Post-Freudian Theory*. New Haven, CT: Yale University Press.

Gedo, J. (1963). A Note on Non-Payment of Psychiatric Fees. *International Journal of Psychoanalysis*, 44, 368–371.

Goodman, D. M. (2016). The McDonaldization of Psychotherapy: Processed Foods, Processed Therapies, and Economic Class. *Theory & Psychology*, 26(1), 77–95.

Guattari, F. (1995/1992). *Chaosmosis: An Ethico-Aesthetic Paradigm* (Translated by P. Bains & J. Pefanis). Bloomington: Indiana University Press.

Guilfoyle, M. C. (2006). *Concealing and Revealing Power in the Therapeutic Relationship*. PhD dissertation, Utrecht University.

Harvey, D. (2005). *A Brief History of Neoliberalism*. Oxford: Oxford University Press.

Haynes, J., & Wiener, J. (1996). The Analyst in the Counting House: Money as Symbol and Reality in Analysis. *British Journal of Psychotherapy*, 13(1), 14–25.

Herlihy, B., & Corey, G. (2001). Feminist Therapy. *Theory and Practice of Counseling and Psychotherapy*, 6, 341–381.

Herzog, D. (2016). Desire's Politics: Felix Guattari and the Renewal of the Psychoanalytic Left. *Psychoanalysis and History*, 18(1), 7–37.

House, R., & Feltham, C. (2015). Counselling Psychology: Critical Achievements, Possibilities, and Limitations. In: Parker, I. (Ed.) *Handbook of Critical Psychology*. New York: Routledge/Taylor & Francis Group, 164–172.

Hurvitz, N. (1977). The Status and Tasks of Radical Therapy. *Psychotherapy: Theory, Research & Practice*, 14, 65.

Hutchinson, M. A., & Stadler, H. A. (1975). *Social Change Counseling: A Radical Approach*. Boston, MA: Houghton Mifflin Harcourt.

Illouz, E. (2007). *Cold Intimacies: The Making of Emotional Capitalism*. Oxford: Polity Press.

Illouz, E. (2008). *Saving the Modern Soul: Therapy, Emotions, and the Culture of Self-help*. Berkeley: University of California Press.

Jameson, F. (2013). *Postmodernism, or, The Cultural Logic of Late Capitalism*. Durham, NC: Duke University Press.

Josephs, L. (2004). Seduced by Affluence: How Material Envy Strains the Analytic Relationship. *Contemporary Psychoanalysis*, 40(3), 389–408.

Kennedy, P. (2010). The Knowledge Economy and Labour Power in Late Capitalism. *Critical Sociology*, 36(6), 821–837.

Krueger, D. W. (1991). Money Meanings and Madness: A Psychoanalytic Perspective. *Psychoanalytic Review*, 78(2), 209–224.

Kupersmidt, J., & Silver, C. B. (2013). The Search for Intimacy. In: Frank, A., Clough, P. T., & Seidman, S. (Eds.) *Intimacies: A New World of Relational Life*. London: Routledge, 225–243.

Layton, L. (2020). *Toward a Social Psychoanalysis: Culture, Character and Normative Unconscious Process (Relational Perspectives Book Series)*. London and New York: Routledge.

Lees, J., & Freshwater, D. (2006). Politics and Psychotherapy in the Context of Healthcare. In: Totton, N. (Ed.) *The Politics of Psychotherapy: New Perspectives*. Maidenhead, UK: Open University Press, 121–134.

Nolan Jr, J. L. (1998). *The Therapeutic State: Justifying Government at Century's End*. New York: NYU Press.

Pollack, C. (2011). Analysis: Between Psycho and Schizo. In: Alliez, E., & Goffey, A. (Eds.) *The Guattari Effect*. London: Bloomsbury, 57–66.

Rubin, J. B. (2003). Psychoanalysis is Self-Centered. In: Spezzano, C., & Gargiulo, G. (Eds.) *Soul on the Couch: Spirituality, Religion and Morality in Contemporary Psychoanalysis*. Hillsdale, NJ: The Analytic Press, 87–102.

Saketopoulou, A. (2019). The Draw to Overwhelm: Consent, Risk and the Retranslation of Enigma. *Journal of American Psychoanalytic Association*, 67(1), 133–167.

Szasz, T. (2003). The Cure of Souls in the Therapeutic State. *The Psychoanalytic Review*, 90, 45–62.

Totton, N. (1999). The Baby and the Bathwater: 'Professionalisation' in Psychotherapy and Counselling. *British Journal of Guidance and Counselling*, 27(3), 313–324.

Totton, N. (2006). Power in the Therapeutic Relationship. In: Totton, N. (Ed). *The Politics of Psychotherapy: New Perspectives*. McGraw-Hill Education (UK). Maidenhead, UK: Open University Press, 83–96.

Zaretsky, E. (2008). *Political Freud: A History*. New York: Columbia University Press.

Zelizer, V. (2005). *The Purchase of Intimacy*. Princeton: Princeton University Press.

Index